MOUNTAIN TROOPS AND MEDICS

(Second Edition)

A Complete
World War II Combat History
of the
U. S. Tenth Mountain Division

In the Wartime Stories of One of its
Frontline Battalion Surgeons

Albert H. Meinke, Jr., M.D.

TRAFFORD

Printed in Victoria, Canada

National Library of Canada Cataloguing in Publication Data

Meinke, Albert H., 1919-
    Mountain troops and medics : a complete World War II
combat history of the U.S. Tenth Mountain Division in the wartime stories of one of its frontline battalion surgeons /
Albert H. Meinke, Jr.

First published: Kewadin, Mich. : Rucksack Pub. Co., 1993.
Includes bibliographical references and index.
ISBN 1-55369-600-X

    1. Meinke, Albert H., 1919- 2. World War, 1939-1945--
Medical care--United States. 3. World War, 1939-1945--Personal
narratives, American. 4. Surgeons--United States--Biography. 5.
World War, 1939-1945--Campaigns--Italy. 6. United States. Army.
Mountain Division, 10th--Biography. I. Title.

D807.U6M45 2002   940.54'7573   C2002-902484-6

TRAFFORD

This book was published *on-demand* in cooperation with Trafford Publishing.
On-demand publishing is a unique process and service of making a book available for retail sale to the public taking advantage of on-demand manufacturing and Internet marketing.
On-demand publishing includes promotions, retail sales, manufacturing, order fulfilment, accounting and collecting royalties on behalf of the author.

Suite 6E, 2333 Government St., Victoria, B.C. V8T 4P4, CANADA
Phone   250-383-6864   Toll-free   1-888-232-4444 (Canada & US)
Fax   250-383-6804   E-mail   sales@trafford.com
Web site   www.trafford.com   TRAFFORD PUBLISHING IS A DIVISION OF TRAFFORD HOLDINGS LTD.
Trafford Catalogue #02-0136   www.trafford.com/robots/02-0136.html

10   9   8   7   6   5   4   3

DEDICATED TO THE MEMORY OF THOSE MEN

OF THE TENTH MOUNTAIN DIVISION

WHO DIED OF WOUNDS RECEIVED

DURING COMBAT

AUTHOR'S PREFACE

MOUNTAIN TROOPS AND MEDICS is a true account of my adventures as a Battalion Surgeon in the U. S. TENTH MOUNTAIN DIVISION, and is at the same time a complete and accurate history of this famous division's military accomplishments in Europe during World War II. To enable me to present each of my personal stories in its proper setting and correct sequence, a certain amount of research was necessary, and in this endeavor I had the good fortune to be able to refer directly to a number of service connected papers that I still have in my possession, and to the unpublished portions of the short bibliography presented with this book. These reference materials were used to confirm names, dates, times, and places, and I was most pleased to find that the information recorded in them corroborated my recollections of events so well that I am confident that the book is historically correct.

My personal stories have been written from memory which has been reawakened and nurtured by reading and rereading the many wartime letters I wrote to my wife and my mother while I was overseas, and by telling and retelling many of the stories to relatives and friends. After hearing some of them people regularly encouraged me to write this book, but I was also motivated by the challenge of trying to accurately convey what it truly means to be a combat infantryman at the front in wartime to the ordinary citizens of our country. This is an extremely difficult task, and surely I have not accomplished it as well as I would have liked. Nevertheless, I hope that my book makes pleasurable, informative reading for all, and perhaps rekindles some old memories for veterans who have "been there."

In the beginning I intended this book to be one of the most humorous ones ever written, but war is not funny, so the book turned out to be a serious one containing humorous anecdotes here and there within it. All of the stories are true narrations of events that actually happened.

Albert H. Meinke, Jr., M.D.

CONTENTS

AUTHOR'S PREFACE 5

CHAPTER I   INTRODUCTION 11
CHAPTER II   DEPARTURE 17
CHAPTER III   PREPARATION IN ITALY 27
CHAPTER IV   INTO THE LINE 49
CHAPTER V   THE STATIC WAR 61
CHAPTER VI   REST AND REHABILITATION 77
CHAPTER VII   RIVA RIDGE & BELVEDERE 83
CHAPTER VIII   MONTE DELLA TORRACCIA 95
CHAPTER IX   THE SECOND ATTACK 115
CHAPTER X   I SPEAK GERMAN AGAIN 121
CHAPTER XI   A WAITING PERIOD 129
CHAPTER XII   TOILET FACILITIES 143
CHAPTER XIII   BATTLEFIELD PROMOTION 153
CHAPTER XIV   BREAKOUT 159
CHAPTER XV   TASK FORCE DUFF 189
CHAPTER XVI   ACROSS THE PO 205
CHAPTER XVII   TASK FORCE DARBY - VERONA 209
CHAPTER XVIII   LAGO DI GARDA 217
CHAPTER XIX   RESIA - THE AUSTRIAN BORDER 233
CHAPTER XX   OCCUPATION PERIOD 247
CHAPTER XXI   CIVILIAN MEDICAL PRACTICE 263
CHAPTER XXII   THE RETURN 273
CHAPTER XXIII   TERMINATION 281

APPENDIX A   APPLICATION FOR UNIT CITATION 289
APPENDIX B   MAPS OF THE COMBAT AREAS 297
BIBLIOGRAPHY   308
INDEX   309

MOUNTAIN TROOPS AND MEDICS

A COMPLETE WORLD WAR II COMBAT HISTORY OF THE
U.S. TENTH MOUNTAIN DIVISION

IN THE WARTIME STORIES OF ONE OF ITS
FRONT LINE SURGEONS

CHAPTER I

INTRODUCTION

The Japanese attacked Pearl Harbor on December 7, 1941, and the following day the United States declared war on the Axis powers. At the time I was still a medical student at the University of Michigan, and was deferred from military service in order to finish. Immediately after graduation I went through an abbreviated nine-month general medical internship, and as soon as it ended I reported for active duty in the Army of the United States.

My first assignment took me to Carlisle Barracks, Pennsylvania to the Army Medical Field Service School where I was obliged to participate in a strenuous six-week course designed to prepare new medical officer inductees for combat duty. Then the Army, in its wisdom, sent me to its School of Tropical Medicine in Swannanoa, North Carolina, where I studied and treated a variety of tropical diseases. My patients were men just returned from the war in the Pacific. Six weeks later I received a ten-day leave of absence, at the conclusion of which I was ordered to report, on November 9, 1944, to the TENTH L DIVISION at Camp Swift near Austin, Texas. When I arrived I was greatly surprised to learn that, just two days earlier, the name of this division had been changed to TENTH MOUNTAIN DIVISION. I had been permanently assigned to the United States Army Ski Troops!

Before Christmas that same year I found myself in Italy, serving as the Battalion Surgeon of the 3rd Battalion of the 86th Mountain Infantry Regiment of the 10th Mountain Division, and commanding its medical detachment. Actual combat began early the next month, and then I found myself living at the front with the infantrymen, sharing many of the hardships, hazards and problems that they faced every day.

Under these stressful circumstances I soon developed a strong empathy for those front line soldiers. They lived under severe and dangerous conditions for long periods of time. Some were killed; some were wounded and died later; a few were permanently disabled; many were wounded and recovered well, but each of those who survived without injury also suffered. They had to endure every long, tense minute of their harsh living conditions and their exposure to danger. As time passed my admiration for these men grew, and I developed a deep respect for them which has lasted to this day and is reinforced, again and again, whenever I meet a veteran of front line combat.

During the course of battle, especially while I was treating wounded men, I would often think of a well-known expression of the time. Referring to the British Royal Air Force, Sir Winston Churchill said it first — "NEVER HAVE SO MANY OWED SO MUCH TO SO FEW."— During the most trying of times, as I treated the wounded, I would often repeat these words over and over again to myself. In my mind the "few" were those soldiers whose duties placed them in close proximity to the enemy, and who were required, directly, frequently and knowingly, to expose themselves to injury and death. They were the wounded that I treated.

Although my battalion aid station operated very close to the front, was often subjected to sniper fire and routinely subjected to enemy shellfire, I honestly didn't consider myself to be one of the "few." I was usually relatively well protected, because much of the time I worked inside a building with stone walls thick enough to protect against bullets and flying shell fragments. Also, whenever we were engaging the enemy, officers and enlisted men alike were most solicitous of my welfare and safety. They saw to it that I was not required to expose myself nearly as much as most of the men in the battalion. One of the line officers summed it up very well when he said, "After all, Doc, you're the only doctor we've got."

The 10th MOUNTAIN DIVISION did not engage in combat as long as most of the other divisions in Europe, but it did participate in a wide variety of different types of warfare, some of which were unusual and highly improbable for ski troops. It is ironic that this division, which had trained so long and so hard to wage war on skis, was hardly able to use them in combat at all. They were only used in the late winter of 1944 in the snow filled valleys of the Apennine Mountains during a static phase of the War, and their use was limited to patrols sent into no-mans-land to seek information and take prisoners. After the snow melted the skis were put away and never used in combat again, but mountaineering expertise and rock climbing skills remained important, and were used to good advantage.

In addition to fighting in the mountains the 10th MOUNTAIN DIVISION also carried its battles across the wide flatlands of the Po Valley, and there I participated in task forces, which penetrated deep behind enemy lines in an American version of what the Germans had named *Blitzkrieg*. I was with the troops in assault boats as they paddled across the wide Po River to establish a beach-head on the opposite shore, and later, in the mountains of the Southern Dolomites, I took part in a very unlikely amphibious attack which was mounted in order to bypass some partially destroyed tunnels along the shore of Lake Garda. No one could have anticipated that actions such as these would ever be assigned to a mountain division, especially one that had gained such wide notoriety as "The American Ski Troops." Nevertheless, circumstances dictated what had to be done, and the division always carried out its assignments extraordinarily well.

I had often been told that it is impossible to describe front line combat accurately and adequately, and after I had been at the front long enough to experience some of the action, and observe the death and destruction at firsthand, I realized that it was true. It is just not possible to make the general public fully understand and appreciate the enormity of the sacrifices that each individual front-line soldier had to make, with a mere description of action at the front. Such things as the anticipation of combat and the physical symptoms such anticipation can cause, the homesickness, the loneliness in spite of being with others, the constant dread and fear of being maimed or killed, the suffering caused by cold, dirty, uncomfortable living conditions, the enemy mortar and artillery shells falling and the vision of one such shell landing directly into someone's fox-hole and blasting him into shreds of flesh and skin and bits of bone, the enemy machine gun fire always probing for someone to kill, the enemy attacking with automatic weapons chattering and grenades exploding, or our men using similar weapons while attacking an enemy position in terrain where there are few places to hide or be shielded from gunfire, — these and many other things in the combat infantryman's life truly defy adequate description. It is my honest belief that the only way for anyone to fully know what front line combat is like is to have participated in it and survived.

Although conditions at the front were always grim, there was humor there too, and it had its place in the daily lives of the infantrymen. The longer I observed its effect upon these men the more I believed that it was important. It was definitely good for morale, and, before long, I became convinced that it also influenced the individual soldier's adaptability and survival. The ability to endure miserable and dangerous conditions seemed to increase with his ability to perceive and recognize a humorous side to the War and his situation in it. The man who was most likely to survive was the one who could see something funny under totally miserable conditions, who would often crack a joke during the worst of times, and who could easily laugh at himself no matter how wretched the circumstances. Humor also contributed greatly to the general morale, and on a number of occasions I noted that the telling of a funny incident, especially one involving the rear echelon, lifted the spirits of the entire battalion.

As my combat experiences continued, I gradually realized that the American soldier was able to understand, appreciate and participate in humor far more easily than the soldiers of all of the other nationalities I had encountered, and perhaps because of this ability he was also far better at adaptation and improvisation. He could "throw away the book" to quickly take advantage of almost any situation, or turn a bad one into something better, or improve his safety or his living conditions, and most of the time he could do it without actually disobeying orders. Soldiers from other armies, including those of the enemy, seemed much more inclined to follow their fixed procedures closely, even in extreme situations in which some other course of action might have ended with a better result.

Once I recognized this superior adaptability of the American soldier, I came to appreciate the work of Bill Mauldin for the cartoons he created while he was a soldier in the U.S. Fifth Army in Italy. In the later months they appeared regularly in the weekly Army newspaper, STARS AND STRIPES, and were later published with covering text material in a book titled UP FRONT. The cartoons clearly demonstrate the adaptability of American infantrymen in combat, and the role that humor played in their daily lives. I still have my copy from the first printing in 1945, and I still read and enjoy it from time to time.

And speaking of military humor, I admit that my favorite all-time television program is M.A.S.H., which has been appearing as re-runs for years. It is true that M.A.S.H. is about a Mobile Army Surgical Hospital, and my unit was only a battalion aid station, and it is true that the stories, written with exaggerated humor for the purpose of entertaining, took place in a different war; but it is also true that this program depicts many similarities to my experiences in World War II. Medically, the presentations are remarkably accurate in depicting typical war wounds. They also demonstrate some of the common psychological pressures and stresses put upon soldiers in combat, and occasionally show realistic scenes involving an aid station under fire, infantry patrols, and soldiers undergoing enemy sniping and shelling. Nevertheless, the prime reason I have for liking this television series so much is that it repeatedly and accurately demonstrates the utter disdain that most drafted civilian doctors felt in their hearts for Army customs and procedures.

My story begins on December 9, 1944, as I am about to leave the continental United States, knowing that I am destined for front line combat. I knew not where I was going nor how long I would be away, and I was certain that my chances for survival were limited. I wondered if I could stomach the conditions of front line combat, but I could only imagine the dire and terrible circumstances I might have to face. I wondered if I would be able to do whatever was expected of me, and hoped that I would not disgrace myself or my country. I realized that I could be heading toward my early demise, and there was little consolation in the thought that there were, after all, worse things than dying.

CHAPTER II

DEPARTURE

As I stood on the dock at Hampton Roads, Virginia waiting to board the ship to which I had been assigned, the sense of foreboding, which I had carried with me for several weeks, turned into a strong feeling of dread. My heart was beating rapidly, my palms were sweating, and there was such a tight knot in the pit of my stomach that it was painful. A first lieutenant in the Army Medical Corps, I was leaving my homeland to face an uncertain future going into combat as an infantry battalion surgeon. Officially I commanded the Medical Detachment, 3rd Battalion, 86th Mountain Infantry Regiment, Tenth Mountain Division. It gave me some comfort to know that this division had attained considerable fame as the elite American Ski Troops, and that it was made up of men in superb physical condition, with more than average education and with extensive training in skiing, mountain climbing and cold weather warfare. Its roster included famous names in mountaineering, and in collegiate and Olympic ski circles, and many people who were familiar with it conceded that the majority of the men in the Tenth Mountain Division were officer material. I was glad to have been assigned to such a division, instead of a unit headed for deployment somewhere in a jungle, but still I dreaded going overseas to face an extremely uncertain future. I knew not how long I would be away, nor what my fate might be, and I especially dreaded the prospect of soon playing a real part in mortal military combat.

Four and a half months had passed since I had been married, and during that time I had only been able to live with my lovely bride for about six weeks. One month had passed since she had come with me to Camp Swift, Texas where I had joined the division, but after our arrival I had only been able to see her twice, before all leaves were cancelled. Our parting had been difficult, and it would have been even worse for me, except that when the time came for us to say our final goodbyes, we couldn't be together. I had to stay in camp; she was in Austin. We said our last farewells over the phone.

The 10th Mountain Division was composed of the 85th, 86th and 87th Mountain Infantry Regiments and numerous support units. In a few hours my regiment, the 86th, would be the first in the Division to leave the continental United States, and eventually it would be first to engage the enemy in combat.

For the past several days we had been stationed at Camp Patrick Henry preparing for the sea voyage, and the preparations had been hectic. All individual and unit equipment had to be stenciled with proper identification markings. The men had to be briefed about what to expect on shipboard and how to behave during the voyage. Records and equipment had to be checked and double-checked. The immunization record of every man in the regiment had to be checked, and it was my responsibility to be sure that all deficiencies were corrected. We kept the aid station open and gave immunization injections at all hours as necessary. I also found it necessary to continue intensive medical first aid training for a group of men who were relatively new to our unit. During these preparations we learned that our battalion would ship out on the luxury liner, ARGENTINA, but this would not be a luxury cruise, and we would be very crowded on board. Nevertheless, I looked forward to traveling on such a nice ship, and was very curious about the voyage, because I had never before been to sea.

This had been a particularly bad day for me. In the morning I had been told that one of the ships in our convoy did not have a medical officer assigned to it, and that I had "volunteered" to fill this void. My footlocker and dufflebag would remain with my unit to be shipped with the battalion baggage on the ARGENTINA. I would need to pick up written orders for this change of plan from a Lieutenant Greenberg at the Camp Personnel Office, and I would also need to make arrangements there for my transportation to the dock.

Immediately after lunch I had set out to see Lieutenant Greenberg, but he proved to be hard to find. He was not at the Personnel Office. I was directed from building to building and place to place for some three hours, and had walked for miles before I finally found him. By this time I was tired and extremely disgruntled by the runaround and the seemingly indifferent treatment I was receiving from the camp personnel. By the time I left it this evening, I was thoroughly disgusted with Camp Patrick Henry and its staff.

Now as I stood at the edge of the crowd of soldiers on the dimly lit wharf, a mist rose into the air that further dimmed the lights from the streetlamps and contributed to the eerie gloom that pervaded the area. At first the scene appeared to be one of subdued confusion, but I soon made out the long lines of soldiers, heavily loaded with gear, waiting to board ship. I also carried a lot of gear. Canteen, gas mask and other required items were attached to my web belt, and I carried a medical officers' first aid kit on a strap over my shoulder. A well-packed mountain rucksack, which was the mountain troop equivalent of the standard Army backpack, was strapped to my back, and I carried a standard officers' bedroll which contained two Army blankets. Although mine was not that heavy, the rucksack, fully loaded, could weigh as much as 90 pounds, a fact which was extolled in one of the Division songs. Enlisted men did not have bedrolls, but each carried a dufflebag, and included in his gear were blankets with which to make a bed. Dufflebags for officers were shipped separately as baggage for them, as were their individual footlockers,

The men waiting in the lines to board the ship were unusually quiet, and spoke to each other in half-whispers, which added to the atmosphere of gloom. It was obvious to me that most of them were as uneasy and anxious as I was. I knew exactly how they felt, or perhaps I felt worse, because I was completely alone, while they would at least be traveling with their own units and among friends and acquaintances. All of my men would be on the ARGENTINA, and I would be essentially alone, not knowing anyone on the ship I was now waiting to board. As I watched and waited near the edge of the crowd, each line of soldiers walked slowly up the gangplank, and the men disappeared, one by one, into the dim hulk of the ship.

Suddenly I was hailed by one of the infantry officers. Would I look at a couple of his men who had developed a rash and were itching? Of course I would. I suspected what the problem was even before I got to them, because there had been several soldiers with such complaints in camp during the previous few days.

As soon as I saw the rash I knew that they had angioneurotic edema, otherwise known as giant urticaria or giant hives. Allergy probably plays a large part in its cause, but it is often precipitated by stress. In those days the usual treatment was an injection of epinephrine (Adrenalin), but a drug with similar action, ephedrine, also worked. Although its onset of its action was slower, it lasted longer, and it could be taken by mouth. Fortunately I had some tablets of ephedrine with phenobarbital in my medical kit, and I passed these out. The phenobarbital, being a sedative, could also be expected to relieve some of the nervous tension which I was sure contributed to the condition. Before the last of the men boarded the ship I had seen at least a dozen more cases. Apparently the treatment I prescribed was satisfactory, because these men traveled on the same ship with me, and I heard no more from any of them. I have never before nor since seen so many cases of angioneurotic edema in one place in such a short time, and I believe that its occurrence in so many men that evening reflects the high level of stress borne by soldiers leaving their homeland for a combat zone.

Finally, as the last of the columns of soldiers were entering the ship, I reached the foot of the gangplank and saw that there were only two of us remaining to board. The other man turned out to be a captain in the Air Force, who had flown a bomber from Europe to the United States, and had been ordered to return to Europe in this convoy, so that he could soon fly another one back. We walked up the gangplank together, and were greeted by an officer belonging to the troop contingent on board.

"Who are you, and why are you here?" he asked.

We explained and showed our orders. The officer looked at them, then shuffled through a stack of papers on his clipboard.

"Well, we weren't expecting you," he said at last. "You'll have to bunk in the sick bay."

We boarded, and quickly found the ship's dispensary below decks in the middle of the ship. There was a modest waiting area next to it, which was wide open at each end to passageways which ran lengthwise of the ship. On the other side of the right passageway was the sick bay, a large room filled with steel bunks which were bolted to the floor and had side rails which were permanently installed on them. They did not look very comfortable, and certainly the room was not at all inviting.

Across the waiting area from the dispensary we spied an open door, and when we looked inside, I was surprised to find that it opened into a typical padded cell. I had seen such accommodations before in a hospital psychiatric wing where such cells were used to confine the violently insane, but I certainly didn't expect to find anything like this on the ship. There were two bunks inside, low to the floor and thoroughly padded with soft materials. They looked comfortable and inviting. The floor and walls of the room were covered with pads that resembled soft wrestling mats, and compared to the crowded conditions in the sick bay, this room looked spacious. We congratulated ourselves on having found it, and moved in.

My new Air Force friend and I then became better acquainted, and exchanged some biographical information. He was sure that as soon as he got back to Europe he would be flying another bomber back to the States, and since I could not write anything about where I was or where I was going because of censorship, he offered to call my wife when he returned to let her know where I had gone and that I was well when he had seen me. I can't remember his name now, but I know that he made the call, because my wife wrote to me about it. She included his name in the letter, but it was one of those that I received, which was lost or destroyed during combat.

My new friend seemed amused by the circumstances, which had brought me into the Army, and by the fact that I had been trained in tropical medicine just before I was assigned to the ski troops. We talked until past midnight, then turned in to our bedrolls on those soft bunks in our plush padded cell quarters, and went to sleep.

Before daylight we were both suddenly awakened by the noise of the door to the room slamming shut. The ship was pitching and rolling, and its engines were running. We were at sea. Then we simultaneously made a startling discovery: THERE WAS NO HANDLE AT ALL ON THE INSIDE OF THAT DOOR! We were trapped! All of the information that I had received about enemy submarines lurking near our eastern shores, and the training about what to do in case we were torpedoed, flashed through my mind. There was a small, barred, glassless window in the door, and we peered through it. No one was in sight. We yelled. We whistled. We hooted and hollered. No one answered. I was sure that if we were to be torpedoed, this would be the time for it to happen.

About an hour passed, while we took turns whistling and yelling, and finally a sleepy-eyed crewman came by and let us out. We promptly moved all of our gear from the padded cell, and moved into the sick bay where we bunked for the rest of the voyage. Neither of us slept any more that night.

Another surprise came a few hours later. A member of the ship's crew came into the dispensary with a huge bundle of medical records and explained that there were 104 Merchant Marine seamen who were undergoing treatment for syphilis on board, and that I was now responsible for continuing their treatment, which consisted of intramuscular injections of an arsenic compound and a bismuth compound. Each sailor had to have three shots of one and one shot of the other each week.

Disposable syringes and needles were not available in those days. We used glass syringes with individually fitted plungers and removable, reusable needles. The medications were suspended in oil which made the syringes and needles difficult to clean. Each syringe and needle had to be meticulously washed. Dull needles had to be resharpened on a whetstone. Then all of these items had to be autoclaved to make them sterile before they could be used again.

This development made a lot of extra work for me. I had expected only to be required to hold a daily sick call for the several thousand men on board. I asked for medical technician volunteers from the ranks to help in the dispensary and got two who later assured me that they had been glad to volunteer, because sleeping in the dispensary or sick bay was a lot better than staying in the hold. I also received some volunteer clerical help, and immediately put these men to work sorting the medical records and preparing a schedule for shots to be given to the Merchant Marines.

Vials of the syphilis medicines were in ample supply in the refrigerator, but the autoclave, needed for sterilizing syringes, needles and instruments, wasn't working. There was apparently no one on board willing or able to repair it. Fortunately there was a tool kit in the dispensary, so I was able to fix it myself. I also personally gave all of the injections of arsenic and bismuth, because these needed to be placed intramuscularly, and no one else admitted that they knew how to do it. We quickly established a daily schedule designating the injections and the men to receive them, and followed it for the rest of the voyage.

The ship we were on was a cargo carrier which had been converted into a troop ship, but I didn't remember her name. Normally, with the holds full of cargo, such a ship would ride low in the water and knife through the waves, but when used as a troop ship there was much less weight on board, and it floated much higher. This gave it a tendency to bounce around on top of the waves like a cork. The voyage went smoothly for about three days, and I had time to go up on deck occasionally. Having never been on the ocean before, I was fascinated by the waves and the deep blue color of the water. The ARGENTINA and sometimes other ships in the convoy were sometimes visible, and there was almost always a destroyer escort in view. One sunny afternoon while I was on deck crew members held gunnery practice from the rear of the ship. Large gas-filled balloons were released and the gun crews shot them down as they rose into the sky. This was the first time that I had been close to a large gun being fired, and the loudness of the noise surprised me.

Only two meals a day were served on board, but there was plenty of good food. The men came out of the holds to go through chow lines, and then ate on deck. During daylight hours music was played over the ship's loudspeakers constantly, and each day a Post Exchange type store, where men could buy cigarettes and other things, was open for several hours. Only a few men reported for the daily sick call, and their problems were minor.

Then our convoy ran into heavy weather. Waves were 15 to 20 feet high, and sometimes seemed higher. Fine salt spray blew across the decks constantly. The crests of the big, dark waves were capped with a brilliant white foam. The ship pitched and rolled constantly, and as a consequence, seasickness became a major problem. The medicines we had for it did not work very well. Most of the men stayed in their bunks in the holds and suffered through it. Only a very few reported to sick call. While the problems with seasickness were at their worst I went into one of the holds to see how things were. The bunks were stacked six high from floor to ceiling, and there was barely enough room on each one for a soldier to lie down with his equipment. Almost everyone was seasick, and some were retching and vomiting. The lucky ones had the top bunks, because they avoided the intermittent vomitus which rained down from above. The passages were slick with it and the smell was horrible. On another day I was called down to another of the holds to see a victim of this slippery condition who had fallen and injured himself. Being a physician I had had exposure to stench such as this, and worse, during my training, so it didn't bother me much, especially since I didn't have to stay in it. I did, however, feel sorry for the men who had to live in those holds.

Sick call increased during those seasick days, and I saw more patients each day. The program for administering the syphilis shot continued and was working very well. I was too busy to be seasick myself, but I admit that I didn't have my usual hearty appetite for a few days. I couldn't help but wonder if things were as bad for the men of my medical detachment on the AR-GENTINA. I hoped not.

After three or four days the seas calmed, and the men began to eat again. The holds were cleaned out, and life on the ship became much more tolerable. More boat drills were held with everyone donning a life vest and reporting to his proper lifeboat station. There was also more gunnery practice.

Before we were halfway across the Atlantic Ocean we learned from members of the ship's crew that our destination was Naples, Italy, so no one was surprised when the Straits of Gibraltar came into view. The weather was clear as we passed through, and the seas were calm. Many of the men went up on deck to catch a glimpse of this famous landmark, and I went up too. I viewed the straits from the African side of the ship, and was impressed by the narrowness of this famous waterway. "The Rock," however, did look like its pictures.

Shortly after we entered the Mediterranean Sea I received an invitation to dinner at the ship captain's table, and this caused quite a stir among the Army officers on board. They, as well as some of the ship's crew, assured me that such an invitation was a great honor. Of course I accepted, and I anticipated a pleasant dinner with the ship's officers.

Allowing plenty of time in order to be sure that I would not be late, I went up to the deck where the ship's officers lived and where the Captain's dining room was located. As I made my way along the passageway, I was stopped short at an open door to one of the cabins by a sign which read:

CAPT. XXXXXX XXXX, MC

ARMY TRANSPORTATION CORPS

I looked inside, and there, seated in a chair with his stockinged feet propped up on a small table that folded out from the wall, was a man in Army uniform wearing captain's bars and the Cadeuceus of a Medical Officer. An open whiskey bottle stood on the table. It quickly dawned upon me that I had just stumbled upon the regular ship's surgeon, and that I was yet another greenhorn medical officer who had been officially conned into doing his work while he rode back and forth across the sea nursing his bottles of booze. I suddenly became very angry,—mad beyond caring what I said or did,— so mad that I was blinded to the fact that he outranked me, and I emphatically spoke my mind. I don't remember now exactly what I said, but I am sure it wasn't nice.

There were no words between us throughout dinner that we attended a few minutes later at the Captain's Table. I was still so mad that I hardly remember anything that happened at dinner, but I must presume that I was courteous and went through all of the proper motions. I certainly hope so.

For the scant rest of the voyage this Transportation Corps Medical Officer, whose name I remember but have deliberately omitted, spent a good share of the day in the dispensary helping with the work. I turned the entire treatment of the syphilitic sailors back over to him, and spent my time running the sick call for the troops on board.

The next day our ship entered the harbor at Oran, Algeria, and anchored close enough to the shore so that I could clearly see the shoreline and the buildings in the city. The reason for this interruption in our voyage wasn't apparent since no one boarded or got off of the ship. I remember the large quantity of garbage floating in the water all around and two youngsters swimming about in it,— a girl about 12 years old and a boy who looked younger. It occurred to me that they were a long distance from shore. However, they were excellent swimmers, and after about an hour they swam back toward shore. Some of our men watching them wondered out loud how they kept from getting sick in the filthy water. Then after only a few hours at anchor, the ship's engines started up and we were under way again.

On December 23, 1944 we entered the harbor at Naples and anchored. Our ship could not dock because the harbor facilities were severely limited by the effects of the War. Access to dock space was blocked by the hulks of numerous half-sunken ships resting on the harbor bottom with their super-structures showing above the water. Some of the docks had also suffered damages form bombings.

Although our ship had to wait its turn to reach dockside so we could disembark, it had anchored close enough to shore for me to clearly see the many damaged buildings and the dirt and rubbish in the streets. A few poorly dressed people were walking about. Olive drab military vehicles were lined up along the waterfront, and from time to time soldiers could be seen disem-barking from their ships and marching to them. This was certainly not the Naples I had read about in school, nor the sunny Italy described in travel brochures. This was wartime Italy, a grim time for the Italian people; and I was acutely aware that this was foreign soil.

As I gazed at the gloomy scene, I wondered, with anxiety and forebod-ing of bad things to come, what would happen to me in the days ahead.

CHAPTER III

PREPARATION IN ITALY

Although our ship had arrived in Naples Harbor on the 23rd of December, we could not disembark until the next day. The ARGENTINA docked first, and it was some hours later, as the last of her troops were marching down the gangplank, that my ship also docked and began to disgorge troops. Because I was among the last off, it was the middle of the afternoon before I stepped ashore and marched past some booths where Red Cross workers were passing out doughnuts to our men. A line of waiting Army trucks was strung out along the street parallel to the dock, and I climbed aboard one of them near the rear of the column. These were quartermaster trucks which were normally used for carrying supplies and equipment, and now, loaded with troops, they were so crowded that everyone had to stand upright during the ride to the staging area at Bagnoli, a few miles to the North. As our motor convoy pulled away from the docks, I looked again at the harbor in Naples, and what a dreary scene it was! It was windy, and the sky was gray and overcast. Low clouds were everywhere, and the temperature was near freezing.

During the ride I tried to see as much of Naples as I could. Some of the buildings showed war damage, and the rest looked neglected and dirty. In the shadows, here and there, I could see people indistinctly. I saw streetcar tracks in some of the streets, much like those in our cities at home, but no streetcars were anywhere to be seen. In a little while I saw the first child that I clearly recognized to be a child. He was boy about 10 years old, standing between the streetcar tracks in the middle of the street in plain view of everyone, and urinating in a magnificent stream. A few minutes later I saw a second youth, pants lowered, squatting between the tracks and defecating. These scenes were a distinct novelty to our troops, and gave rise to many ribald comments and remarks. I had never seen anything like it in the U. S., but this was only the first of many similar performances I would see during my stay in Italy.

Bagnoli was the site of an orphanage and school, which had been under construction when the War began. Construction had then ceased, leaving many of the buildings uncompleted. However, enough of them were far enough along in the building process so that a lot of German soldiers could use them during their occupation of the region. Some of the buildings had suffered war damage, and some appeared neglected, but there were still enough usable ones available to shelter our troops. The buildings were dirty and dingy on the outside. Crude attempts at camouflage and the scars and accumulations of wreckage from bombings and shellings did nothing to improve their appearance. Most had polished marble floors inside, but were without furnishings. Window openings were large, but, with few exceptions, contained no windows. There as no heat, electricity or running water.

Christmas Eve, the day we arrived in Bagnoli, was my first day on Italian soil. I was assigned to sleep on the floor of one of the marble-floored buildings, and it turned out to be one of those with the large window openings but without window frames, sash or glass. The weather was cold and rainy, and the dampness was bone chilling and pervasive. I was cold and uncomfortable most of the time. However, there was one building available to me that was heated. It was the Red Cross Building, which had a large reading room furnished with chairs and tables, where I could sit and write letters. I had not written on shipboard because I knew that my letters could not be mailed until the end of the voyage, and then all of them would be sent off together, so this Christmas Eve I made several trips to the Red Cross Building to write home and to warm myself. I wrote three separate letters to my wife and one to my mother, all at different times.

That night I slept in my bedroll on the hard marble floor, and it was cold! Even after I had put on everything that I could wear, including extra socks, field jacket and lined trench coat, my two Army blankets weren't enough to keep me warm. I was also wearing khaki colored long winter underwear, but still I shivered and my teeth chattered most of the night. It wasn't until the following morning, Christmas Day, that I was able to warm up again, inside the Red Cross Building where I wrote yet another letter to my wife. Never before nor since have I spent such a lonesome and miserable Christmas Eve as this one.

Field kitchens were set up outdoors between buildings and under canvas to feed the troops. For each meal we went through the "chow line" holding mess kits and canteen cups into which food and drink were served, and after eating we went through another line to clean our utensils in the manner prescribed by Army Regulations. For this procedure three large garbage cans were set in a row, each one standing on top of a lighted gasoline burner to keep the solution in it hot. The first contained hot soapy water with a dish mop and a brush with which to clean the gear; the second contained a disinfectant rinse, and the third contained a clear hot water rinse. After going through these three steps the utensils were supposed to air dry.

I don't remember what we had for supper that first night, nor for breakfast the next morning, but I do remember that at about noon we had a typically American Christmas dinner, with roast turkey and dressing, mashed potatoes, cranberries, squash and all of the usual trimmings. Portions were generous and my mess kit was heaped full as I reached the end of the serving line. There the soldier manning the last station in the serving line deftly placed a slice of vanilla brick ice cream atop the pan full of hot food that I had received. I always had an excellent appetite, and mixtures of food didn't bother me. This mixture of melted ice cream over turkey, dressing and gravy didn't bother me either, and I ate heartily. However, some of the men didn't like it and objected emphatically, even to the extent of not eating at all.

This worked out well for the poor Italian children who scrounged food scraps from our Army garbage. I saw this now for the first time as I went through the dishwashing line. My first stop was at a series of large garbage pails into which we were to scrape whatever food scraps were left in our mess kits. Standing on the other side of these cans were several skinny, dirty, hungry-looking children dressed in ragged clothing. They carried old, well used institutional size tin cans with makeshift homemade wire bale handles, and they were begging for leftover scraps from the soldiers' mess kits. Usually the men were not able to scrape their leftovers into the garbage cans at all, but instead scraped it from their mess kits directly into the children's tin pails. There were no complaints from the children about the admixture of foods.

During the War this scene was repeated over and over again all over Italy wherever the Army had kitchens set up. Soldiers would often take an extra bit of food, a slice of bread, or a cookie that they knew they wouldn't eat, just to give it to one of the children at the end of the meal. Sometimes adults were involved in this scrounging, but not often. Usually it was only children. Bill Mauldin deftly captured this scene in one of his cartoons on page 66 in the original edition of his book, UP FRONT. It shows a steel helmeted infantryman with mess gear in hand, and a small girl holding a tin can bucket, facing each other. The title of the cartoon? THE PRINCE AND THE PAUPER. The caption really wasn't needed. The picture tells it all!

During the whole of the time I spent in Italy I don't remember ever seeing a fat child. Occasionally there was a plump adult, but they were few and far between. The food shortage was not so bad for people in the rural areas, since in spite of the War there was always a local harvest. In many places there were still potatoes, carrots and turnips still in the ground waiting to be dug. Scarcity of food was a much bigger problem in the cities, and was partly the result of lack of transport to carry food in from the countryside.

While the whole regiment was in Bagnoli none of the three Battalion Aid Stations were set up, because the entire regiment was so close together. We operated only the Regimental Aid Station to take care of sick call for the whole regiment.

Our first casualties on foreign soil occurred on the day after our arrival, but I had no direct contact with them. I heard about them from one of the other medical officers. It seemed that some of the men bought "cognac" from an Italian street vendor, and had a party. The "cognac" turned out to contain very little real liquor, but was mostly high octane American aviation gasoline with wood alcohol added to it. By the time I learned of the tragedy there were six men in the hospital who were not expected to live. After that day I never heard anything more about them.

Upon our arrival at Bagnoli we were told that we would probably stay about two weeks for more training, in order to give the balance of our equipment and the rest of the division (the 85th and 87th Regiments) time to catch up with us. The whole Division would then move up close to the front for still more training before going into the line. Now these plans suddenly changed. Shortly after noon on Christmas Day we were told that at the front our American 92nd Division had been routed, and the Germans had broken through the gap with three divisions. There was nothing to keep them from driving all of the way to Rome except our regiment!

Instead of remaining a component of the 10th Mountain Division, the regiment now became a part of a task force named Task Force 45, which also included some British artillerymen, some American antiaircraft personnel, and a few other miscellaneous units, all of which had been quickly converted into infantry. There would be no more training. We were going into battle as quickly as we could get there! Our regiment was ordered to move up to the front as fast as possible!

Headquarters and the 1st Battalion boarded a train and headed north immediately, and the rest of us were trucked back to Naples to board an Italian freighter which had been turned into a troop ship. The name of the ship wasn't important to me, and I don't believe I knew it at the time, but learned much later, after the War was over, that her name was the SESTRIARE. Those men who had come to Italy on the ARGENTINA did a lot of grousing and complaining about this ship, but to me she did not look much worse than the ship on which I had crossed the Atlantic only a short time before. The biggest difference was in the toilet facilities, and the arrangement on the SESTRIARE deserves detailed description.

All of the toilets to be used by the troops were located on the top deck, which was at least two stories above the level of the sea. Amidship on both sides of the ship two sets of parallel wooden two-by-fours had been erected and were supported at about chair height. They ran literally from the cabin wall across the deck to the deck rail. There were about eight inches of space between the paired two-by-fours, and in this space, a little below their upper surfaces, a long piece of metal eavestrough had been suspended. These troughs were longer than the two-by-four pairs, and protruded through the rail about three feet beyond the side of the ship. Salt water from the sea was pumped through them constantly, and it ran from the cabin wall out through the deck rail, then fell back into the sea. One could urinate into the trough from either side, ride the rails sidesaddle, or sit astride them as in riding a horse,— whichever way one preferred. Crude as it was this system seemed to work satisfactorily in the calm shelter of the harbor, but as soon as the ship reached the open sea, strong winds constantly lifted the overflow, and whatever it might contain, high into the air to rain down upon the ship as a more or less fine spray!

This sea voyage lasted overnight, with about 18 hours on the open sea, during which time we had at least two meals that I am able to recall. Usual field kitchen routine was followed. The men went through the chow line, then up on deck to eat. I remember that most of the diners crowded into the extreme ends of the ship, the bow and the stern, to get as far away as possible from the spray created by those crude toilet facilities. A few found sheltered areas in some of the passageways off of the deck in which to eat.

During one of the meals I overheard two soldiers who were sitting on the floor in one of those passageways with backs against a bulkhead. Their conversation accurately summed up the situation. It went something like this:

"Want some salt?" said soldier number one, offering his companion an individually portioned packet of it.

"Hell No!" said soldier number two, casting a meaningful eye at the spray outside of the passageway and only a few feet from him, since I've been on this tub I've eaten more salt and more shit than I ever wanted."

The day after we left Naples the SESTRIARE docked at *Livorno*, a city known to Americans as Leghorn. Here we disembarked and were immedi-

ately trucked to a new staging area. Our route took us very close to the famous Leaning Tower of Pisa, and we all had a good look at it as we passed. A
few miles beyond it we stopped and set up our bivouac, finishing about at
suppertime.

We set up camp in an open area which contained some trees and looked
like a large park, where people perhaps took walks and held picnics before
the War. Company areas were designated, and two men put together their
canvas shelter halves to make two man pup tents, just large enough for two
men to shelter their gear and sleep inside. These were erected precisely in
neat rows, then as soon as the pup tents were in place each man had to dig his
own fox hole to the prescribed dimensions, at the prescribed distance from
his tent, and in the prescribed manner, using the small, shovel-like entrenching tool which he carried. Headquarters tents, field kitchens, latrines and aid
stations were established in tents and there was a motor pool. Drinking water
was sterilized in large Lister bags, and it became one of my duties to see to it
that camp sanitation measures were strictly observed in our battalion area.

We set up the aid station in the large tent included in our equipment for
that purpose, and when we had finished erecting the tent, every piece of equipment was cleaned, shined, and put in its proper place according to the training manuals. Records were in order, and each man in my medical detachment could recite his duties. The daily sick call was held in the tent. Routes
of evacuation to the rear were established, checked and rechecked. Everything was done "by the book." We followed the Army manuals as closely as
we could, and were ready for the inspections which followed.

It seemed that we were now ready for combat. Our medical detachment
had improved vastly from what it had been at Camp Swift. I felt that we
could function well and do our work satisfactorily. Most of the uneasiness
over my ability to command, when I was first introduced to my men, had
now been dispelled, but the gnawing dread of going into combat was still as
intense as ever.

With combat preparations now nearly complete, I had time to think back
upon the rapid succession of remarkable events which had befallen me since
I joined the division. My wife and I had arrived at the small railroad station in
Bastrop, Texas, to learn immediately that there was no place in that small
town for her to stay. As soon as I had seen her off on a bus headed for Austin,
Texas, I phoned the camp, announced my arrival, and asked for transportation to report for duty. A Jeep soon arrived to pick me up, and as I climbed
into the front seat next to the driver, I tossed my baggage into the back. From
the wording in my orders I knew that I would be joining the 10TH L DIVI-

SION. I had learned from several Regular Army officers that an L division was a "Light Division," i.e. a division without heavy vehicles or equipment. Such a division would be great for sloshing around in some distant jungle, and since I had left the Army School of Tropical Medicine to accept this assignment, I expected to be assigned to a unit destined for jungle warfare somewhere in the Pacific.

As we were driving toward the camp, I contemplated the countryside. The land was flat and dry, almost like a desert with only a few scrubby trees here and there. I missed the large green trees which I had been accustomed to seeing in Michigan. The soil was reddish-brown and very dry. Dust clouds blew up easily almost everywhere. The thought crossed my mind that this was odd country in which to be training soldiers for jungle warfare. Then, when the entrance to Camp Swift came into view, I saw a sign made up of large individual letters formed in a large arc and suspended high above the gateposts, which read: "THROUGH THESE GATES PASS THE BEST DAMN MULES IN THE WORLD." These are perhaps not the exact words, because I am not completely certain about my memory of it, but the message was clear.

That there were mules there, I could believe, for on company streets, between barracks and service buildings, on lawns and in flower beds, on the parade grounds ——everywhere the eye could see —— mules were running loose. And they didn't look like just ordinary mules. They were huge, long-eared beasts, as big as horses, and as they were running all over the camp in all directions, they were braying and kicking and making motions as if to bite. Soldiers wearing fatigues (uniforms) were chasing them, most of them yelling and cursing the mules as they tried to round them up, and it appeared that the men had to take care to avoid being kicked or bitten. It didn't appear that they were making much progress in capturing the animals. I thought to myself, "Good God! What kind of a circus is this outfit I'm joining?"

After we passed through the gate the driver made several detours to avoid running into mules, and eventually dropped me off at the entrance to the Division Headquarters Building. As soon as I entered I was enthusiastically greeted by a number of officers and men. Everyone seemed genuinely glad to see me. One of the officers explained that the mules had broken loose by accident, and assured me that what I had seen outside was not normal camp routine. The mules were the division's transport system in wild and otherwise inaccessible mountainous terrain. With a number of these animals and a gun crew, a 75 mm. Pack howitzer could be carried in, set up, and fired from a mountaintop where it was impossible for mechanized transport to go.

Now, for the first time, I learned the nature of the division to which I had been assigned. Just two days before my arrival its name had been changed to the TENTH MOUNTAIN DIVISION. I WAS IN THE SKI TROOPS !!!! These soldiers were skiers and mountain climbers trained in winter warfare, — trained to survive for long periods of time in sub-zero temperatures.

I was completely happy with this assignment, and felt greatly relieved not to be going into combat somewhere in the tropics. I liked the idea of being on high ground, and of having convenient hills in which to hide. My worries about jungle warfare had been unnecessary, for I was never to see a jungle nor treat an acute case of any tropical disease during the rest of my Army career.

Next I was directed to the Division Personnel Officer's desk, and he, too, greeted me warmly. He told me that the Division was going overseas very soon, and was being brought up to full strength.

"We're filling in all of our medical officer vacancies," he said, "and you're the first new doctor to arrive. You'll be assigned to the 86th. I guess you can have your choice. Do you want the first, second or third battalion?"

By this time in my Army career I had received much confidentially given advice from many sources as to how I should conduct myself: "Don't volunteer for anything; don't be pushy or make yourself conspicuous; keep a low profile; etc." I had always been adept at hanging back, staying on the fringe of activities, and avoiding the limelight, —— traits which were hangovers from my early school days. Then, too, I was fully aware of my own mortality, and kept self-preservation constantly in mind. For an instant I pondered that a field commander in a combat situation with three battalions to manipulate would think sooner of number one and number two, while number three was more likely to remain in reserve. It took only a few seconds for these thoughts to race through my mind.

I didn't hesitate. I said, "I'll take the third."

That was how it happened that I received my present assignment, command of the Medical Detachment of the 3rd Battalion of the 86th Mountain Infantry.

As things turned out later my battalion was not in reserve any more than the others. In fact it was the only battalion to be chosen three times to participate in combat task forces deep into enemy territory, and it was regularly chosen to lead some of the important regimental attacks. Before the fighting ended we had become quite accustomed to watching for enemy soldiers to our rear, as well as forward and on our flanks.

I have never regretted choosing the 3rd Battalion. As time in combat passed, I became very proud of it, its officers and its men!

For readers who are not familiar with military organization it seems appropriate to briefly explain a few things about the structure of the Division and the role of its medical personnel. The Division consisted of three mountain infantry regiments, the 85th, 86th, and 87th, plus division artillery units, a medical battalion, and a number of other support units. Each infantry regiment was made up of four companies, three of which were wholly made up of infantry squads, and the fourth made up of men who operated mortars and heavy caliber machine guns, which was called the HEAVY WEAPONS COMPANY. The companies in each battalion were designated by letters. Companies A, B and C were the infantry companies, and Company D was the Heavy Weapons Company of every 1st Battalion in the Army; Companies E, F and G were the infantry companies, and Company H was the Heavy Weapons Company of every 2nd Battalion; Companies I, K and L were the infantry companies, and Company M was the Heavy Weapons Company of every 3rd Battalion. There was no such designation as J Company. Each regiment had a Headquarters Company, which was responsible for all regimental operations, and among other support units attached to it was a medical detachment which was split out from the Division Medical Battalion and provided medical services. Other support units supplied such things as artillery support, ammunition and supplies, communications, intelligence data, transportation, and other things.

Although the Regimental Medical Detachment still belonged to the Division Medical Battalion, it operated as a separate command entity because it was "detached" from the Medical Battalion. The Regimental Medical Detachment was pared down in number of men by detaching three Battalion Medical Detachments from it, and assigning one to each of its battalions. Each of these battalion medical detachments operated as a separate command entity, with the Battalion Surgeon in command, because it was "detached" from the Regimental Medical Detachment. Each battalion medical detachment operated a battalion aid station. The remainder of the Regimental Medical Detachment was commanded by the Regimental Surgeon, but it also had an Assistant Regimental Surgeon, a Regimental Dental Officer and an Assistant Dental Officer. The Regimental Medical Detachment also operated an aid station which was always available to anyone in the regiment.

My command, the 3rd Battalion Medical Detachment, served Companies I, K, L and M of the 86th Mountain Infantry Regiment, and also served the 3rd Battalion Headquarters. I worked closely with battalion headquarters, and usually had a field telephone hooked up to the battalion communications system. Consequently I had much more contact with the men there than I did with the Regimental Officers and men. In spite of our designation as a part of the Regimental Medical Detachment, and ultimately of the 10th Mountain Division Medical Battalion, my men and I considered ourselves to belong and be a part of our 3rd Battalion.

Each battalion medical detachment had a complement of 41 men: a battalion surgeon, a medical administrative officer, and 39 enlisted men. The enlisted men were divided into three categories: company aid men, aid station personnel, and litter bearers.

Company aid men treated the wounded in the field where they fell, and were normally the first medics to make contact with them. Each individual infantryman carried a first aid packet on his belt that contained bandages and sulfa powder. It was to be used first. If additional supplies were needed they came from the company aid man's kit which contained various additional supplies and medications, including extra bandages, sulfa powder, and styrettes containing morphine. Each styrette resembled a miniature toothpaste tube, but with a hypodermic needle instead of a cap on it, and each contained one quarter of a grain of morphine. In order to use it the protective sheath over the needle had to be removed first, then the sterile needle pushed deeply into the patient's skin; then by squeezing the tube the morphine was injected through the needle. Each company aid man lived with the company he served, went wherever it went, and normally returned to the aid station only when he needed to replenish his medical supplies. His duty was to render immediate first aid, then enough further treatment so that the wounded soldier could, without suffering any further harm, walk or be carried to the aid station. Among other things he was trained in the control of bleeding, the proper application of bandages, and the application of temporary splints, using whatever materials were at hand.

Aid station personnel came in two categories: (1) medical/surgical technicians who directly assisted the surgeon with actual medical work, kept medical (treatment) records, and were responsible for the medical instruments and supplies, and (2) administrative and service people who kept the non-medical records required by the Army, managed the non-medical supplies, drove and maintained the vehicles, tended the mules, and generally were required to see to it that the unit ran smoothly and according to Army regulations.

Litter bearers were exactly what the name implies. Organized in teams of four men, their job was to carry, on their litters, those of the wounded who were unable to walk, and to bring them safely from the battlefield to the aid station. They also had the duty of guiding the walking wounded to treatment and safety. In extremely rugged terrain they were also occasionally used to carry a casualty out of the aid station to the rear to some place where he could safely be picked up by a vehicle for further transport out of the combat zone. Most of the time the litter bearers handled casualties who had already been treated by a company aid man, but this wasn't always the case. Therefore they, too, carried first aid kits and were trained in first aid procedures.

When I first arrived at my new command in Camp Swift, I found that only seven of the 39 authorized enlisted men were present at the dispensary.

"Where are the rest of the men?" I asked the sergeant in charge whom I had just met. His reply worried me a bit.

"The company aid men are out with their companies," he replied, "and Headquarters says that the litter bearers should be here in a couple of days, but they've been saying that for a while now."

The men that were there that afternoon were the aid station complement, and I met them all right away. Some time later when I called the whole medical detachment together, I also met the company aid men. I liked every one of these men immediately, and after I had spoken with each one individually, I felt much better about my new job.

Two days later the missing men, the litter bearers, arrived, and a major problem became immediately apparent. They had all just graduated from the Army Cooks and Bakers School. Now, suddenly they were medics, expected to carry medical aid kits and treat casualties. None of them knew anything more about first aid than the average infantry private, and most had never even seen a splint, a triangular bandage or a morphine styrette. They certainly needed some rapid retraining before they would be adequately able to do what would soon be required of them! They had come from widely separated parts of the country and varied ethnic backgrounds. Some had only minimal education, but all appeared to be reasonably intelligent and capable of learning. Among them were several older men, whom I suspected were infantry rejects, either because of age or some physical limitation. One was 42 years old and said he was having trouble with his knees. This was very evident, for when he walked everyone in the room could hear them creak and grate, and when I examined him I found the typical gross changes of advanced osteoarthritis.

In the beginning my men had all been total strangers to me. Now as we were bivouacked in the vicinity of the Leaning Tower of Pisa, I felt that I knew most of them fairly well. I didn't know the company aid men as well as I knew the rest because they were out with their respective companies most of the time, but I knew that they had all been well trained and were capable of doing their jobs. Our litter bearers had received extra training from our own medical technicians, and I felt that now each one could adequately do whatever might be necessary in the field. I felt confident that every man in my detachment would perform well.

By now I had grown to know and like the key people in the aid station. Actually they had become "best friends," and remained such until after the end of the War. As time passed I felt that our friendships among each other grew continually stronger as we went through the trials of combat together and our dependence upon each other increased. These key people were:

Lieutenant Byron P. Summers, M.A.C., our Medical Administrative Officer, was a Regular Army career officer who had enlisted as a private and had worked his way up through the ranks. He had gone through Officers' Candidate School, and had completed a course in medical administration at Carlisle Barracks. He knew both the official and the unofficial side of the Army, and was easily able to take most of the responsibility of running the Medical Detachment from my shoulders. He had already been invaluable in guiding me through the mazes of red tape and regulations, and he would continue to do this throughout the rest of the War. He was known familiarly as Barney. He grew up in Missouri, still had a little bit of Missouri accent, knew Army slang, and his repertoire of cuss words was the envy of many of his friends. However, to his credit, I can truthfully say that during the time he and I spent together he did not swear much, and I never once heard him swear when a woman was present.

Sergeant Arthur Draper was first sergeant of the Detachment and the highest ranking non-commissioned officer in it. He was perhaps ten years older than I, and had been a newspaper correspondent and journalist whose home was in New York State. He had been active and prominent in skiing in New England, and that was why he had joined the ski troops. He was an excellent journalist, and later took it upon himself to write many of the citations for decorations which men of the 10th Mountain Division received. He was a tall man, intelligent and capable, and he ran the aid station smoothly. He handled people extremely well, was courageous and dependable, and functioned especially well during the most stressful of times.

Sergeant Irving "Chuck" Miller was the chief medical technician for our unit. In addition to directly assisting me with sick call and the care of casualties, he was in charge of all of the medical equipment we had. He was about seven or eight years older than I, was Jewish, and his home was somewhere in New Jersey, not far from New York City. Since I spent most of my growing up years living in a Jewish neighborhood in Detroit, we hit it off really well from the beginning. I remember that he thought it was strange that I, a gentile from Detroit, should know about schmalz herring, lox and other typically Jewish things.

We had left the U.S. without much of our mountain gear, and had also left the mules behind. We didn't know it then, but the mules were on the way to Italy, and should arrive in time for us to use them in the most mountainous of the battlefields in which we would soon find ourselves. Additional equipment was now issued to everyone. Because the weather was colder that anticipated we received extra blankets, and I added two more to my bedroll. There were mountain stoves on which to cook or heat rations. These operated on the same principle as a gasoline blowtorch, but had a baffle of heat resistant metal to spread the flame. For light in the aid station we used gasoline lanterns which operated on the same principle, and had a mesh mantle which glowed white-hot, and produced a bright, white light as it hung in the flame. The aid station tent was made of very heavy canvas, and was heavily impregnated with waterproofing. Light did not penetrate through it, so blackout rules could more easily be observed.

We also received motor vehicles. The battalion medical detachment was allotted one Jeep, a short, open vehicle, modifications of which are still being produced and used by both the armed services and the civilian populace, and a 3/4 ton weapons carrier (truck) with a trailer. This was enough transport to carry all of the aid station equipment plus six or eight men, including the drivers. When the aid station was not being moved I could consider the Jeep as my personal vehicle, but officers were ordered not to drive, so wherever I went, I always had my Jeep driver with me.

At about 2:00 a.m. on one of the nights while we were still camped near Pisa there was an air raid alarm. Sirens sounded up and down the coast, and we were out of our pup tents and into our foxholes in a flash, donning our steel helmets as we went. It was cold in those holes! I can remember seeing my own breath when I exhaled, and also the breaths of others rising from nearby foxholes. I don't remember exactly how long we were out there, but it was long enough to become thoroughly chilled. After a time we learned that this had been a false alarm, and with a lot of grumbling, crawled back into our pup tents for a little more sleep. Some officer among the higher brass had decided that an air raid drill would be good for the troops, and gave the alarm. His action had apparently alerted the entire west coast of Italy.

Some of us were now wondering about the German breakthrough in the North. Why weren't we being overrun? If the Germans were headed back to

Rome, why were we sitting here in camp instead of "out there" stopping them? The explanations we received seemed odd but plausible, and they involved the way the German Armies were fed.

Our men ate C or K rations while they were at the front. A soldier could easily carry C rations for one or two days, since a day's ration consisted of six cans. Three contained wet food that could be easily heated or eaten cold. Varieties included frankfurters and beans, meat and noodles, spaghetti and meatballs, lamb and rice, and meat and vegetable stew. The cans usually arrived by the case, each case containing all of the varieties available, and each man got to choose from whatever was left in the box when he got there. Enlisted men were supposed to be fed first, and most of the time they were, so I got to eat a lot of the least popular variety, which was meat and vegetable stew. The second can for each meal contained dry food. Each one contained thick, heavy crackers, which we called "dog biscuits," a packet of powdered coffee, bullion or lemonade, from which a canteen cup full of warm or cold drink could be made, some candy and three cigarettes with matches. I actually liked the K rations better. A day's ration of these consisted of three oblong cardboard boxes, and a man could easily carry K rations for several days with him in his pack. The breakfast box contained a small, flat tin of scrambled egg and ham, some "dog biscuits," coffee powder, hard candy and cigarettes. The noon meal box contained a small tin of cheese with bacon bits in it, and bullion or lemonade powder instead of coffee; and the evening meal box contained a tin of veal loaf and hot chocolate drink powder. The dry contents were the same in all three meals. There was also a D ration which we saw only occasionally as a supplement to the other rations. Each D ration meal consisted of a chocolate bar into which raisins, nuts and chopped dates had been molded. They were so rich and concentrated that men who ate them without taking in abundant fluid at the same time often complained of stomachache.

The German soldier ate differently at the front. Menus were not standardized. Yes he had chocolate bars, dehydrated foods, preserves and other things, but he foraged a lot, and did much of his own cooking. In most situations there was a military kitchen not far behind him at the front, in which case a hot meal would be delivered, possibly as far forward as his individual foxhole. Later we found that many of the German prisoners carried large sausage skins filled with lard which they used for cooking. Many of the prisoners to whom I talked as they passed through our area to the rear thought that our C and K Rations were terrible.

With these differences in mind the debacle of the Christmas breakthrough becomes a bit more understandable. The War at the front had been static for some time with the two sides, situated long distances apart, watching each other from the hilltops and ridges, across valleys which had become no-man's-land. These valleys were devoid of soldiers, but were filled with farms in which the natives lived and worked as best they could. In these valleys military activity almost always occurred at night and consisted of patrol activity from both sides. These patrols were not a part of any battle strategy; they merely sought military intelligence information and hoped to capture prisoners.

For centuries Christmas had been a traditional and important holiday for the Germans. One of their traditions was to have an exceptionally fine Christmas dinner, so instead of sending out the usual small night patrols on December 24th, they sent out a number of 80 and 90 man foraging patrols in broad daylight to try to collect food for their Christmas dinner at the front. The story then goes that the outposts of the 92nd Division, seeing these patrols coming toward them, misinterpreted them to be a full-scale attack. They spread the alarm, and the personnel of the division broke and ran for the rear. Meanwhile the German patrols, meeting no opposition, merely walked through our lines into the rear areas, and found field kitchens set up but unmanned, all kinds of military equipment and supplies, and even abandoned motor pools. The Germans helped themselves with business-like efficiency, then returned to their own lines to celebrate. Actually there had been no breakthrough at all, and Rome was never in danger.

I must believe that this story is true because later that spring in the Po Valley I had the chance to talk to many German prisoners. A few of them said that they had been there, and told this same story. We were also capturing German military vehicles which were equipped with tires bearing American brand names.

As soon as the final process of equipping and supplying the Regiment was completed, we made another move. I was surprised because we went south instead of North toward the enemy, and I finally decided that perhaps the higher command just wanted to see how we handled ourselves during a move. Actually, moving in this direction didn't bother me, for at no time was I enthusiastic about going to the front. Our destination was *Quercianella* on the coast South of Leghorn. We were to establish a new, model bivouac there, and our aid station was to be located just across the coastal road from the Ligurian Sea. When we pulled in to our destination, it was raining hard.

The aid station tent had to be set up once again, but this time it had to be "dug in" to protect it from "enemy fire." With everyone available in the detachment helping, we dug a large hole in the hillside in which to erect it. The work was difficult and took a long time, because we had only two short handled spades and our individual entrenching tools. In addition we had to dig a long, deep drainage trench toward the downhill side, so that the aid station would not fill up with water. The rain continued all day long, and we wallowed in a sea of mud. When the tent finally went up, I was glad to see that only a small part of the top showed above ground level.

Now, for our next big job, every man had to dig his own individual foxhole to strict Army specifications: 3 feet by 4 feet, and 48 inches deep. We had been ordered to dig our individual foxholes in a designated area that was uphill from the aid station tent, and there we soon ran into a problem. The soil was only a foot deep over a large area of what seemed to be a huge slab of white marble. Since foxholes had to be 4 feet deep and ours had to pass inspection in a day or so, I requested permission to dig in another area. My request was denied, most likely because we were in an area which had been heavily mined by the Germans, and any part of it which had not yet been specifically cleared of mines was strictly off limits. I explained our problem at Battalion Headquarters, and was told to hold things as they were until clarification from higher command could be obtained. Some hours later a messenger arrived, tongue in cheek, with the information that if we dug the foxholes as deep as we could, then cleaned and polished the marble bottoms, they would pass inspection.

That night in the aid station tent I wrote a letter to my wife, being careful to avoid the drops of rainwater that came through the roof here and there. It was damp and cold, and the floor inside the tent was a quagmire. Lieutenant Summers, Sergeant Draper, the medical technicians and I slept in the aid station. The rest of our men were outside in pup tents, but, inside or out, nobody was comfortable.

Although we stayed at Quercianella for a week, and it rained much of the time, that first night was the worst. During the following week we did a lot of "soldiering," and passed multiple inspections. Most of my work involved holding sick call for our 3rd Battalion, the inspection of kitchens, latrines, water supply, and reviews of sanitation procedures used in camp. Additionally, because I felt responsible for the readiness of my men, we held more training sessions for our litter bearers in first aid and other medical subjects.

While we were thus occupied, the Regiment suffered its first casualties caused by the enemy. Shortly after lunch one day a soldier, who had been assigned guard duty at the periphery of the bivouac area, wandered off of his assigned path into a slightly sunken area containing some railroad tracks, and stepped on a mine. The resulting explosion caught the attention of many in the area, and several men, including one of the chaplains, Lieutenant Clarence Hagan, went to his assistance. There was at least one more explosion a little later when another mine was stepped on, and in the end eight men, including the chaplain, were dead and four were wounded. As I remember it, some of the wounded were evacuated directly to a hospital, and some may have been treated at one of the other battalion aid stations. There were still more mines present which had to be disarmed and removed before the dead could be taken from the rail bed.

I was some distance from the scene of this disaster on my way to an officer's staff meeting, but close enough to hear the explosions and see some of the peripheral commotion. Later, after everything had quieted down, I walked over and, from a safe distance away, looked at the area carefully. The tracks were located in a railroad bed which was several feet below the surface of our bivouac area. There was the wall of a building on the far side, and a narrow, paved area from which the ground rose sharply upward to the level of our bivouac area on our side. On the building and in several other places signs in large, bold letters were posted, which warned about mines and declared the area "Off Limits." These signs had been written in both English and Italian, and they prominently displayed the symbol of the skull and crossbones. To this day it is difficulty for me to understand what happened there. The sentry wandering on to the tracks may have been thoughtless or heedless, but I feel that so many others rushing into the area after the first explosion was stupid and unnecessary.

Quite some time after I had written the above two paragraphs I received a surprise telephone call from California from Bill Ferguson, who in January 1945 was T/3 William E. Ferguson, a part of the complement of the 2nd Battalion Aid Station. Bill was trying to renew old Army acquaintances, and when I told him I was writing this book, he brought up the minefield incident. He told me that he was one of the medics involved in it, and in the spring of 1945, after censorship had been lifted, he had written a letter to his parents describing the incident in detail. He immediately sent me a copy of this letter, and gave me permission to use it here.

He was able to add much to my sketchy account of the incident, which has served to make what happened more understandable. He explained that his 2nd Battalion Aid Station was located next to the railroad tracks, but some distance away from the road crossing from which the guard had wandered to detonate the first mine. When it exploded the medics at the aid station ran to the scene along the railroad tracks rather than taking a longer, roundabout route to enter the tracks from the road crossing. The signs warning about the minefield were not visible to anyone coming to the scene from this direction, and since these medics were stepping on the bare surfaces of the railroad ties, they did not set off any other mines until after they had arrived and were grouped around the fallen guard. Only the medics who had come along the tracks were in the minefield; the chaplain and the other men who were killed by the second explosion were not in the railbed as many had been led to believe, but were up on the bank to one side. No one had actually ignored the signs.

Bill Ferguson's letter to his parents is an excellently written, first person account of this tragedy, which in my opinion is an important incident in the annals of our regimental medical detachment. I therefore quote it in its entirety, exactly as Bill sent it to me. The words in parentheses are Bill's added in 1990 for purposes of clarification.

Northern Italy
April 7, 1945

Dear Family,

At last it can be told, for it has been three months and one day since the mine explosion in which Russ was injured. It's probably the incident to which Norm Bennett (Norman H. Bennett, C-87) was referring when he mentioned "hearing of Ferguson's doings."

On the afternoon of January 6, an infantryman who was walking guard along the edge of a minefield, strayed from his tour and set off a German S mine which killed him instantly. Whoever was nearest at the time saw him lying there, when attracted by the explosion, and yelled for a medic. It so happened that all of us medics were together at the time, so several of us grabbed our aid kits and others grabbed a litter and ran off toward the man. About six of us were at his side in a couple of minutes, but I was the first to find out he was dead. I stood up and shouted that the man was dead and told the assembling crowd to leave before another mine went off and hurt somebody else. Russ (Russell L. Keene), Bob (Robert L. Allen), and a couple of others repeated it and cautioned everyone in the minefield to freeze to prevent stepping on another mine. I could see the prongs of a mine sticking through the gravel, a couple of feet away. It was our first experience with a minefield, or obviously we wouldn't have had so many medics in the minefield, nor would we have had a crowd of spectators on the bank above.

No sooner had the words of caution left our lips when there was a deafening explosion. I hit the ground and waited a couple of seconds before looking up. There lay Jim (James O Wilkins) with a couple of holes in his head and blood running out. Jeeter (William U. Walter) lay a few feet away so I checked his pulse and his pupils, but didn't bother with his smoldering clothing because he was dead. Out of the corner of my eye I saw Russ dragging himself away with blood running down his face. Three other bodies lay motionless but I couldn't tell who they were then (Harry Malonas) and another medic whose name I can't remember, dead, and the third man I referred to was either the dead minefield guard or perhaps H. J. (Jay) Alders wounded.

I glanced behind me, and Bob Allen said, "Fergy, I'm hit. There's pain in my back." There was blood running down his face, too, but he didn't feel anything there. There was only one other man left in the mined area with any sign of life in him. He was a medic too (Howard H. Schless), and was also unscratched. He and I were the only men actually at the site of the explosion and unscathed. He was too far inside the mined area to risk getting out, so he didn't move his feet, but did all he could for Jim, since Jim was lying at his feet. I was at the first dead man's head all this time, but near enough to the edge of the mine field to jump out to safety (into a concrete ditch). I helped Bob part way up the bank and he went to the aid station. At the top of the bank were three more men bleeding like stuck pigs. (I guess I meant visceral wounds.) I had them put on a couple of trucks that were handy, and sent them right off to the hospital. When they were gone we still had to get Schless out of the middle of the mine field with all of the dead men. He was beginning to crack up. The mine detector crew arrived and started into the field to get out Schless and the bodies, so I left and returned to the aid station to see what I could do. Russ, Bob Allen, and another medic (Alders) were the only wounded there, so I got into the ambulance and went to the hospital with them. (I don't remember where Capt. Modlin and Lt. Stovich were all this time, nor why the three mortally wounded men were not receiving plasma by the time we put them in the trucks. Perhaps the two officers had been working on Allen, Alders and Keene at the aid station.)

At the hospital, while Bob was waiting to be x-rayed, I donned a mask, cap, and gown and went to the OR to watch the doc fish around for the shrapnel in Keene and Alders. It was the first time I'd seen anything like that, so I told Keene and Alders exactly what the doc was doing to them. (They couldn't tell because of the abundant local anesthetic and maybe morphine.)

Bob and I had become good friends, and he was most seriously wounded so I returned to him and helped hold him up for the x-rays, etc. I think it did him a lot of good to know I was there, even though he was under the influence of morphine most of the time. The pictures showed a fragment had hit him in the back, glanced off his shoulder blade and lodged near his spine. (As I remember it in 1990, it was in a tight place more or less between the aorta and vertebrae, so it was deemed unwise to try to remove it at the time.) One lung was puncture and contained about a quart of blood. I went with him to another ward, but they weren't going to work on him for some time, so I said so long and went back to the aid station, hitchhiking on anything that came along.

Back at the aid station , the final count was four medics killed, three medics wounded, one chaplain killed (on the bank above) and three infantrymen killed (the minefield guard and two at the top of the bank, near the chaplain). We reconstructed the scene and found that Jeeter was closest to the mine, for it practically exploded in his back when it hopped up out of the ground. I was about 6 feet away from the explosion but not hit because Jeet took all of the shrapnel that would have come my way. Schless was about 8 feet away from the mine but was saved by Jim, who was between him and the explosion.

It was horrible to think that these two fellows (Jeet and Jim) were killed under such circumstances, but on the other hand, the fact that they each saved a life doesn't make it seem quite as bad, and in addition it taught a lesson to an entire Battalion in regard to rescuing men from mine fields.

Russ has been back for some time, as you know, but Bob will probably not rejoin us. (After recovery from his wounds, he was assigned to serve in a prisoner of war camp.) I miss Bob very much because we were such good friends, but I think we all miss Jeet more than any. He's missed mostly because his dry, keen wit doesn't pop into our conversations any more.

That was the closest call I've had so far, and I really thanked God that I wasn't scratched.

Love, Bill

As we continued training our litter bearers at Quercianella, the infantry officers and their men were being educated in the subject of patrolling in the mountains, and were being briefed about the terrain and snow conditions in the Apennines just to the North of us. None of the medics had skis, but we were told that there would be snowshoes and toboggans available later if they were needed.

My Jeep now officially became a medical vehicle and had a huge red cross on a white background painted on it. It covered the entire surface of the hood. A similar one covered the entire front over the radiator grill. Smaller ones were painted on each side of the body above the rear wheels, and on the left and right sides of the rear end. Anyone seeing it from any angle should know without any doubt that this was indeed a medical vehicle. Our truck and trailer were similarly marked. We painted large white circular areas on the front and back of all of the medics' steel helmets, then painted bright red crosses in the center of each. Every medic also had white armbands with a similar red cross on each one. No one on either side should have any good reason to mistake an unarmed medic for an armed infantryman.

Saluting was now forbidden, and at first this seemed strange. Many of the men had been so accustomed to saluting for such a long time that it was automatic. However it only took a day or so to break the habit, and everyone seemed to like the idea. External insignia of rank were also removed. Until now officers wore their insignia on shirt or jacket collar and on their steel helmets, front and center, painted in white. Non-commissioned officers also removed the stripes from their sleeves and the insignia paint from their helmets. These measures were normal at the front, and were taken to avoid pointing out troop leaders to the enemy during combat.

On January 8, 1945 the whole regiment left Quercianella by truck for the front lines. I watched as our aid station tent was carefully folded up to be taken along, and that turned out to be the last time I saw that tent, for after that time we never used it again. After all of the misery connected with it at Quercianella my memories of that tent are not good ones, so I have no regrets about not setting it up again.

So far my worst experiences of the War had been at Quercianella, so I was not sorry to leave the area, although I admit that in good times and in good weather this part of Italy was probably very beautiful.

CHAPTER IV

INTO THE LINE

It was raining again as the regiment left Quercianella for the front in a convoy of quartermaster trucks and battalion vehicles. Before we left I assigned a regular driver to each of our vehicles, and these men kept those positions for the rest of our stay in Europe. Three of us rode in the jeep; our aid station went with our medical technicians in the 3/4 ton truck; and the housekeeping equipment was carried behind it in the trailer.

As we entered the foothills of the Apennines the rain turned to snow, and the road became slippery. This slowed the progress of the column considerably, but otherwise caused no problems. The mostly forested countryside remained quiet. The air was completely still as huge snowflakes settled slowly to the ground. A little bit higher into the hills, snow covered the leafless trees, the large flakes clinging to each little twig. The valleys were dotted with open fields, and here and there we could see small, picturesque clusters of buildings. The snow covered landscape appeared quiet and serene. This was truly the most beautiful country I had ever seen.

Eventually we arrived in the town of San Marcello, and the Battalion Command Post was promptly established in a house, which had apparently once belonged to someone quite well-to-do, because it was nicely furnished and had landscaped gardens that had at one time been well kept. It was unusual for houses in that area because it had a central heating system with a furnace. There was wood to burn, but the furnace had apparently been designed burn coal, and the wood didn't produce much heat, so the house remained cool inside, but not as cold as outdoors. There was enough space available for us to set up our aid station inside, and we held sick call there for the personnel stationed in or near the town.

The 1st and 2nd Battalions moved directly into foxholes on the defensive front, replacing the units which had been holding it. Our battalion was designated to be the regimental reserve, and was broken down into many small units which were scattered over a large area throughout the mountains in order to provide immediate support anywhere along our front. Most of these small units were too far away for the men to be able to come to sick call in San Marcello, so I had to visit them, and see individuals in many different places, much like a rural doctor at home might make house calls. This meant that I had to make daily trips of about sixty miles in the Jeep through mountainous country. Only a portion of these trips could be made during daylight hours, because wherever the enemy had direct observation of the roads and trails, he was able to shell them with remarkable accuracy. Most of the route had to be traveled at night, in darkness and without lights. Therefore I worked every night as well as much of the day, and got whatever sleep I could, whenever I could.

At this time we were warned that the enemy had a mean trick in which his patrols would stretch piano wire across a road at neck height for a man riding in a Jeep. These wires were very strong and practically invisible, even in the daytime, and there had been some decapitations as the result of driving into them in a Jeep at high speed. We promptly adapted our Jeep to avoid this kind of disaster by welding a heavy iron bar, sturdily braced in the upright position, to the front bumper. It extend well above head height, so that in case we ran into such a wire, it would be cut by the bar without injuring anyone. At the same time we also welded a rack made of angle iron on to the back of the Jeep in such a way that we could conveniently carry two litters with patients on them.

The territory in which our battalion was deployed was approximately 27 miles along the front and 2 to 3 miles deep. Whenever I made the rounds of the units, one of the medical technicians came along, and of course my driver was always with me too. Not all of the men I had to visit were accessible by road. We sometimes had to leave the Jeep and climb a mile more or less up an often-steep mountain trail to some cluster of buildings which was occupied by only a few soldiers, and which served as an outpost or observation point. This often involved receiving challenges from a sentry along the way, and it was imperative to know the correct daily password to be recognized as a friend and avoid being fired upon in the dark. Occasionally the soldier with the medical problem would come down the trail to meet me for a roadside consultation, and this saved a lot of time. Sometimes I would be asked by a civilian to see a sick friend or relative, and I always did this gladly, as long as it didn't interfere with my primary duty to the battalion. Before long I found that I was building up quite an extensive civilian practice, and I soon had to take my interpreter with me whenever I made these rounds.

We had been established in San Marcello for only a short time when it became apparent that life could be made easier and more pleasant for all of us if we did some bargaining with the natives. Such dealing required an extensive use of the Italian language, especially if there were to be any haggling. It was also becoming more and more important to be able to use the language in the treatment and instructions to civilian patients. Although I had studied Latin in high school for three years, and often recognized and knew the meanings of isolated Italian words, I could not speak Italian at all satisfactorily.

There was an excellent solution to this problem, and I soon put it into practice. It involved the previously mentioned 42 year old man who had arrived at Camp Swift to be a litter bearer with the obvious problem with his knees. His full name was **Vincenzo Consiglio**, but most of us called him Vince or used only his last name. He was born and raised in Sicily, then emigrated to the United States and made his home in Chicago. He spoke fluent Italian, and when I questioned him about this, he said that he had no problem at all with the Italian language, but admitted that he could not read or write English. In spite of an accent and some difficulty with grammar, his spoken English was quite adequate, so I told him that, while he would still officially be a litter bearer, I wanted him to be my aide and interpreter. I would have him deal with the natives whenever we needed anything such as living quarters, space for the aid station, fuel, information, directions, etc. I also told him to keep his eyes and ears open and report to me anything that he might learn from the natives that might help keep us out of trouble. He seemed pleased with this assignment. He always did an excellent job, and as time passed he seemed to become more and more proud of his part in the operation of our medical detachment. I am sure that he gave extra time and effort to his role as my liaison with Italian patients.

Occasionally Consiglio would obtain a particularly nice place in which to set up the aid station, and would tell us how he managed to obtain it. This happened often enough that his tactics eventually became familiar to us. It seemed that mainland Italians were generally afraid of Sicilians, because of their reputation as gangsters, so he would begin by telling the hapless landlord to be that he, Consiglio, was *"Siciliano."* This announcement, accompanied by a proper amount of swaggering, usually frightened the man, and with a little reinforcement, produced a satisfactory level of awe and deference. Then Consiglio would explain what was wanted, and if the man protested he would say to him, "You want me to do like Mussolini and take your wife and daughters too?" If he ever did anything more threatening than that, I don't know about it. Even though I believe that many Italians let us use their rooms and their houses reluctantly, I can say, with a sense of pride, that our medical detachment treated all of the premises as they would have treated their own, and to my knowledge we did not ever cause any damage to any of them.

Consiglio also became indispensable to me in the medical treatment of native Italians. He translated the medical history of each for me, and explained my medical instructions to them in detail. He also seemed to find and bring to my attention a lot of natives who needed medical help, and I believe he was part of the reason that I was so busy with civilian practice much of the time. He was a kind and gentle man, and although not well educated, he had attained a remarkable, practical wisdom which he frequently demonstrated. After the Division returned to the United States I never saw Consiglio again, and I regret that I have not taken the time to look him up.

Now that we were established in our defensive positions, I realized that we had become the first regiment of the Tenth Mountain Division to enter into combat. The arrangement of the 1st and 2nd Battalions manning the forward positions while my 3rd Battalion acted as the Regimental Reserve was much to my liking, because it meant that I should not receive many casualties right away. Once again I was glad that I had been given the choice, and that I had volunteered to serve the 3rd Battalion.

Our territory stretched from Bagni di Lucca in the Southwest through La Lima, San Marcello and Maresca, to Oorsigna in the Northeast. The terrain was extremely rugged, with snow filled valleys between steep hills and rock outcroppings. The snow lasted for about six more weeks, and this was the only period in the history of the Division in which skis could be used, and they were only used for patrol activity. No major assaults on skis were ever made.

As I studied the map in connection with my daily Jeep rounds, I became interested in learning about the situation on the whole front from coast to coast, and I gradually picked up much of this information at battalion and regimental staff meetings, but also asked questions here and there at other times and places. I already knew that we were in the Mediterranean Theater of Operations and in the Fifth Army commanded by General Mark Clark. I soon learned that we were also a part of IV Corps, commanded by General Willis D. Crittenberger.

It appeared that IV Corps was a sort of catch-all where units were placed that didn't quite fit anywhere else. It included our regiment as a part of Task Force 45, but later, when the rest of the 10th Mountain Division arrived in

Italy and went into the line, we were removed from the task force and placed under the control of our own division again. The whole division then became a part of IV Corps. Other units included the Brazilian Expeditionary Force, which was deployed on our right, and the all black 92nd Infantry Division, which was deployed on our left. There was also the 1st Armored Division, composed of tanks, tank destroyers and other armored vehicles, all of which were of limited use in the mountains, but became most important later on when we broke into the Po Valley. The 6th South African Division, which I believe held the front West of us, probably all of the way to the coast, completed the IV Corps roster. Occasionally we would see some strange and exotic appearing soldiers, and I usually assumed that they belonged either in this latter division or the British Eighth Army on the East side of the Italian peninsula. On our right, between us and the British Eighth Army, was II Corps, composed of four American divisions.

Prior to our arrival in Italy, IV Corps had also included a very famous unit about which we had already heard a lot, even before leaving the United States. This was the 442nd Infantry Regiment, also knows as the Nisei Regiment, because it was composed entirely of Japanese Americans. It was an outstanding unit, famous for its efficiency, and it had a long list of accomplishments. Casualties in it had been higher than average, and many of its men had been cited for bravery and heroism. The families of many of these men had been put into internment camps in the United States, because there was great concern that the west coast might be invaded by Japan at any time, and therefore these people had been declared a threat to national security in time of war. This being so, these Japanese-American soldiers probably felt that they must be extra courageous in order to prove their loyalty to their country. We didn't meet any of them because, by the time we had reached the scene, they had already left. They had fought their way up the boot of Italy and were occupying their segment of the front in territory which they had wrested from the enemy, when their unit was withdrawn to fight again in Southern France. In my opinion it amounted to tacit praise for the 442nd Infantry Regiment, when it was replaced in the line by an entire division.

The 92nd Division had a very different story. Except for a few white officers, it was composed entirely of black soldiers. After the war was over I occasionally came across references to this division, and they usually lacked any words of praise, often describing the division as having "a miserable combat record." The Christmas Day fiasco, which had brought us so quickly from Naples into Northern Italy, and which has been detailed in the previous chapter, occurred on the 92nd Division front, and the incident had soured most of our men on it. Most of us questioned its capability in combat, and more than once I heard line officers express concerns over the security of our left flank while that division was in the line just to the left of us. Some of our units were required to keep contact with some of their units, and these were the only times in which we worried that passwords would not be remembered or would be overlooked.

That the problems of the 92nd Division were also recognized by the higher echelons of command is well documented in the book, COMMAND MISSIONS, written by General Lucian K. Truscott, Jr. General Truscott was the Corps Commander who later took command of the American 5th Army from General Mark Clark. His book details some of the problems of this division and the less-than-successful solutions, which were tried in order to overcome them. Eventually, some years after the war was over, the Army made the announcement that there would be no more racial segregation, and that from then on all units would be racially integrated.

Then there was The Brazilian Expeditionary Force. I don't remember exactly how large it was, but it was on our right flank much of the time. We saw quite a lot of the Brazilians. They had a reputation for driving recklessly and too fast, and also of stealing anything they could lay hands on. They spoke Portugese, which none of us understood, and they did didn't understand English. Since many of our outposts had to keep up contact with theirs, both used what can honestly be described as "pretty awful Italian," but it seemed to suffice.

One day, early in the spring when things were relatively quiet and our aid station was located high up on the shoulder of a mountain peak, we had an excellent view of the mountainside opposite us across the valley, and on it we could see the whole of a winding road which snaked down into the valley and ran off into the distance. At the top, which was closest to us, we recognized a Jeep carrying four Brazilian soldiers starting down the hillside, and at the bottom we saw four of our tanks just beginning their climb up the hill. The Jeep appeared to be traveling much too fast for road conditions, and we speculated that when it met the lead tank there would be a crash. We were right. The Jeep rounded a curve and smashed head on into the lead tank. One man was thrown from the Jeep but didn't seem to be badly hurt, and in a few minutes all four were up and walking about the wreckage. In the meantime men emerged from the tanks, and we watched as a group of men rolled the wrecked Jeep off of the road and down an embankment, so that the tanks could proceed on up the mountain.

Some of the men from our motor pool also witnessed this accident, and began to complain bitterly that, although the Brazilians were poor drivers who wrecked a lot of vehicles, all they had to do was requisition a new one and they would get it. At the same time our units could hardly get replacement parts for our vehicles and couldn't get replacement vehicles at all. Our motor pool men were making all kinds of repairs with scrounged parts and baling wire.

A little later in the spring we had an episode with the Brazilians, which has remained on my mind a lot. Our aid station was set up and in operation in an old barn located in a grove of chestnut trees, and our vehicles were parked inside the fenced barnyard which was connected to the country road by a fenced lane perhaps 100 yards long. Early in the morning one of my men awoke me, saying that some Brazilians were stealing things from our trailer. I told him to wake up the rest of the men and ran out into the yard to find a Brazilian Major, wearing the Cadeuceus of a medical officer, and three of his men, loading their Jeep with some of our housekeeping items, which we had not unpacked because we didn't expect to be using them at this location. There now began a vigorous argument, with a lot of yelling and arm waving, but I don't think either side understood the other. It was probably a good thing that no one was armed. As the argument progressed, more and more of our men appeared on the scene, and we began to get the better of it. It didn't end, however, until I threatened the Brazilian officer with great bodily harm, and literally chased him out of the barnyard and halfway down the lane. While I was thus occupied, my men unloaded the things from the Brazilian Jeep, whereupon the Brazilian soldiers drove off in it, picking up their major in the lane on their way.

The Army Tables of Organization and Equipment authorized our medical detachment to have a field radio, called an SCR-300. In the beginning we were issued one, but soon lost it to one of the line companies when one of theirs was found to be inoperable. Not having the radio didn't bother us much because we stayed close to the Battalion Command Post and usually had a field telephone line from there to our aid station. Now after this incident with the Brazilians, lo and behold, we had an SCR-300 field radio again. We carried this radio with us throughout the rest of the War, although I only went on the air with it once during the whole time, and that was to relay information to one of the companies whose reception from the Battalion Command Post was apparently blocked by a hill. I did however listen a lot to keep abreast of what was going on, and I believe that listening to the battalion and regimental messages during combat situations often helped to keep us out of trouble.

There is also possibly a sequel to this story. Some ten or fifteen years after the War, I was engaged in general medical practice in my home town of Eaton Rapids, Michigan, when a new doctor, an obstetrician-gynecologist, moved into the neighboring town of Charlotte. Our paths did not cross much, but I met him several times at county medical meetings and other medical functions. He was a foreign graduate from Brazil, and his English was very difficult to understand. His practice apparently did not do well, because after only a few years he left the area. After he had departed I learned from the nurse who had worked in his office that he had been a doctor in the Brazilian Expeditionary force with the rank of major. His size and height were about right, and I often wonder if he was the Brazilian major I had chased down the lane in Italy that day. I still am not sure.

One day I learned that there was a Hebrew battalion operating not far from us. I became very interested in meeting some of these men because I had been brought up in a Jewish neighborhood in Detroit. Many of my child-hood friends and their families spoke Yiddish, which I could understand very well because it is so much like German. So I went over to the Hebrew Battal-ion area one afternoon, expecting to be able to speak at least a little with those men, but this turned out to be a big disappointment. They spoke only Hebrew, which might as well have been Greek as far as I was concerned. A few of them knew a word or two of English, but not enough to be able to hold any significant conversation. They seemed industrious, were well disciplined and polite, and their unit appeared to be smoothly and efficiently run. I liked these men, but never again tried to contact any of them.

Then there were the Sikhs from India. I believe they fought somewhere to the East of us in the British 8th Army. They were tall, fierce looking, had beards, wore turbans, and all of them carried huge, long knives. Although we had no direct contact with them in the line, I occasionally saw some of them, in groups of two or three, at various times in the rear areas. They had a repu-tation for being fierce fighters, and of eschewing their guns for the knives they always carried. The story was told that they liked to patrol at night, silently creep up on enemy positions and cut the throats of enemy soldiers as they slept. One story, often repeated, was that a Sikh patrol had gone deep into enemy territory, found a small group of German soldiers asleep, and silently slit their throats. Then they beheaded them and placed the ten or twelve heads in a circle on the ground, each facing the center, to be found by their comrades in the morning.

We had not been at the front very long before I knew pretty much about the nationalities of the units of the Allied Armies in our sector, and by this time I had also learned a great deal about my own Tenth Mountain Division.

It was an unusual, one-of-a-kind division that had had an unusual origin. The 87th Mountain Infantry first came into being shortly before the Japanese attacked Pearl Harbor, and was the first mountain infantry unit of its size to be organized. At first it contained a skeleton compliment of enlisted men who were mostly skiers and mountain climbers, and a group of officers who were neither. Recruiting to fill the ranks became urgent and was taken over by the National Ski Patrol, a civilian organization of skiers who had banded together nationwide prior to the War to provide first aid and teach safety on the ski slopes in the United States. In order to join the 87th, applicants for enlistment had to be either skiers, mountain climbers or outdoorsmen experienced in cold weather camping, and each was required to submit three letters of recommendation, which were reviewed and approved before he could be accepted.

Some of the early training that the men of the 87th had received had been in the shadow of Mt. Ranier in Washington State, and the rest at Camp Hale near Aspen, Colorado. In the summer of 1943 the 87th, now officially a Mountain Infantry Regiment, was sent to Alaska as part of a task force which had been ordered to attack and take the island of Kiska which was occupied by the Japanese. They found no Japanese on the island, but during the assault, suffered some casualties, when several units engaged each other, because they could not recognize each other in the fog and bad weather. Although the 87th stayed on Kiska for a while, by January 1944 it had returned to Camp Hale where extensive winter training was under way once again.

The 86th Mountain Infantry Regiment was activated by a cadre of officers and men from the 87th plus a few men who had had mountain training with other smaller units before the 87th was established. Recruiting for the 86th was a bit different. Although skiers and mountain climbers were still being sought, the recruiters were also looking for large men with a high degree of physical stamina, above average intelligence and an education. I was told that before my arrival, qualifications for admission into this elite regiment included a physical height of 6 feet or more, and completion of at least one year in a college or university. After mingling with them, it was easy for me to believe that every man really did have a year or more of college education, and it was obvious that most of them were tall. Later, during combat, when litter casualties started to come into the aid station, many of them were in fact taller than our six-foot long litters were long.

The 85th Mountain Infantry Regiment was the last to be activated, and, as a consequence, had the least mountain training. It, too, began with a skeleton cadre of officers and men from the 87th, but when I arrived at Camp

Swift, many of the ranks had been filled from replacement depots, without strict adherence to the requirements for enlistment. I am not sure if any screening process was used. Time was short and the regiment had to accept more or less what was sent to them. Several times I heard that some of the Division Officers had misgivings about this and wondered if the 85th could handle its load under combat conditions. As things turned out this was a needless concern. This regiment clearly distinguished itself very well.

The three regiments were first organized into the 10th L Division, and a shoulder patch to be worn by the men of the Division was authorized. It consisted of crossed bayonets in red and edged in white, on a blue "powder keg," which was also edged in white. The shoulder patches were in short supply, but I somehow managed to obtain all I needed. Subsequently, when the division was renamed, an addition was authorized which consisted of shallow arch of the same blue as was in the powder keg, with the word, MOUNTAIN, embroidered in white across it. This arch was to be placed across the top of the powder keg, and thus evolved the official 10th Mountain Division shoulder patch as it remains today. These additions were not available to us at Camp Swift, so we sewed them on later, after leaving for overseas. The addition of the word, MOUNTAIN, gave the patches a distinctive appearance, and the significance was quite clear. However I still wonder about the powder keg and the crossed bayonets. Perhaps the crossed bayonets were meant to represent the Roman numeral X.

In the early months of mountain warfare training the skiers and mountain climbers were all enlisted men, and problems arose because their officers had no training in these fields. In order to try to correct this, enlisted men from the mountain troops were sent to Officer Candidate School, expecting to return to their units, only to be reassigned to other, flatland divisions after they graduated. After this had happened a few times, dedicated mountain men refrained from applying to become officers, although many of them were eligible on the basis of their Army General Classification Tests. In my regiment 64 percent of the enlisted men scored high enough on the test to be eligible to attend Officer Candidate School, while the average of men to achieve this level in eleven other divisions was less than 30 percent. Fortunately one large group of officer candidates from our division did receive special treatment, and the newly commissioned officers were returned to the Division, but this was accomplished only after much fuss and friction in the higher echelons of the Army and in Washington, D.C.

So when the Division was ready to leave the United States an unusual condition existed. While some of the officers were skiers and mountaineers who had been trained by the Army to become officers, many were officers who had been trained in skiing and rock climbing by the men they commanded.

The identity of the German units facing us never did concern me much. We were often told that there were more German divisions lined up against us than we had in the line, but that the enemy had severe problems keeping them filled with men. However, the specific identification of enemy units didn't seem important to me. I thought it was enough to know that anyone in a German uniform was an enemy.

CHAPTER V

THE STATIC WAR

During our early weeks at the front my battalion suffered hardly any battle casualties. I expected this because we were the reserve battalion, and our men were generally a few hundred yards behind the actual front line. But the two battalions, which were manning the forward positions, didn't suffer many casualties either, and although this was something I didn't expect, the reasons for it were soon obvious.

At this season of the year combat activity on both sided was primarily defensive. Large field units didn't move, and the situation at the front remained static. In most places no-man's-land was a wide valley in which there were no soldiers at all, but civilians still lived in the farmhouses there and could be seen moving about from time to time. The opposing armies assumed positions on the hills and crags and watched each other across the valley. Both sides seemed content to minimize the fighting in order to preserve as many of their conveniences and creature comforts as possible. This is well illustrated by the following story:

One day during my Jeep rounds we approached a tiny village from the rear. I could see that it was located on a high outcropping of rock, which extended well out into a very wide, flat valley like a peninsula. The valley floor extended for a long distance forward and to both sides, and was dotted here and there with farmhouses and other smaller buildings. On the other side, in enemy territory, a long range of mountains was clearly visible. Upon learning from the natives that some British soldiers were manning an artillery position nearby and were staying in the village, we asked where they were living and were quickly directed to their quarters. When we arrived we found that they occupied one whole floor of a house which not only was heated but also had the luxury of indoor plumbing. The five or six British soldiers in the house were having afternoon tea, and I noticed immediately that the housekeeping was terrible. Dirty mess kits, opened food tins, and all kinds of trash lay about. There was a large bathroom at the rear of the house, which contained a modern looking flush toilet which looked as though it could be made to work by supplying water to it, but the room was poorly ventilated and carried a stench worse that any outhouse I had ever before encountered. It occurred to me immediately that, when the rest of our division arrived, our artillerymen might be assigned to relieve this position, and if that were to happen I was sure they would clean it up promptly. Our men would never willingly tolerate living in conditions such as these. One of the British soldiers invited us to share tea with them, but I refused and thanked him without saying anything of my misgivings about the sanitation. The British told us that there were no Americans in the town, and there was no medical work for me there. Then as we were preparing to leave, their sergeant looked at his watch and announced that it was time to fight the war. He invited us to observe, so we all trooped outside and walked about one hundred yards to where their artillery piece was hidden under its camouflage covering.

As the gun crew started to work, the soldier in charge explained that when they fired we should be sure to cover our ears, because the blast could injure our eardrums. After the camouflage materials were removed there stood a cannon which I thought had an unusually long barrel. Its bore diameter appeared to be about five inches. I watched with interest as they loaded it. They warned us when they were ready to fire, and I covered my ears with the palms of my hands, but in spite of this precaution the explosion startled me. It was much louder than I had expected. The man in charge looked intently at the hills across the valley with field glasses, and soon expressed satisfaction with the shot. He explained that nothing of significance had been hit, because there was a tacit agreement with the enemy not to blow up each other's comfortable living quarters and limit the war to retaliation in kind. If they had hit the German billets over there, the Germans could, and would, destroy his comfortable quarters and much of the village on this side. An answering round arrived almost as if on schedule. It landed high in the hills well beyond the village. The British fired two more rounds, and each time the Germans replied. Each side had been careful not to hit anything which might cause discomfort to the other.

As the crew replaced the camouflage materials, one of the men announced again that this had been their war for that day. The British walked back to their quarters and I to my Jeep, and as we drove out of that village I tried to imagine what would happen when the enthusiastic 10th Mountain Division Artillery took over these positions. I was certain that they would shoot to inflict as much damage to the enemy as possible. The intensity of the war must then increase, and the casualty rate was bound to rise.

I remember a daytime visit to another small village that was similarly located in view of the enemy. From this village our men could watch enemy positions across the valley, and with spotting scopes or field glasses could often see German soldiers sunning themselves, walking about and carrying out their daily activities. I saw them clearly myself when one of the men let me look through his field glasses. It seemed to me that those enemy soldiers were two or three miles away, but I was assured that the distance was only about two thousand yards.

A number of our soldiers had special, single shot Springfield rifles mounted with special sights, and were acting as snipers. They traveled back and forth along the front, scanning enemy territory with their scopes and binoculars and looking for opportune targets. Whenever a German soldier was seen out in the open, they would fire across the valley at him. Apparently some of these shots hit their intended target, but I suspected that this sniping activity produced a lot more bragging than damage to enemy personnel.

One day I received an urgent message to see a very sick youth in another small village, the name of which I have forgotten. When I arrived I found the patient to be a 14-year-old boy, critically ill in the nephrotic stage of advanced renal disease. He had a pale, pasty appearance, was bloated from head to toe with massive pitting edema (fluid in the tissues), and had a very high blood pressure. This was indeed a serious, life threatening illness, and there was little I could do for him there, so I explained to the family through Consiglio, my interpreter, what the problem was and that the outlook was grave. I told them that I would try to get hospital treatment for him.

Then another civilian asked me to see a relative who lived nearby in the same village who was also very sick. This second patient was a younger boy, and he too was very ill. He had a very inflamed and swollen throat covered with a typical diphtheritic membrane. His illness appeared so far advanced that I feared he would need a tracheostomy soon, in order to prevent suffocation. I asked, and other people then told me that there were many sick people with very sore throats in the village, so I started examining throats. I believe I looked at most of the people in that village, perhaps one hundred in all. An occasional older person and about half of the children and young adults had Diphtheria!!!!! I reported this as quickly as I could going through channels, and, within a short time, managed to have the nephrotic youth and the child with the impending respiratory problem evacuated by ambulance to a rear area hospital. I also was assured that the American Military Government would arrange to have a team of doctors and nurses sent up to the village to handle the epidemic.

The Army had neither given nor required diphtheria immunizations for its personnel. Some of our men had spent a lot of time in that village, and I worried that some, particularly those who had actually lived there, might have been exposed sufficiently to contract the disease. I had no doubt that a lot of our men had been immunized during childhood, as I had been, but I had no idea how many. Eventually my worries proved to be unfounded, for, to the best of my knowledge, none of our soldiers came down with Diphtheria. I never had an opportunity to go back to that village, and know nothing about the outcome of the epidemic, but I still occasionally wonder how it was handled.

Because our troops remained healthy, and military casualties remained very low, I had free time. The numbers of sick and ailing civilians kept increasing, and gradually more and more of my time was devoted to a civilian medical practice. Most of these patients were ordinary Italian people, and I felt sorry for them, especially the little children. I was glad to do what I could for them, and most of my men felt the same way.

The aid station didn't stay in San Marcello very long. With the approval of 3rd Battalion Headquarters, we made several moves in order to stay as close as possible to our companies in the front line. In spite of the fact that ours was the reserve battalion, it wasn't long before two of our companies, located North of Bagni di Lucca, were frequently participating in night patrols into no-mans-land and enemy territory, so we moved the aid station several time in order to be closer to them. This did not alter the need for the day and night Jeep trips for sick call, and they continued as before.

Those early moves proved to be good training for us. They afforded experience in packing and unpacking, functioning while on the move, and adapting our aid station to the various types of local buildings available. They were not made under duress, nor with any great sense of urgency, but they did teach us how to move quickly and efficiently. We still carried the aid station tent with us, but did not unpack it, preferring to stay in a building. In fact it never became necessary for us to set up or use that tent again.

Italian farmhouses made good places in which to locate an aid station. They were not at all like the farmhouses we had at home. The typical one was four stories high, and built of stone and mortar. Some of the older ones were smaller, but built with stones so well shaped and so well fitted together that mortar wasn't needed. The ground floor was invariably used as a barn and stable area, but near the main entrance there were always two or three separate rooms which were used as storage and workshop areas. These provided excellent space for an aid station, and the extra thickness of the stone walls at the base of these tall buildings afforded excellent shielding from enemy bullets and shell fragments. In most of these farmhouses the walls were four or five feet thick at ground level, and the windows were small, making it easy to black them out for nighttime operation. In some of them the walls were actually so thick that the windows seemed to be set into tunnels.

The main entrance typically had double doors, some wide enough to drive a team of horses with a wagon through a central passageway leading to the back of the barn area. Opening into this passageway, were the several small rooms, which we often used to house the aid station, and there would also be a stairway which went up to the second floor. On the ground floor at the back of the house was where the farm animals, such as horses, cattle, sheep, goats, geese, ducks, rabbits and chickens, were kept, and from this area another wide door opened out into the barnyard and the fields beyond. **At the very back of the barn area, situated against the rear wall, was always a substantial manure pile.** In most houses this pile was surrounded by a low stone and mortar wall, capable of holding water and designed to keep the manure liquids from flowing all over the barn area. There was a four or five inch overflow pipe which ran out through the back wall of the house and allowed any overflow to run out into the barnyard. This location for the manure pile was most likely deliberately planned, because manure produces heat, and warm air rises, in this instance keeping the whole building from being quite so cold in the winter. However, with warm air, odors also rise, and inside these buildings the smell of manure was ever present.

The second floor and above contained living quarters, each level designed to house two to four families. This is where the people who worked the surrounding fields lived, but now, in wartime, many additional people lived there. Each of the upper floors had a central hall running from front to back, with doors opening into the living quarters. The stairwell from the second floor to the top floor was at the back of the building and opened upon each of the floors.

Next to the stairwell, at the very back of the building, each floor had a toilet room which was always located against the back wall of the house to allow for outside window ventilation. There was also another very good reason for placing it there. Stacked one on top of the other, exactly over the manure pile in the barn area below, this location afforded the effluent soil pipe a straight vertical drop to the indoor manure pile, and human excreta from each floor could easily pass down that pipe to the manure pile to be added to that of the animals. The stairway was always located adjacent to the toilet rooms, and in many farmhouses access to the toilets came from the stair landings between floors rather than from the halls. However, no matter which of these locations had been chosen, the operating principles controlling the flow of sewage were the same.

In most of the farmhouses the toilets themselves were crude. Each consisted of a stone slab, as long as the room was wide, which was set horizontally upon another piece of stone of the same length, so that it was supported at chair height. Thus a stone bench, usually located opposite the doorway against the outside wall, was created, and it gave the toilet room an appearance somewhat similar to an American outhouse. One difference was that it was built of stone, and the other was that there was only one, unbelievably small hole in the stone seat. The hole was only about four to five inches in diameter, and always, whenever I looked at one, it seemed much too small for its intended purpose. Occasionally, in order to shield the user's rear end from the cold marble, there was a doughnut shaped pad, made of braided straw, in place around the hole, and once I saw a much more elaborate arrangement that had a basket-like sling designed to hold one's rear up away from the stone. In most places, however, that cold marble slab with its pathetically small hole was all that there was.

The method of handling the wastes was also primitive. Attached to the underside of the slab, and connected to the hole in it, was a collecting duct of similar size through which any excreta deposited there must pass. These ducts (one from each toilet hole) all slanted steeply downward and ran into a single long shaft of a larger diameter which ran vertically for the entire height of the building. Since the lower end of this shaft was poised directly over the indoor manure pile on the ground floor, all of the human excreta produced in the entire building ended up in that pile. This duct system not only carried wastes down, but also acted like a chimney, and carried the gases and odors up the shaft and into the toilet rooms, continually and in copious quantities. Many of our men joked that the could enter a farmhouse blindfolded and make their way up to the top floor using only their sense of smell. Later, when the entire Italian countryside smelled of it for several weeks, we learned that the farmers spread this manure, human and all included, on their fields every spring.

While we were still in reserve and operating our aid station close to Bagni di Lucca near the western end of our sector, I had the opportunity to take my first real bath since leaving the United States. Consiglio, my interpreter, had discovered that there was a bathhouse in operation in town, so from time to time a number of us went there to bathe. The name, Bagni di

Lucca, translates into "The Baths of Lucca," and the town had received its name because there were hot springs there, flowing constantly from the mountainside, and bathhouses had been built around them to take advantage of the endless supply of free hot water.

The day was January 18, 1945. A jeepload of us went into town specifically to avail ourselves of the bathing facilities. I remember entering the bathhouse and the proprietor asking, "*Bagno*?" which meant something like, "Do you people want baths?" Consiglio did the talking for us. The cost was five lira, which in the lira issued to us by the Army was five cents. If we wanted soap and towels we had to bring our own.

Once all arrangements were completed, the proprietor led me along a dim hallway into a room which was perhaps 10 by 12 feet in size. There was a small window or skylight close to the ceiling so there was daylight in the room. I could see that the wall opposite the door was actually the stone of the side of the mountain, and pouring from a spout, which appeared to have been driven into the rock, was a steady stream of water. It steamed as it emerged and ran into a huge, sunken, marble tub which had been set below the level of the floor. The tub was much larger than a standard bathtub, about 3 feet wide, 3 feet deep and a bit more than 6 feet long. It seemed to have been carved from a single block of marble. At the right end of the tub was a drain opening in the bottom, and another opening was located above it near the top to take care of any overflow that might occur. The floor and walls of the room were covered with multicolored ceramic tiles arranged in various designs. As soon as we entered the room the proprietor knelt down and placed the stopper into the drain opening to allow the tub to fill. He smiled, said something in Italian which I didn't understand, then hastily departed, closing the door behind him.

Over five weeks had passed since we had left the United States and Camp Patrick Henry, where I had had my last real bath (a shower to be sure). During all of this time I had been separated from my dufflebag and footlocker, and the only extra clothing I had with me was a single pair of socks, which I changed occasionally. I carried the extra pair in my pocket, washed them whenever the chance to do so presented itself, and changed into the clean pair whenever I thought it necessary. Because I had no clean clothing to put on, I now carefully dusted my dirty long underwear with the DDT powder furnished by the Army. I had been following this practice for several weeks, and would continue to follow it routinely during the rest of the fighting in Europe, in order to avoid the infestations of body lice and other vermin which occasionally afflicted one of our soldiers, and which I found much more frequently on civilian patients.

That DDT powder was effective is well illustrated by an incident which occurred sometime later during our sustained advance in the foothills of the Apennines. Our battalion had just overrun a large area, and near the end of the day we moved our aid station into a small town which had been taken with only minimal damage. Lieutenant Summers and I came upon a family living in a house with an extra bedroom, and we were invited to sleep there overnight. We were delighted to accept, and spent some time that evening with our host, after which we went upstairs and crawled into a big, soft double bed with a pair of feather tick comforters to cover us. Both of us, being very tired, slept soundly. In the early light of the next morning, after the roosters in the neighborhood had begun to crow, I became aware that Barney was doing a lot of moving and scratching. We were both sleeping in the long winter underwear that we wore all the time, but I had powdered mine regularly with DDT, and he had not. We looked. Sure enough, there they were, BEDBUGS BY THE DOZENS! There weren't any on me, but Barney was loaded, and the bedding on his side of the bed was teeming with them. DDT powder quickly took care of the situation for him, and I believe that after that he also dusted his underwear religiously, at least until the fighting ended. As for me, I didn't have a single bite then, and was never bitten at any time.

After I had finished powdering my underwear in the bathhouse, I put my clothing down on the stone bench that was the only piece of furniture in the room. Then I tested the water temperature with my toe. The water coming from the spout was not scalding hot. I think it steamed only because the room was cool. Although the water in the tub was quite warm, it was still comfortable, so without hesitating, I jumped down into the tub. Then as I was lying down stretched out and literally reveling in my first tub bath in many weeks, the door opened and I heard a feminine voice say, *"Buon Giorno."* A middle-aged woman exploded into the room and came up to the edge of the tub. She spoke rapidly in Italian which I didn't understand, but I recognized a few of the words: *lavare* (wash), *saponetta* (soap) and *oggi* (today).

I had never been so embarrassed in my life! I am sure my jaw dropped and my facial expression must have been one of utter astonishment. I blushed from head to toe, and sat up quickly trying to cover up as best I could, whereupon the woman quickly knelt down by the side of the tub, snatched the bar of soap I had placed there, and started to wash my back vigorously. She spoke rapidly in Italian all the while, but I didn't understand any of it. After she finished I didn't stand up, nor did I volunteer to let her wash anything else, and she finally left the room, still chattering in Italian all of the way to the door.

After regaining some composure, I finished bathing, toweled off, dressed in my previously worn clothes, and left the bathhouse feeling much refreshed. When I compared experiences with some of the other fellows later, I learned that they had all received similar treatment, and so had others of our men whenever they had gone there to bathe. Most of them, however, described the woman who did the back washing as appearing considerably older than the one who had startled me so thoroughly. We all agreed that we had been introduced to one of the customs of the time and place.

My dufflebag, but not my footlocker, finally caught up with me a few days after this bathing experience, and I had some clean clothes again. After bathing and shaving, this time out of my steel helmet, I changed into completely clean clothing for the first time since we left the United States. We were operating our aid station in a local farmhouse, and I had no trouble finding a woman living there to do my laundry. I furnished a bar of Fels Naptha soap which my wife had mailed to me, and the price for washing all of my dirty clothing was a package of American cigarettes. The washing was actually done in a cold mountain stream, and the clothes were pounded on the rocks. We often saw women doing laundry in this manner in this part of the country. The clothing came back to me in a short time. It was clean, neatly ironed and folded. Even the khaki colored long underwear had been ironed. When I paid the woman, I gave her a couple of Hershey chocolate bars as a tip. She immediately seemed pleased, almost ecstatic, and thanked me repeatedly.

By this time it had become regimental policy to periodically rotate the battalions into the reserve position, in order to give the men at the far front some rest and even out the "dirty work." When it became my 3rd Battalion's turn to move up into the forward foxholes, I wasn't particularly worried or concerned, because I knew that so far the front line battalions had suffered hardly any casualties in this static phase of the War. We relieved the 1st Battalion in the "hot spot" in the line, which was the Monte Mancinello-Belvedere sector, and we moved our aid station into an Italian hospital in the town of Lizzano, which was very close to enemy lines.

This hospital was not like the ones we had in the United States, but more like the sanitaria in which we treated tuberculosis and other chronic diseases. It was located near the edge of town on a paved street, but was hidden from direct observation by the Germans by a substantial hill. The hill also blocked out some of the sounds of combat from the nearby front, and while we were inside the building, we were not aware of the noise of small arms or machine guns, but could still hear the explosions of the mortar and artillery shells of both sides.

The building was one of the larger ones in town. It had a wide driveway leading up to the entrance. Inside there was a large lobby from which a wide stairway led up to a similar lobby on the second floor. This second floor lobby became our aid station, and we set up housekeeping in some of the adjacent rooms. Civilian nurses and other hospital workers were present, all of them Italian. I think that some Italian doctors occasionally visited, but I don't remember meeting any of them. Neither do I remember seeing any of the civilian patients, for they were housed in portions of the building that we didn't use.

Once we were installed in these new quarters the living was certainly easy. It was hard to believe that we could be so comfortable and at the same time be officially engaged in front line combat. We were far more comfortable than we had been when we were the reserve battalion. We slept in beds and ate at tables with tableware and china. The toilets were inside and there was running water; sometimes there was even hot water available. Occasionally we had electric lights, but they were not as bright as those at home. The voltage and alternating current cycles were different here than they were in the United States, but I suspected that the dimness was really due to low voltage due to overloaded circuits. Electricity was scarce and the Italians were trying to make it go as far as possible.

Until we moved into that hospital building I had still been cold quite often, in spite of having four Army blankets and wearing clothes to bed, so when I found a thick, white woolen blanket with wide colored stripes at one end, I added it to my bedroll. After that I slept much warmer. I kept this blanket for the rest of the War, and there were times when I was glad I had it, because there were occasions when I gave up my Army blankets to litter wounded who were being evacuated.

Things were not so cozy and comfortable for the infantrymen who were facing the enemy directly and manning the defensive positions on the other side of the hill. Their operations were typical of infantry units serving in the Apennines that winter, and were typical of the way most infantry units were employed in winter defensive situations.

Most of our front positions were in plain sight of enemy soldiers situated high on the crags and ridges in front of them, and to move about in the daytime was to invite enemy fire. Those men who manned outposts and forward strong points had to remain in their foxholes or dugouts for long periods of time, stay constantly alert, and eat cold rations. They couldn't be relieved during daytime hours because to be seen in the open in daylight was to risk sudden death from an enemy shell. The weather was still cold; the ground was still covered with deep snow, and the forward foxholes were cold, damp and mercilessly confining. Our night patrols into enemy territory had been small, and had mostly been carried out on skis. There was still ample snow on the ground to continue patrolling on skis, but the snow would soon be gone, and after our battalion left this position in the line, no one in it ever put on a pair of skis in combat again.

Our battalion had been assigned to hold and defend a specific portion of the front. Since we were relieving the 1ˢᵗ Battalion, we merely moved into their positions and manned their foxholes, dugouts and other structures. If this had been newly captured ground, we would have had to build these dugouts, dig the foxholes, lay the field wire, and newly prepare all of the defenses. We did plenty of this later on when we were moving forward daily.

As was common military practice, our battalion front was divided into two portions, each assigned to one of our infantry companies to defend. Spread out in foxholes and other shelters, immediately behind these forward companies, was the third infantry company. These men were the reserves that could quickly be committed to close any gap that might be developing in the line. The fourth company, the heavy weapons company established firing points all across the front, in which they set up their heavy mortars and 50 caliber machine guns. They tried to choose locations that were protected from enemy fire by the terrain, but still allowed good observation and direct fields of fire against the enemy. Usually they would be firing their weapons from higher elevations in the terrain, over our infantry positions at the enemy beyond. Often these positions would lie within the area where the reserve company was located.

The far forward foxholes and other points from which the enemy could be observed were usually connected to their company command post, and sometimes they were interconnected with other observation points and heavy weapons strong points. From anywhere in the system and alarm could quickly reach everyone in the area. Company command posts were connected with their respective battalion command posts, and through them to their regimental headquarters. More importantly, all across the front the company command posts were hooked up to each other laterally, so that lateral communication was possible in case of an enemy attack on any unit's flank.

Artillery and mortar fire was also included in all defense plans. Artillery pieces were usually located well behind the front line because they had a long range. Their targets could not be seen by the gun crews, and therefore their fire was called for by forward observers who initiated and directed it, usually over a field phone, but occasionally, in some circumstances, by radio. Artillery fire was effective in striking the enemy on his front side, or bursting in the air over his head to rain shell fragments down upon him at high velocities. Timing of the explosion, distance and direction could be corrected and adjusted by the forward observer who was always in a position to see where each shell exploded. Effective airbursts were accomplished by pre-set timing fuses in the shells, which cause the shell to explode at a predetermined point in the trajectory. In some locations enemy positions were shielded from direct artillery fire by high hills. Such areas were more accessible to mortar shells, which had a high arching trajectory and could be made to rain down from nearly overhead on any target near enough for such a shell trajectory to reach. Because of these high trajectories mortars had much shorter ranges than artillery pieces, and had to be fired from positions much closer to the target. The explosions from mortar shells could often be seen by the mortar crew that had fired them, and necessary adjustments and corrections could quickly be made to put the next shot directly on target. The larger mortars had longer ranges, and it was comforting to know that they were available when needed.

It was customary for all mortars and artillery pieces to fire practice rounds, whenever they were set up in a new location. This was done in order to record the range settings for many local terrain features such as hidden draws and approaches to our territory which the enemy would be likely to use if he attacked, and allowed many guns and mortars, sometimes within seconds after a report from a forward observer, to simultaneously plaster the approach of an enemy patrol with myriads of exploding shells. This was called "firing for effect."

Artillery was usually not under the direct control of a battalion or company, but fired in support of these units when requested. Mortars, on the other hand, being much closer to the front line, were usually under the control of the battalion, and on occasion, under special circumstances, were assigned to the control of a specific company.

In portions of the front like this one, which were static for long periods of time, it was possible to set up even more elaborate defense mechanisms which included mines, booby traps and trip wires set across the paths and trails out in front of the outposts. Some trip wires were designed to detonate explosives which were intended to destroy whoever or whatever stumbled across the wire. Some wires were designed, when tripped, to send an illuminating flare up into the air to light up the whole area for the machine gunners on guard in the strong points. Often whenever such a flare went up, it was followed by much shooting.

Until we moved up to Lizzano, Captain Thomas A Egan, the Regimental Dental Officer, was with us much of the time. He worked in the aid station and elsewhere, using portable equipment. I remember him as being older than I was, a quiet person who worked unobtrusively and did not participate much in the kidding and joshing that often occurred in the aid station. I think he chose to stay with us because we were the reserve battalion, and it was much more convenient to work with us than with the front line battalions. But now that we were actually manning the front, we had a new dental Officer, the Assistant Regimental Dental Surgeon, Max H. Raabe, First Lieutenant, Dental Corps. He had graduated from the University of Michigan Dental School in Ann Arbor, Michigan in February 1944, some four months after I had graduated from the medical school. He knew some of the same people I had known when I was in school there. Not long after he arrived we began reminiscing about our school days.

From the very first time we met I liked Max very much. He was an enthusiastic, friendly, out-going person who had been well trained in his profession. He liked to talk about dentistry, particularly the newest developments, and in my conversations with him I learned a few things about teeth and tooth care that were new to me. Without much urging Max reviewed a lot of dentistry, and later on I was grateful for this, because many of the things we discussed were useful later, in situations where no dental officer was available. Among the surgical tools we carried was a dental kit containing a few basic dental tools among which were several pairs of odd shaped forceps used for extracting teeth. Max showed me how they were used, and later this knowledge also came in handy.

I never did pull a tooth for a soldier. Among our soldiers dental problems were few and far between, and whenever a problem occurred there was generally a dental officer available. At other times I was always able to satisfactorily treat the toothache long enough to refer the man to the rear for specific treatment.

Within the civilian population it was a different story, and as time went on I did pull a number of teeth. The recipients of this service always seemed truly grateful, for they had all suffered the agony of severe toothache for an extended period of time before they came to me. As far as I know, toothbrushes and toothpaste could not be bought in Italy during the later years of the War, and the Italian peasants seemed to have a tendency to neglect their teeth. They generally had poor ones with many in various stages of decay. I am certain that none of the teeth I pulled could have been saved. Some were loose and came out easily; others were more difficult, but I feel sure that I did well with all of them and didn't leave any root tips or broken sockets behind.

One incident involving Max Raabe, that I shall never forget, occurred soon after he arrived. The hospital building in which we were running the aid station had a dining room which contained a number of long tables, and there was a functioning, wood-burning, iron stove located at one end. We used it as our dining room, and at breakfast one morning the menu included white bread, which none of us had seen for a while. I don't remember if it was Army bread or had come from a local bakery, but it certainly tasted good, and there was marmalade and canned butter to go with it. The staff of the hospital also used this dining room, and that morning an older woman, who was matronly in appearance and stout in stature, was in charge of the nurses and other workers. Max convinced her to make toast, and took it upon himself to see that everyone got some. She made the toast on the cooking surface of the stove, after slicing the bread with a huge knife at one of the nearby tables. Whenever Max found another customer he would sing out, "More toasta, Mama!!!," and she would add another slice or two to the stovetop. This continued until the bread was gone.

Now that we were established in Lizzano and the whole Battalion was close by, I no longer had to make the long Jeep trips to hold sick call. The trip from the line companies to the aid station took only a few minutes in a truck, but couldn't be made in daylight without drawing enemy fire, so we usually held sick call after dark. It became routine to hold the cases of minor illness and all but the more serious wounds in a protected place at the front until it was relatively safe to travel, and then bring them in to the aid station all at once.

One evening a singular load of patients arrived. One of them had a gunshot wound just above the left wrist on the ulnar side of the forearm. I had previously seen this man during my contacts with the line companies, and I recognized him. Most of the time he was cheerful and outgoing, and prone to making wisecracks. He always talked a lot, and continually reminded everyone that his ancestors came from Russia. He claimed to be able to speak Russian, and often said that he was looking forward to the time when we would join up with the Russian Army, so he could talk to the Russian soldiers. I don't remember which company he was in and I don't remember his name, but I do remember that it had a Russian sound to it.

When I questioned him about his wound, he said that he had received it while on guard duty. As he stood with his rifle butt planted on the ground and with his wrist draped across the end of the barrel, in the manner of the heroes of old Western movies, the gun went off. The wound had been treated by the company aid man. I removed the splint and unwrapped the bandage to examine it. There was very little bleeding, but small bone splinters were visible, and there were powder burns on the skin. I applied more sulfa powder, rebandaged the wound, and reapplied the splint. Then I explained to him that he would be evacuated to a hospital so that his arm could be operated upon that night or at least by the next day.

As I went to a table across the room to complete his records, he said to me, "Sir, do you know what this is called in Russian?" I didn't answer right away because, based upon my previous experience with him, I was sure he wouldn't stop talking. He continued by answering his own question. "It's called tufshitsky!"

I studied him from across the room for a few moments. There was a big grin on his face, which was certainly inconsistent with the facial expressions of the other people in the room. There were about a dozen people there and he was the only one smiling! At that moment the thought crossed my mind.

"You stinker!" I thought to myself, "You shot yourself! This is a self inflicted wound!"

Then in my mind I debated my course of action. Should I report my suspicions immediately? To whom? What procedures must be followed? What paperwork would be required? Who would be responsible for it?

The rest of the patients needed attention too, and while I was caring for them, I thought long and hard about what to do about this man. Hoping to obtain more information about the circumstances surrounding his wound, I kept up a conversation with him while he was waiting to be evacuated. I also tried to obtain information about the circumstances surrounding his "accident" from the other men who had come in with him, but apparently no one had seen the "accident" happen.

In the end I said nothing and sent him to the rear. The wound needed surgical debridement and repair as soon as possible. Time was important at this stage of treatment, and delay could worsen the final result. If infection were to set in the hand could be lost. After all, the history of this wound would be taken again several times, before and after surgery, and if someone later also became suspicious, the matter could be much more easily handled at the rear than I could handle it here at the front. I never saw this man again, and have no idea how well the wound healed, nor what happened to him, but I still wonder occasionally.

Besides the usual minor colds, sprains and strains of the usual sick call, there were two cases of foot trouble in this group of patients. Each had come off of a long period of outpost duty in a forward foxhole. The first one complained only that his feet had gotten very cold and numb, and he feared that his toes had been frozen. They still felt a bit cold when I examined him, but I found nothing to indicate frostbite or vascular injury, and the man admitted that they no longer really hurt. I made sure that his combat boots were large enough, and recommended that he wear two pairs of socks and change them often, at least until the weather warmed up. He appeared greatly relieved, and in our ensuing conversation he told me that what he had feared most was to be evacuated, lie around in a hospital for a while, then go to a replacement depot, and then finally end up in some other unit where he would not know anyone. This was a common concern of many infantrymen. It was important to most of them that they be returned to or remain in their own unit, where they knew and trusted their companions.

The second case of foot trouble occurred after the man had stayed in a forward foxhole for nearly 36 hours. There was water in the bottom of the hole and his feet were cold and wet all of that time. I had never seen a case of Trench Foot, but had studied the condition at length in medical school, in R.O.T.C., and at Carlisle Barracks, and these feet certainly looked like it to me. I evacuated him right away, but never found out what became of him, or even if my diagnosis was correct. If it was, it was the only case of Trench Foot I saw during the entire War.

So the days came and went, one after another, all pretty much the same. I often wondered how long our comfortable situation in the hospital at Lizzano would continue. All kinds of rumors kept circulating: As soon as the rest of the division arrived at the front we were going to attack; we were never going to attack, but just hold the line while our Armies to the North finished the War; we would soon be sent to invade Japan; etc., etc., etc. There were many other rumors, but all became suddenly unimportant when we received official word that the whole Regiment would soon be replaced in the line and sent to a rear area for rest and additional training.

CHAPTER VI

REST AND REHABILITATION

While we were first holding our defensive positions in the line, the rest of the 10th Mountain Division was still some two or three weeks behind us on its way to Italy, but by January 28, 1945 the entire division had arrived at the front. Our regiment was then placed under Division control, and we were no longer a part of Task Force 45. Five days later our battalion was relieved by elements of the 87th Mountain Infantry, and we marched happily away from the front in the dark of night, through deep, wet snow and mud, to a convoy of trucks which carried us to an area near the city of Lucca for rest, rehabilitation and more training.

We soon found ourselves quite far South of the front and at a lower altitude. I remember being surprised at leaving the snow behind and abruptly coming into a spring-like, almost tropical climate. Some flowers were already in bloom, and I noticed trees with oranges and lemons growing on them. The roads were muddy except for those, which were paved, but it didn't rain a lot. In fact, most of the days were so clear and nice that it felt as if we truly were in "Sunny Italy." Actually we had been in this area before when the weather had been much colder and we were acting as battalion reserve. Two of our companies were doing some active patrolling near Bagni di Lucca, and at the time we were moving our aid station often, so we had not stayed long. That first time Consiglio had found a very nice country villa in which we could stay and operate the aid station, and this time he made arrangements for us to occupy the same place. It was located on a modest estate well out in the country and not near a main road. The manor house was three stories high, and had a central stairway rising upward from a large entrance hall. Each floor had indoor bathrooms and flush toilets, but there was no electricity and therefore no running water with which to flush them. However, because we had a lot of manpower, which was not being kept very busy, it was no problem to have some of the men carry water from the well in the yard upstairs to the toilets in five gallon cans. Several such cans were kept filled and standing nearby, and the toilets could be flushed by merely pouring a gallon or two from a can into the bowl. This worked well, and we used the system throughout our stay.

We were living on a family estate. The Italians called the manor house a villa. It was located in a large yard fronted at the road by a high fence made of sections of stonework covered with a light, beige colored, smooth mortar. The wide driveway was paved with crushed stone, and led from the road through a wrought-iron gate and a formal garden to the entrance of the house. The garden contained roses, some of which were already in bloom, several other kinds of flowers, some evergreens, and citrus, and palm trees. Several smaller, one story outbuildings stood nearby, one of which was a small winery and also housed the water pumping equipment for the well which normally supplied water for the entire premises. The others were garages and tool storage buildings. Most of the rest of the land was planted to grapes used for making wine, which was fermented, aged, bottled and labeled right there on the estate.

The young man in charge of running the estate was a member of the family that owned it. He had stayed behind with a younger brother to look after the family's interests, while all of the other members of the family left the country to avoid the War. I met him soon after we moved in on our first visit, and I liked him very much. I think he liked me too, but could never be sure because he did not speak English or German, and our conversations were always carried out through Consiglio who translated for both of us. His name was Louis, which he pronounced as Lewis, and he was about my age, which at the time was 25. He told us his last name and several other names that he had but I don't remember them, nor do I remember his younger brother's name.

Louis explained that his family was very wealthy and owned cotton mills and factories in Egypt and Mexico. They belonged to the peerage, and he was titled, but I didn't clearly understand what his title was. I thought he might be a Count or a Duke, so we usually called him Louis to his face, and referred to him as "the Duke" when he was out of hearing range.

As was our custom by now, we set up our aid station in one of the large first floor rooms close to the main entrance of the villa, and kept an adjacent room for a storage and living area. By spreading their bedding out on the floor, the men made sleeping quarters out of a couple of rooms and a hallway on the second story. The officers also had a couple of rooms on the second floor, and because there were only three of us, and I was the ranking officer, I had one of them all to myself. The room had a nice bed and a writing table with matching chair, which stood, in front of a West window. I remember writing letters and censoring those written by the men as I sat at the table and watched the setting sun. I liked the room very much because it resembled one in my grandmother's summer home where I had spent a lot of time, and sometimes slept as a child.

On this second visit Louis treated me as his special guest, and proved to be a most gracious and charming host. On the second day of our stay he invited the officers of the aid station to have dinner with him the following evening, an invitation which was promptly accepted.

After cleaning up as best we could for the occasion, we arrived at his door and were ushered in by an elegantly dressed servant who looked and acted like a butler. We were in the part of the villa where "the Duke" and his brother were living. It was immaculately kept, and tastefully and expensively furnished. After a few minutes of conversation we were ushered into a formal dining room and seated at an elegantly laid table. I, as the guest of honor, was seated at the head, and the other two officers, Lieutenant Summers and Lieutenant Raabe, the dental officer, were on my left. Louis and Pfc. Consiglio were on my right and Louis's brother sat at the foot of the table. Consiglio was needed as an interpreter in order to carry on a conversation, because neither Louis nor his brother spoke English. There were flowers on the table, and each place was set with rich looking silverware, a cloth napkin, stem crystal and a large plate of fine china. Each plate was exquisitely decorated in great detail with a picture depicting an historical event that had occurred in Italy.

The dinner was delicious, and was elegantly served, European style, by a manservant dressed in a white coat-jacket, white vest, white tie and white gloves. Everything was spotlessly clean. The courses were served separately, and everyone received a clean plate and new, clean silver for each one. The waiter served us individually from large serving dishes and platters, using a serving spoon and fork which he manipulated together in one hand, all the while wearing immaculately clean white gloves. Between courses large picture plates were placed before us, and there seemed to be such a great variety of them that no picture appeared before anyone twice during the whole meal. Red wine, dry and clear, the best I had ever tasted, was served throughout the meal, and we learned that it was the wine made for export right there on the estate.

I recognized the first course as Westphalia ham. My Grandfather and my father had occasionally brought some of it home from the delicatessen when I was a boy. It was highly salted, smoked, and sliced paper-thin like chipped beef, to be eaten without further cooking. It was accompanied by delicious dark bread, which we learned was made partly with rye flour and partly from flour made from chestnuts. There were a lot of chestnut trees in Italy, and chestnut flour was used by Italian cooks in many ways.

The second course was macaroni, which was no thicker than the spaghetti we were accustomed to at home, and came in longer segments than the macaroni we knew. I recognized it immediately, however, because there was a tiny hole down the length of each piece. It was cooked exactly right, and served with a sauce made of meat, tomatoes, spices and a special Italian cheese. The taste was delicious, but there was something peculiar about the texture. When chewed, there was a grating sensation between one's teeth, as if the macaroni contained scouring powder. I suspected that this might be due to the flour from which it was made, and asked Louis if the macaroni had been made with chestnut flour. He said it wasn't, but the flour in it was stone ground and was "grainy" because there actually was stone dust in it.

The third course appeared to be the main one. It consisted of braised beef cutlets in a garlic sauce that was ever so slightly sour, so the overall effect was that of eating roast beef with a slight salami flavor. We were surprised that such meat was available in wartime Italy, and asked Louis about it. He assured us that there were still many things in his country that money could buy, and that he and his family had plenty of money. The meat and all of the other scarce items served had been obtained on the black market. Served with the meat course were crisp french fried potatoes, which had been cooked in olive oil. They too were delicious, and tasted only slightly different from the ones we were used to at home.

The next course was a salad made from a green vegetable, which was new to me. I cannot remember its name, but I remember that it tasted a lot like watercress. It was served with a delicious wine vinegar and oil dressing. There were also ripe olives, which I didn't like very much. Compared with the canned ones grown in California, these were tough, had much larger pits, and were quite bitter. I can also say the same thing for the Italian green olives that I later tasted from time to time. Olive trees seemed to grow everywhere in Southern Italy. Tending them and harvesting the crop seemed to be almost a year around operation. After we had come down from the mountains I saw small groups of people harvesting olives almost every day.

The final course was dessert, which consisted of dried figs from Sicily. They were served with more wine. Louis then offered us an Italian cigarette which I thought was at least as good as any of our American brands, and after a few more minutes at the table, we all went into the sunken living room for coffee which was served strong and black in demitasse cups. Instead of cream and sugar we were invited to add a strong, sweet liqueur to it. The resulting mixture tasted very goon indeed.

The living room was Tastefully and expensively furnished, and there was a beautiful grand piano in it. No one in our group played, but I had had some lessons as a boy, and had also memorized a few classical piano pieces for my own pleasure while I was in college and medical school. So I sat down and played these for a while. The piano was of concert grand caliber, in excellent condition and precisely tuned, so even my poor playing sounded great.

When the party broke up soon afterward I realized that during the course of this miserable war, I had just had a totally unexpected experience, and had had a very good time. I went to bed feeling guilty because I had not yet censored the outgoing mail for my men, so I resolved to rise early the next morning to do it. I did, and after the chore was done, I felt better.

About a week later on consecutive evenings and at his invitation we ate dinner with "the Duke" twice more. These affairs were almost repeat performances of the earlier meal except that the seating arrangements and menus were a little different. I remember spaghetti instead of macaroni, veal cutlets instead of beef, and fancy cake for dessert. After the second of these dinners we listened to phonograph records on a record player, which didn't run on electricity, so it had to be wound up from time to time. This time we smoked our American cigarettes, and I left some with Louis because he said he liked them. While the records were playing I slipped upstairs and brought down my monthly bottle of Post Exchange whiskey, which officers were allowed to buy and which had arrived just that day. It was one of the well-known and less expensive American brands. We opened it, and all had a couple of drinks. Somehow the whiskey tasted much better when served in "the Duke's" fancy glassware. He seemed to like it very much, so I left the rest of the bottle with him.

Earlier in the week still more evidence of wealth became apparent to me when the servants opened one of the outbuildings and pushed out a shiny automobile, a Fiat, I believe. They had been putting gasoline into it from a large can when "the Duke" came out of the villa to drive into town on "business." Not having seen any civilian gas stations in operation in all of the time we had been in Italy, I asked about the gasoline. Louis said the it too came from the black market, and explained again that if one knew the right people and had enough money, almost anything could still be bought in Italy. This evidence of his wealth certainly impressed me. Louis didn't deliberately flaunt it, nor did he apologize for it. He seemed to me to be a genuine "regular fellow," and I found myself liking him more and more as we became better acquainted.

In all we spent about two weeks with Louis while our line companies did a considerable amount of training. My people in the medical detachment, by now already well trained, had little to do. Even our litter bearers seemed by now to have mastered the basics of first aid in the field. Our main duty was to hold sick call for the battalion, and because this usually did not take much time, I was able to devote more time to an ever-growing civilian medical practice. But this is a subject I will deal with separately later.

Throughout our stay with "the Duke" I attended staff meetings at both Battalion and Regimental Headquarters, and it became apparent that our life of ease would soon come to an abrupt end. Higher headquarters were busy making plans for our division to go on the attack, and there was much speculation in the ranks about what the mission might be. Wild rumors were rife, and we joked every day about the "Rumor of the Day."

Finally on February 15, 1945, the day after our last dinner with "the Duke," the field order, which settled all speculation, arrived. The division was to take and hold Monte Belvedere and Monte della Torraccia, and the 86th Mountain Infantry Regiment would lead the attack!

CHAPTER VII

RIVA RIDGE & BELVEDERE

The arrival of the order to prepare for an all-out attack started a flurry of activity. The scope of the division's assignment was considerably wider than it had at first appeared, because in order to take and hold Monte Belvedere it would also be necessary to take and hold a considerable amount of surrounding territory to deprive the enemy of his ability to launch any successful counterattack. Much of the early planning had already been done in the higher echelons, and now the information had to be passed on to all unit commanders in the field in order to allow each one to form a compatible battle plan for his troops to follow in carrying out the specific mission assigned to his unit.

Lieutenant Summers and I attended a lot of regimental and battalion staff meetings. We received most of our information about the overall battle plan during these sessions. I was often surprised by the amount and depth of the information given out. The deployment of all units in the division was discussed and re-discussed as necessary minor changes were made. It was reassuring to know that a large number of competent officers would be familiar with the overall battle plan, but it was also somewhat disconcerting to realize that I was expected to be one of them.

Although I always listened carefully to everything that was said at these meetings, visualizing and understanding what was about to happen militarily was difficult for me. I couldn't muster any real enthusiasm for learning the roles of the other regiments and the neighboring units in the action to come, but I was very deeply concerned about what my battalion and our medical detachment would be doing, and I worried a lot that we might not be able to keep up, or that we might get lost, or blunder into a minefield, or even into an enemy unit and be captured or wiped out. Occasionally military terms were used that I didn't properly understand. Then I would become confused, and while I tried to figure out what was meant, I would lose concentration and miss some of the information that followed. However, I never left a briefing without asking about everything I didn't fully understand. However, I never interrupted a briefing to do so, because I always remembered the old adage,

"It is better to keep one's mouth shut and appear a fool, than it is to open it and dispel all doubts."

This led me to wait until the end of the session before directing my questions more or less informally to one or more of the staff officers present.

Our battalion officers knew I was a greenhorn, and they were particularly supportive, especially Major Hay, the battalion commander, and Captain Drake, the executive officer. In the early weeks after I had arrived at Camp Swift, one or the other of these men often went out of his way to provide reassurance and see that things were going well for me. That helped a great deal, and I was grateful. At first one or the other of these officers made it a point to speak to me, at the end of each briefing, to make sure that I knew what was expected and to explain anything that I needed to have explained. In time, as I gained confidence and knowledge from the many briefings, they didn't need to explain much to me any more. The rest of the officers were also helpful in raising my confidence, although they probably didn't realize it. In this regard I particularly remember Captain Everett Bailey, who commanded L Company, Captain Frederic Dole, who commanded K Company, and a Captain Watson, who commanded I company before he was evacuated with a serious abdominal wound during his company's first major attack. There were others too, whose names I don't remember now, but I definitely remember a coherent group of extremely competent officers who inspired confidence in their men.

Our battalion commander was Major John Hay who came from Montana, and had been a National Park Ranger before he entered the Army. At first I wondered why he was only a Major while the other battalion commanders were Lieutenant Colonels, but I soon decided that it was because he was the youngest, by far, of the three. He appeared to be only about five or six years older than I. (*Long after the War I learned that he was only three years older.*) I also decided very soon that he was the best battalion commander in the division, and once again was glad that I had chosen to serve his battalion.

It now pleases me very much to know that my judgment was correct. In recent years I have learned that John Hay remained in the Army after the War, and achieved many noteworthy accomplishments. They included command of a task force that stayed in the Arctic for many weeks to test cold weather gear, command of combat divisions in the Korean and Vietnam Wars,

and command of the 101ˢᵗ Airborne Division, during which time he made
over one hundred parachute jumps with his men. He eventually retired with
the rank of a three-star general. In October of 1986 my wife and I drove from
Michigan to California, and stopped on the way to see him at his home in
Colorado. I was happy to see that he was still very active and seemed physically fit. It was a true pleasure to be able to visit with him once more. We
spent a most pleasant evening with General and Mrs. Hay, as guests in their
home, and this marked one more event in my life that I shall always remember.

My confidence in the officers and men in my battalion grew steadily
from the time I had first joined it, and by the time we entered combat I felt
quite comfortable about belonging to such a great group. This is perhaps best
illustrated by quotations from three of the many letters I wrote to my wife:

December 30, 1944 - "I have a big job and a lot more actual responsibility than ever before. However, I have everything under control, including
myself, and I am with a swell bunch of officers and men. I'm sure I'll make
out alright."

January 29, 1945 - "All I can say now is that this is a wonderful Army,
and that the men under me are just about the best in it."

February 12, 1945 - "Today is miserable, wet and rainy, but the work
goes on in spite of the weather; and I am busy as always. I guess that the
"Doc" hears all kinds of the men's little problems that the other officers never
hear about. I'm glad of one thing though; I'm with one of the best groups of
soldiers in the world, and I have a lot of confidence in them."

As I attended more and more briefings and passed on more and more
information about the impending attack to my men, I began to get a clearer
idea of the general battle plan. The main division objective was to take and
hold Monte Belvedere, the largest and highest mountain peak in the area.
This peak was crucial to the German defenses, and we could not hope to
successfully break into the Po Valley without first securing it. Its importance
was evidenced by the fact that it had been previously taken three or four
times by other Allied units, each time at great cost, only to be quickly lost
again in the vigorous counterattacks that inevitably followed immediately.

In order to take and hold Monte Belvedere with the least difficulty and
the least cost, the Division planned to first assault and take a chain of four
mountain peaks to the West of it. These peaks were part of a long, high ridge,
which gave the enemy superb observation of the entire South and West sides
of Belvedere. From it the enemy had direct observation of and could directly
fire heavy artillery onto the rear of any force attacking Belvedere. As soon as

our men had taken and were holding this ridge, a direct assault upon the peak
of Monte Belvedere from the Southwest was planned, which, in the absence
of enemy artillery fire from the ridge should be successful and easier than the
previous attacks on Belvedere had been. Then as soon as Belvedere was in
our hands, it would also be necessary to capture and hold the mountainous
areas to the East, including Monte Gorgolesco, several smaller hills, and finally Monte della Torracia, because the previously successful counterattacks
had come from these areas. Taking and holding all of this territory was extremely important because it would significantly deprive the enemy of his
ability to counterattack and successfully regain Belvedere.

So the first division objective in the overall battle plan was to take and
hold these four peaks. They stood in a straight line, approximately equidis-
tant apart, with high saddle areas between them. They ran approximately
from Southwest to Northeast, with the easternmost peak in the row standing
almost due West of Belvedere. Beginning from the West, and in order, their
names were *Monte Mancinello, Monte Serrasiccia, Monte Cappel Buso and
Pizzo di Campiano*. Collectively they became known as **Riva Ridge**, a name
that soon became well known, not only to the military in Italy, but also later
in news releases to the world. Many years after the War a racehorse was
named after it, and the name, Riva Ridge, was further perpetuated when that
horse won the Kentucky Derby.

The back side of Riva Ridge sloped downward quite gently to the Northwest. The enemy would have no difficulty bringing up heavy equipment and
reinforcements from that direction. In contrast to the enemy's easy slope, the
side, which our troops faced, was about 1500 feet high, was very steep, contained many rock faces, and had a small river at its base. For a man to climb
this cliff in daylight would be a difficult feat, and, until now, it had been
conceded by both sides that it would be impossible to launch a successful
attack up this façade. We were quite sure that the Germans were not expecting any action there, and we knew that they didn't guard it heavily. Our mountain troops were planning to surprise them by beginning their attack with an
assault up the steep side of Riva Ridge at night, under cover of darkness,
relying heavily on the element of surprise for quick success. Mountain Infantrymen, burdened with weapons and heavy loads of ammunition, were not
only expected to make the climb, but were expected to do it in the dark, and
perhaps fight even before they reached the top.

Some of the best rock climbers in the division had already explored the
cliff facings, and taking factors into consideration such as the difficulty of
the climb, the desirability of stealth, the avoidance of rock slides, available

cover, etc., they had picked out four routes of ascent, one for each of the peaks. To aid the climbing infantrymen they had also securely fastened ropes to the rocks at the steepest and most difficult places along these routes. These ropes were mainly high up, and none were within direct view of the enemy. All of this preparation had been accomplished with no sign that the enemy had detected any of it.

The 1st Battalion of the 86th Mountain Infantry plus Company F of the 2nd Battalion were chosen to make the assault. As soon as I learned this I was once again glad that I had chosen to serve the 3rd Battalion.

Once Riva Ridge was secure in our hands, the rest of the Division was scheduled to attack Belvedere from the Southwest, with the 85th Mountain Infantry going first over the peak, then the peak of Monte Gorgolesco, and finally taking Monte della Torraccia farther to the Northeast. The 87th Mountain Infantry was scheduled to attack alongside of the 85th to take the forward slope of Belvedere, then continue on to protect the left flank of the 85th. The 2nd Battalion of the 86th, less Company F, which would be up on Riva Ridge, was to stay in the vicinity of Vidiciatico as the Division Reserve, and my 3rd Battalion was scheduled to follow along on the right flank of the 85th to protect that flank, and clear the Southern slopes of all enemy soldiers. Company K would sweep the foothills, while Company L would operate higher up to protect the flank of the 85th.

Everyone seemed to agree that this was a good battle plan, but there was yet one possibly very large problem that worried me. I didn't know if it was truth or rumor, but unofficial word had come down, presumably from Division Headquarters, that a ninety percent casualty rate was anticipated for the force attacking Riva Ridge. I didn't take a mental giant to calculate that if four companies of 200 men each were participating, a 90 percent casualty rate would amount to over 700 casualties. I wondered if the men of the 1st Battalion and F Company were aware of this, and if it was having any serious effect on their morale. It certainly was a topic of conversation in our 3rd Battalion Aid Station. We worried because casualties of that number in a single day would swamp all of our aid stations and dangerously overload all medical installations in the theater, all of the way back to the base hospitals.

Because we knew that the entire 1st Battalion was included in the attacking force, we knew that its aid station would be supporting it, and we assumed that the 2nd Battalion Aid Station would also back up the assault since its Company F would also be participating. Then, just before we left for the front, I was told the we too would be setting up in an area at the base of Riva Ridge, and would probably receive casualties from the action. This convinced me that at least someone in the higher command was expecting a high casualty rate.

Late in the evening on February 17, 1945 we left the rear area near Lucca in the dark. At the end of the journey, in the early morning hours, we pulled our vehicles off of the road. It was still dark. We followed a narrow lane in the direction of Riva Ridge, which appeared high and menacing in front of us. After a short distance we were directed to set up our aid station in a small building the back of which had been built into a hillside so that most of the building was buried. After daybreak everyone had to stay under cover, because we didn't want to tip the enemy off to the fact that there was a large troop concentration in the area. The movement of a huge amount of supplies and equipment, and a large number of men had occurred under the cover of darkness, and when daylight came the roads were deserted. We fervently hoped that the Germans had not become suspicious that anything was afoot.

We stayed under cover in the aid station all day, and after darkness fell, we watched Riva Ridge, which was not very far in front of us, with tense anticipation. The attacking forces moved out soon after darkness fell, but we didn't know the exact time. As we watched, our searchlights were still moving their beams about on the ridge top as usual, but the rock faces, where our soldiers were climbing, remained in darkness, and we could see nothing of them. As the hours passed everyone became increasingly tense and edgy. Midnight came and went, and still we heard nothing. We knew that the men were carrying heavy loads, of which only a canteen and some K Rations were not weapons or ammunition. Were the routes too steep? Were the loads too heavy? Certainly, by now enough time had gone by for them to have reached the top. One o'clock passed and still we heard nothing. What could possibly have happened? What was going on?????

Shortly after 1:00 a.m. we heard sounds of combat. It sounded as if it began with machine pistols, but rifles, grenades and mortar rounds soon followed. The sounds seemed to come from high up, so it appeared that at least some of our assault forces had reached the top. Now our searchlights were shut down, leaving the peaks above in darkness. Was this a good sign, or was it bad?

Intermittently, for the rest of the night, the sounds of combat came down to us from the top of Riva Ridge, but we weren't receiving any news of progress, and we knew nothing about what was happening. The hours dragged on, but finally, in the middle of the morning on the 19th of February 1945 we received a report of the progress made in the fighting up above, and the news was good. All of the attacking companies had reached their objectives before daybreak, and some of the expected counterattacks had already been repulsed. Casualties had been astonishingly light, and we would be getting some of them soon. Of course we could not know how many there had been, but we knew then that it was far, far less than the 90 percent estimates we were thinking about beforehand.

Some idea of the number of casualties sustained in the assault and in the subsequent defense of the ground that was taken is found in the 86th Mountain Infantry Regimental History, which includes in it the information that an estimate was made at about 7:00 p.m. on February 20th of casualties suffered in the previous 48 hours. This would include the assault on Riva Ridge and some 36 hours of successful defense against the many vigorous enemy counterattacks that immediately followed. The numbers reported were: one officer killed and two officers wounded; six enlisted men killed and twenty-five enlisted men wounded. This represents about four percent of the attacking force, and in view of the enormity of the mission accomplished, is a remarkably low casualty rate. When considering these numbers one should also realize that over 98 percent of the wounded who made it to a hospital alive would survive in good condition.

Our litter teams were now called forward to pick up casualties. A few minutes later they sent word back that evacuation would be possible by Jeep, so we sent the Jeep forward, and it soon came back with some walking wounded. In the second trip it brought two litter cases, and our driver, Pfc. Charles Argyle, told us that the driving in the lane up ahead was very bad. At one place in the trail the men had to unload the litters from the Jeep, so that he could back up some distance and make a run toward a large shell crater in the wagon trail and literally leap the Jeep over it. Then they carried the litters across the gap, reloaded them on the Jeep, and drove the rest of the way to the aid station.

It had taken eight to ten hours and a number of special procedures to bring these wounded men down off of the ridge, so it was fortunate that there weren't many. We learned later that a couple of days later the Division Engineers stretched a cable from the top down to the valley floor, and with a basket type litter and ropes and pulleys, a casualty could be brought down in a few minutes. On the return trips much needed supplies and ammunition went up to the men now dug into defensive positions on the peaks.

While we were treating these casualties Major John Seamans came into the aid station. I knew him then only well enough to recognize him, and at the time I assumed that he was a regimental staff officer who had come to observe how well we, as medics, were operating. I asked him if he had come to inspect us. He didn't answer directly, but just smiled and said he liked what he saw. It wasn't until sometime later that I realized he was not a part of the regimental staff, but was a 2ⁿᵈ Battalion staff officer. Then I wondered why he had visited us, and eventually concluded that it was because F Company of the 2ⁿᵈ Battalion was participating in the attack, and our aid station was where F Company casualties were likely to come through. I will have more to say about this officer later.

We promptly evacuated our casualties to the rear, using the Jeep to take them out to the main road where the collecting company ambulances could accommodate them. With our troops now occupying the ridge above, there was now much less enemy shelling of the area, and traffic was getting through without enemy harassment. From time to time, all afternoon long, we continued to hear the sounds of combat above, and we assumed correctly that the Germans were mounting multiple counterattacks on the newly won positions.

After dark that evening, February 19, 1945, we packed up again and moved to a staging area just South of Monte Belvedere. From there, later that night, our 3ʳᵈ Battalion would launch its main attack, and it was there that we made our final preparations. As long as the 1ˢᵗ Battalion and F Company could hold Riva Ridge, our 3ʳᵈ Battalion attack was scheduled to coincide with the attacks of our other two regiments upon Belvedere, beginning about an hour before midnight.

All of the essential aid station equipment went into our rucksacks, and we left our vehicles behind. They would be of no use to us, since there were no roads where we were going. I carried a few cigarettes, some K Rations and my toilet articles in the top compartment of my rucksack, and the rest of it was filled with packages of freeze-dried blood plasma paired with bottles of sterile distilled water, because the plasma had to be reconstituted by dissolving it in the water before it could be administered intravenously to the more seriously wounded for the treatment of hypovolemic shock. I remember anxiously sitting with many other men on the floor in an old building, in a dim light, with my back against a wall, waiting tensely, and worrying because I did not know what to expect.

At about 11:00 p.m. word was passed along to move out in single file, five yards apart. We all knew that these instructions meant that we were likely to be fired upon. There were some broken clouds in the sky, and a bit of moonlight from time to time, and our searchlights were still lighting the peak of Belvedere, so there was light enough for us to see the trail quite well. Under these conditions a man standing up out in the open was conspicuous, and I wondered how well the enemy above would be able to see us. Just thinking about this caused the knot in the pit of my stomach to tighten. Most of the men seemed to have similar thoughts, and almost all showed signs of nervousness as we anticipated marching out into the open in view of the enemy under these conditions.

We, medics, followed M Company, the heavy weapons company. I watched as the men marched past, walking five yards apart, carrying mortar tubes, machine gun barrels and other pieces of equipment. When my turn came I stepped into the line as it marched out into the large open field on the southern shoulder of Monte Belvedere. I stayed five yards behind the man I was following. We crossed the field at a brisk march, still keeping five-yard intervals, and then turned a little to the right. From there it looked like a long way up to the distant woods which would offer us concealment, and now the trail became steep, rising at a 45 degree angle, more or less. Parts of it were sloppy with mud, and patches of snow here and there created some very slippery segments. Regardless of whether it was mud or snow, each step forward up the slope resulted in the foot sliding half a pace or more backward down the slope, and it took a lot of effort to make any headway. In spite of these conditions, we crossed the open area in good time, glancing frequently over our shoulders at the peaks above where the Germans were, and hoping they wouldn't see us. I soon became breathless and gasped for air. My chest ached. I thought that perhaps my good physical condition had deteriorated, but when we finally reached the shelter of the woods, it was obvious that the exertion had affected all of the men in this manner. It was reassuring to learn that I wasn't the only one winded.

I don't remember much about the rest of that night. We kept moving for quite a while, and I didn't know exactly where we were, but in retrospect I believe we were on the western slope of the southern shoulder of Monte Gorgolesco. Accounts of the action in my references state that our 3rd Battalion had gained its objective, San Filomena, by 3:45 a.m., sustaining only one casualty, that the 1st Battalion plus F Company were still holding Riva Ridge against all counterattacks, and that the attacks of the 85th and 87th Regiments had started on schedule. At this hour the 87th was fighting on the reverse slope of Belvedere, and the 85th had crossed the peak of Belvedere and was fighting in the saddle area between Belvedere and Gorgolesco, where it was having difficulty with fierce enemy resistance.

Shortly before daylight we set up our aid station in a barn-like building somewhere on the mountainside. One of my letters indicates that it was near a place named Gabba. At about the same time orders were received at the

Battalion Command Post for L Company to move up the mountainside, make contact with the men of the 85th, and attack alongside them to help take the peak of Monte Gorgolesco. This advance began almost immediately and produced casualties. Walking wounded and litter cases began to arrive at the aid station and were promptly attended. Most of them had already been treated in the field by a company aid man. I was surprised that they were generally in good shape, and there was little that I had to do.

Our biggest problem now was getting the wounded out of the aid station and to the collecting company. There were no roads so the litter cases had to be carried down to where they could be loaded into ambulances. Wounded soldiers began to pile up in the aid station, and soon there were so many that litter teams from the collecting company were called up to help. Non-medics from some of the service units were also used to help carry stretchers to the rear, while the collecting company litter teams were sent forward to the battle area to bring out wounded men who were still lying where they had fallen.

Sometime soon after daylight had arrived, a group of walking wounded came in to the aid station, and I remember one of them very well. He was Walter Hyry of Company L. He had been struck in the front of his helmet, but in the excitement and stress of the attack had not realized that he had been hit until one of his buddies pointed it out and he saw the blood that was dripping from his face splash into his hand. He had left his rifle in the field, but had his helmet with him when he arrived, and in the middle of the front of it there was a hole about two inches wide, four inches long, and vertically oriented. The hole was ragged; spikes of metal were bent inward at various angles all around its edge, and some of the metal seemed to be missing. When I examined the wound I found a ragged piece of metal embedded in the bone of the skull at about the hairline in the middle of his forehead, and I couldn't be sure whether it was a shell fragment or a piece of the helmet. It was firmly embedded, like a nail driven into a block of wood, which made the wound the equivalent of a compound skull fracture. I decided that the metal should be left undisturbed until it could be removed and the wound properly repaired in an operating room under sterile conditions. Walter didn't like this idea at all. He had been given morphine out in the field, and felt no pain, but the narcotic had also loosened his tongue; he kept insisting that I should remove the metal from his head. I had to explain several times about the dangers of bone and brain infection, but before he settled down I had to tell him emphatically that I didn't want his brains hanging out of his skull in the dirty old barn we were using as an aid station.

On the 45th anniversary of this battle for Monte Belvedere, February 19,

1990, I had lunch with Walter and his wife at a reunion of some 10th Mountain Division Veterans, and heard his side of the story and its sequel. He remembered that we were very crowded with serious casualties at the aid station that morning, and there was a problem getting them down off of the mountain. He remained at the aid station for some three or four hours, then walked down, leading another soldier who had succumbed to combat fatigue. When he got to the collecting company, the doctor there uncovered his wound, looked at it, and covered it right back up. The same thing happened at the next stop, and the fragment wasn't removed until he got all of the way back to the hospital, where it was removed in an operating room. He still doesn't know if the fragment came from a shell or from his helmet, but the wound healed well. In due time he was able to return to duty, and finished out the war in his original Company L. He still carries the scar high in the middle of his forehead, but it is no longer very conspicuous.

Sometime in the middle of the morning one of the company aid men from L Company came in to the aid station to replenish his medical supplies. He told us that he thought the men of the 85th had had successfully taken the peak of Gorgolesco, and that L Company had crossed over the crest of its Southeast shoulder. There they had been held up by the worst artillery and mortar shelling they had ever received. At this point there had been very close air support for our ground troops, which had been critical in relieving the situation, but not before one of the bombs had landed among the men of L Company, adding to the casualties. He also announced that early in the attack Paddy had "gotten it." I didn't know Paddy and assumed that he might be a soldier of Irish descent. My men knew who he was, however, and explained to me later that he was known for his acts of bravado, even to the point of recklessness. It was not until quite some time later, when I read about his posthumous award of the Silver Star Medal, that I learned his correct name, Pfc. Thomas J. Patti.

As soon as Monte Gorgolesco was secured, the 85th continued its advance, and our L Company advanced with it on its right flank. Then toward the end of the day, following new orders, L Company swept downhill in a southerly direction to take its original objective, Mazzancana, and link up with K Company in a defensive position for the night. I can't remember how many times we moved the aid station to follow the action that day, but we ended up near the Battalion Command Post near Mazzancana, and under cover in a building.

I had seen Mazzancana on our map, and thought it was a small village, but that was not the case. It was only a single large farmhouse, which had been fortified by the enemy and used as a strong point. I learned later that it was the custom in Italy to give place names to such farmhouses, and even to other single buildings.

Once the Battalion had established its defenses around Mazzancana for the night, we expected to be relieved the next morning by the Brazilian Expeditionary Force, which had advanced with us on our right flank. We looked forward to this relief, but early the next morning orders arrived requiring us to stay where we were for another day. We wondered what had caused this change in plan. Then at a briefing later that day we learned that the 85th had not taken Monte della Torraccia as was first believed, but was still some 400 yards short of it. The attack had bogged down when the lead battalion, the 2nd, after fighting through the night and all of the next day, and suffering heavy casualties, had become short of ammunition and supplies. It was unable to reach its final objective. Nevertheless, in spite of it being late in the day, it was able to dig in and hold all of the territory it had taken.

Within the hour we received new orders. Our Battalion was to have the honor of passing through the 2nd Battalion of the 85th Mountain Infantry to take and hold Monte della Torraccia!

Now there was a problem getting supplies into the area because the roads in the region had been badly broken up by the spring thaw and a lot of heavy traffic, which included tanks, so we did not know yet when this switching of units or the attack was to take place. The situation now seemed a lot less urgent, however, because by this time the enemy counterattacks were less frequent, and the division was no longer sustaining a lot of casualties.

Emergency road repairs were made, and after arrangements for transport and supply had been completed, we received the final orders. We were to relieve all of the positions of the 2nd Battalion of the 85th Mountain Infantry during the night of February 23-24, and attack the peak of Monte della Torraccia at 7:00 a.m. on February 24, 1945!

CHAPTER VIII

MONTE DELLA TORRACCIA

Late in the evening of February 23, 1945 we were preparing to relieve the troops of the 2nd Battalion of the 85th Mountain Infantry, who were still occupying the same foxholes on the approaches to Monte della Torraccia that they were occupying three days previously when their attack had been halted. Once we had taken over their positions, our battalion had orders to attack on the morning of February 24th, and take Monte della Torraccia from the Germans.

We would again be going where vehicles could not travel, so, as we had done for our previous advance, we packed up the essential aid station equipment and supplies to be carried in our rucksacks and in hand. Each man was assigned as much as he could reasonably carry, and, in addition, carried K Rations for two days. Most of the items we normally carried in our rucksacks were left behind to be brought up to us later.

We waited quietly in a forward assembly area near Mazzancana for the word to move out, and as we waited, evidence of the tension among our troops began to appear once again, as each man contemplated the prospects for his survival through the coming action. No one knew exactly what to expect. Our intelligence reports indicated that della Torraccia would be strongly defended. We all knew that our attack would be one of all out proportions against major opposition, and the fighting would surely be fierce.

The order to move up came shortly after midnight, and the battalion immediately set out toward the heights on foot. The night was dark, and the march was made quietly under strict blackout conditions. Men were heavily loaded with weapons and ammunition, and keeping five-yard intervals between them, they marched in single file along a narrow trail, which led to a large hill. The trail went part-way up the hill, then circled steeply to its forward side and passed through the yard of an abandoned farm building, which had probably been a small farmhouse.

The name of this building was "Carge," and the battalion aid station we were to relieve was set up in it. It was a single building, but, like Mazzancana, it had a place name. Our battalion's forward fox holes were only a short distance farther ahead, and not far beyond them, presumably well dug in on the forward slope of della Torraccia, were the Germans.

Our aid station personnel once again marched near the end of the battalion column behind M Company, so the night was nearly over by the time we arrived at Carge. Most of the infantrymen were already in place in the foxholes up ahead. There were no casualties under treatment in the aid station, and the medics we were relieving had already packed up their gear. They wished us luck, said that they were ever so glad to be leaving, and departed promptly.

We started to move in and set up our equipment before they completely cleared the building. First I inspected it inside and out as thoroughly as I could. It had the thick stone walls of the typical Italian farmhouse, and, even though it was still dark and I couldn't see it very well on the outside, it appeared that only the upper stories had been slightly damaged. On the inside I could see that the walls on the ground floor were intact and sturdy and blackout measures had already been adequately taken. The large room in which we would operate constituted the entire first floor of the building. In the center, arranged in a large square, stood four sturdy wooden posts, which supported a heavy, strong ceiling, which appeared to be intact and undamaged. Toward the back of the room were the remnants of animal stalls or pens and some straw. No people were living in the building. No animals were present. There were no other buildings nearby.

We set up our working area in the central square delineated by the four posts. There were some boxes upon which we could set two litters to serve as makeshift operating tables, and there were also some crates and bins upon which we could set up our instruments. We hung the single gasoline lantern overhead near the center of this working area to shed its bright, harsh light over the operating tables. We also had flashlights and candles if we were to need them.

As one entered through the door the left one third of the room would serve as living quarters, where we could cook and store food and water. In the far rear where the stalls were located, the straw there was used to prepare sleeping spots. The entire right side of the room became the area in which we would take care of the wounded. Everything considered, this made a satisfactory aid station, and in a short time we were set up and ready to receive casualties.

In the fighting to reach Mazzancana we had lost some company aid men and litter bearers who had been wounded and evacuated, but I do not remember that any of our medics were killed. We received replacements just before we left Mazzancana, and now assigned them to the existing vacancies. Our aid station personnel had also changed again. We no longer had a dental officer, and had with us instead, Lieutenant William E. (Ed) Rogers, the Battalion Graves Registration Officer, and a small squad of his men. This group traveled with us for most of the rest of our time in combat, and were the only soldiers with the aid station who were armed. They carried only carbines, and did not have grenades or other special weapons. They worked unobtrusively, and did an excellent job in one of the most unpleasant, distasteful, disagreeable duties of the War, that of collecting and registering the dead from the battlefields. Whenever they were not busy doing this, they helped care for the wounded, helped carry litters, and later acted as guards for the litter teams made up of German prisoners that we often used.

There also was a chaplain with us, who was older than the rest of us, and although I remember him well, I don't remember his name. He was Catholic, and because of his background and training in Latin, he did very well with the Italian language. I remember that he always carried multiple canteens. We could always be sure that one of them contained water. He also stayed with us during the attack phases for the rest of the War, but when things were quiet, he spent a lot of time at regimental headquarters where there were other Chaplains present.

Sergeant Miller's post was inside the aid station. He had laid out the equipment and supplies we would need, and he would also be supervising the other two medical technicians. Sergeant Draper, Lieutenant Summers and I completed the aid station complement. The four litter teams were with us too, although they didn't remain inside for long. Once the battle began we saw them only whenever they brought in a stretcher case. As usual, the company aid men were not with us because they were out in foxholes with their respective companies.

Once we were completely set up and ready, there was nothing more to do but wait. It was still dark. Everyone in the aid station remained solemn and sober, and things were so quiet that we only whispered or spoke very softly to each other. We sat around in the aid station waiting for daylight and the battle to begin, and mostly kept our thoughts to ourselves. I am sure that we all hoped that the events soon to come would not be too terrible. Twice I heard some quiet prayers in the back corner of the room. No one slept. Everyone was dreading what they thought was about to happen.

After a time I stepped outside and saw the faint rosy glow in the Eastern sky, which signaled that dawn would soon be here. More of the nearby terrain was now visible, and I noticed that the ground toward the front sloped gently downhill for about fifty yards, then quickly rose again. Farther in the distance I could see the outline of della Torraccia. Our building was on the northeast side of the large hill, which we had circled in order to reach it, and the trail along which we had moved was steepest over the fifty yards or so just before it reached our dooryard. I noticed that it was trampled and muddy as it passed through on its way forward. I knew it was the only route into the area, a mere footpath trail, impossible for vehicles to negotiate. Much of the surrounding area was open ground, but I could see many small patches of trees and scrub growth in all directions. Behind and above us the top of our hill was wooded.

As it began to get lighter birds began to stir and twitter, but except for these slight sounds, all remained very still and quiet. There was no wind. Not a tree or bush moved. Nothing seemed to be stirring in the whole countryside. No one said anything when I returned inside. We all just sat there nervously awaiting the artillery barrage, which we knew would precede the attack.

Division Artillery began firing exactly on time, and shells immediately began passing directly over us. They arrived in groups of several at a time, and soon one group followed another so closely that it seemed that there were always shells in the air above. While in flight they made a peculiar, indescribable noise, which was so loud that it surprised me. Our shells landed with heavy explosions, which seemed to be so close to us that I feared for our men in the forward foxholes. Sitting inside the aid station with artillery shells flying overhead was frightening enough, but it must have been awesome to the men up forward. We all hoped that it was having the desired terrifying effect upon the enemy soldiers, for this shelling was intended to "soften them up" and stun as many as possible just prior to our infantry attack.

This was the first time I had been underneath a major bombardment, and what was most surprising to me was the unusual sound that the shells made as they passed overhead. I have heard it many times since, but still find it almost impossible to describe. I know of nothing else quite like it, and find it hard to think of anything with which to compare it. One might perhaps experience a similar sound if he were to lie face up, parallel to and between the rails, under a long, rapidly moving railroad train, while loud explosions were occurring all around. Big artillery shells have often been described as sounding like an express train passing overhead, and I now knew why such comparisons easily come to mind.

After twenty minutes the barrage ended abruptly, and there followed a few seconds of stunned silence. I looked out of the door of the aid station and saw that daylight had arrived. Nothing moved or stirred. It seemed as if time and sound had ceased to exist. Then an authoritative voice came booming up the hill.

"Clap or no clap!!! You're going on this attack!! You can see the doc later!"

This was overheard by a number of people, and it subsequently became the subject of some humor, which circulated among the troops for a while, but it didn't strike me as being funny. I anticipated one of the men coming through the aid station with gonorrhea, but none appeared, and it was several weeks later before I saw any one with symptoms even remotely suggesting this disease. I still sometimes wonder what happened to the soldier who received this direct order. I wonder if he really did have gonorrhea. If he did, I must speculate that he was killed during the attack.

In another minute or so the sounds of rifle and machine gun fire began, and before long we could hear the mortars and artillery joining in. The infantry attack had begun. At first the sounds were very close to us, but as time passed they became more distant and seemed to be coming from higher up on the mountain. Early in the attack enemy mortar and artillery shells began falling into our aid station area. At about the same time we heard our planes diving from overhead as they bombed and strafed enemy positions just ahead of our troops. I was thankful that they were ours, and that we weren't being attacked from the air in this manner. The participation of those fighter-bombers must have been frightening to the enemy, because of the devastation they could inflict. Just their unopposed presence in the air above must have been very disheartening.

The initial enemy response included heavy shelling which inflicted the most casualties on our reserve units while they were still stationary in their forward assembly areas where they were not very well protected by the terrain. These troops were to follow the attacking companies, but had not yet moved forward, and were sustaining casualties at a faster rate than expected, while up ahead the attacking companies were also suffering casualties, but fewer than expected. Before any serious enemy shelling began, the attacking companies had moved rapidly and were well forward of the assembly areas. Although they were encountering grenades and small arms fire, it appeared that facing these weapons was not as lethal as being trapped by enemy artillery fire.

Later on I often observed that, in an attack in this kind of terrain, it seemed to be safer for infantry to keep moving forward than to hesitate and allow itself to be trapped in enemy counter-fire. I feel sure that our field commanders were aware of this, because it was a priority, at least in our battalion, never to allow an attacking unit to be pinned down because it hesitated or held back. If by accident an attacking unit did become pinned down, it immediately became a high priority to relieve it and get it moving again.

This pattern of casualties made a lasting impression upon me. I gained a great respect for the lethal capabilities of German artillery, and from then on I paid a lot of attention to keeping my aid station and my men away from areas where enemy artillery counter-fire might be expected to fall.

Only minutes after our infantry attack began, walking wounded and litter cases began arriving at the aid station. The first litter teams to arrive reported that they had been momentarily held up several times by enemy shelling, and that there were many more casualties "out there." All of these early cases had shell fragment wounds, which had already been treated by the company aid men, and they were in remarkably good condition. I was once again surprised to find that there was very little I needed to do before they could be evacuated to the rear. Those who could not walk had to be carried back down the trail to where vehicles could be used, and soon there were enough of such cases that litter teams from the collecting company were again called up to help. Later, as the numbers of litter wounded mounted, volunteers from various other service units were again pressed into service as litter bearers, and our litter teams were split up so that at least one, and preferably two, of our medics were included in every team that went out. This system worked well and allowed us to keep up an orderly flow of casualties, first to the aid station and then to the rear.

As the morning wore on and our troops kept advancing, the casualties had to be carried for longer and longer distances through areas into which enemy shells were still falling. Shells were also frequently coming in all around the aid station, making the entire trip hazardous for both litter team and casualty. It became common to have a litter team arrive exhausted and completely winded, because they had run the last fifty yards up the slope to the aid station with their burden.

In the middle of the morning I was momentarily dismayed when one of our company aid men was carried in on a stretcher. I recognized him immediately as one of the new men we had sent out as a replacement early that morning. He was unconscious, and there was a very obvious round bullet hole in the center of the red cross on the front of his helmet. The bullet had pierced the steel helmet and the helmet liner, and had entered the center of his forehead. There was, however, no apparent exit wound and no evidence of damage to the back of the helmet liner, so I concluded that the bullet was still inside his skull. A neurosurgeon would be needed to explore the wound for possible removal of bone fragments and perhaps the bullet. Even though the prognosis was not good, time was important. His pulse and blood pressure remained satisfactory, and after we arranged for airway support to relieve his stertorous breathing, we evacuated him immediately ahead of other cases that were waiting.

Many of the men in the field had seen this unfortunate casualty being carried on the litter, and more saw him later at the aid station. The litter team had bandaged the wound and replaced the helmet on his head, so that the bullet hole in it was in plain view. It was obvious to anyone close enough to see it, that it was indeed a bullet hole, and the men were outraged by this apparent atrocity. At the time many were vocal about it, and some of the accounts of the battle for della Torraccia, which I later read, mention the incident of the medic who was shot through the red cross on his helmet as an example of an atrocity committed by the Germans.

However, in this case simple logic does not support such a concept. There was no doubt that this was a bullet wound, either from a rifle or a light machine gun, and the bullet which caused it must have traveled through the air for a long distance, losing a lot of its power before it struck the helmet. If it had been deliberately fired at the red cross, it would have had to have been fired from a close enough range for this four inch target to be clearly seen, in which case the bullet should still have had ample velocity and energy to pass completely through the head and come out somewhere in the back. The shocking power of such a bullet would very likely be great enough to literally explode the brain, and cause instantaneous death. At the time we were all so busy that I couldn't explain this to the men, and after things had quieted down, our medics at least didn't want to talk about it any more.

In another hour we learned that I Company had taken the main objective, the peak of Monte della Torraccia, but had then received orders to continue to attack and take the hills and ridges to the North and East of it. So the advance continued into the early afternoon, and, when all of the additional objectives were in our hands, new orders were received for the troops to dig in and prepare to defend all of the newly won territory. This was exceptionally rough terrain, and our litter teams now faced a much longer and more arduous trip each time they went to these new forward areas to retrieve a casualty. They still had to remain alert every step of the way because the enemy was intermittently shelling their routes throughout the afternoon and evening.

We were still removing casualties of the day's action from the field when at about 4:30 p.m. the first enemy counterattack in force came at us against the K Company front, which was on our left flank only a very short distance forward of the aid station. Once again a multitude of artillery shells landed in our vicinity, and this time many were so close that I could hear the shell fragments whizzing through our dooryard and slamming into our building. I now realized for the first time that our battalion forward positions were much farther away from us than were the enemy positions on our left flank, and this worried me. If the German counterattack were to break through here, our forward companies would be cut off, and the enemy would control the only route to the rear. Worse yet, such a breakthrough could easily overrun our aid station, and this was a prospect that I didn't relish at all.

As the counterattack continued there were more casualties, and they were now occurring closer to us. The shelling became so intense that for a while the evacuation of casualties from the field to the aid station had to stop, but in time it abated, and we were confident that the attack had failed. Casualties were brought in from the field once again, and with them came the report that the counterattack had indeed been successfully repulsed. By mid-evening the medical situation appeared to be quite well under control again.

Then, at about 11:00 p.m., the K Company front began receiving another heavy concentration of enemy shelling, and our aid station again came under heavy fire. Shells were exploding in our dooryard and fragments were once again striking the stone walls of the building. This time the shelling covered a larger area and appeared to be on a much larger scale than the one before, and it was soon obvious that the Germans were about to launch another, much larger counterattack against the same area in which they had failed that afternoon. Although I didn't know it at the time, more litter squads were needed on the battlefield that night and were requested by Major Hay who was at the Battalion Command Post. Litter cases were arriving at the aid station in rapid succession, and I was so busy that I didn't pay much attention to the men who were carrying them. In addition to the four litter teams we had in action, I now know that at least four more were sent forward from the Division Medical Battalion, and these also were eventually expanded in number by the addition of non-medic volunteers.

As the shelling increased, the route to our rear came under fire of such intensity that it became impossible to evacuate casualties to the rear. It would have been suicidal for anyone to expose himself out there on the trail. However there were occasional short pauses in the shelling, and because the travel distance from the K Company front was short, more casualties kept arriving at the aid station. Some of them were serious and required my full attention to such things as the control of bleeding and the control of shock caused by excessive blood loss. Wounded soldiers rapidly piled up inside, and soon litters with casualties on them covered much of the floor space, even including that which we had thought would be reserved for our housekeeping area. There were also walking wounded in larger numbers, many of whom appeared relieved that they weren't fatally wounded and would be evacuated.

The shelling continued unabated; the aid station became increasingly crowded, and the medical situation soon became critical. Several of the litter patients were shocky and were receiving intravenous plasma. Bloody bandages were in view all over the room, and I was having problems controlling the bleeding in two of the most critical litter cases. Their litters had been placed upon the boxes in our central area, under our gasoline lantern. Both were in shock, and were receiving plasma. They were pale and pasty in appearance, bathed in cold sweat, and their extremities were cold and clammy. Their blood pressures were alarmingly low and their pulses rapid. With the stark, white light of the lantern shining on their pale, cadaverous faces, I am sure they presented a frightening picture to the rest of the men in the room. I couldn't change this, however, because I had to keep working to try to control the bleeding quickly, or both would soon die.

Other litter cases were in better condition, and were crowded together on the floor. The walking wounded were not so visible because they remained in the darker areas of the room. Many sat on the floor, watching the proceedings with their backs propped against the wall. Occasionally one or two of the wounded would moan or groan, and from time to time one would ask for something more for pain, but I never saw anyone cry. All of the men in the room, whether wounded or not, appeared strained and anxious, and many were obviously frightened, particularly during the periods of most intense shelling. The only ones who were relaxed were those of the litter cases who had received enough morphine to dull their senses.

I remember one man in particular who had been struck in the leg and shoulder by shell fragments. His wounds didn't appear to be life threatening, but they were painful, and he was clearly frightened. He kept repeating,

"I'm going to die! I'm going to die! It hurts! It hurts!"

In a short time the generous dose of morphine he had received began to take effect and he no longer complained of pain, but he continued to repeat over and over again,

"I'm going to die! I'm going to die. I'm going to die!"

His pulse and blood pressure remained stable, and he didn't appear to be going into shock. I didn't expect him to die and repeatedly told him so, but no matter how much I tried to reassure him, he just kept loudly repeating,

"I'm going to die! I'm going to die! Oh God, I'm going to die!"

As his cries continued and the exploding shells continued to fall all around us, I became concerned that this carrying on was having a bad effect upon the others in the room, so I knelt down beside his litter once more to try to calm and reassure him. I checked his wounds again and found no evidence of any immediate problem. I told him that I thought his wounds were more painful than serious, and that he should recover nicely. He wasn't listening. The harder I tried, the louder his cries seemed to become. My efforts at reassurance were not having any effect upon him at all.

At this time the Chaplain knelt down on the other side of the litter, and began to speak to him in religious terms. Almost immediately this approach appeared to be more quieting than my efforts had been, so I arose to turn my attention elsewhere, leaving the Chaplain with the patient. In a few minutes the cries stopped, and I turned to see that the man was receiving the Last Rites. When we evacuated him several hours later, he was still in good condition and peacefully asleep on the litter. I remember the Chaplain administering the Last Rites several times in the aid station during that battle, and occasionally at other times later, but I don't remember that any soldier ever died inside our aid station.

While the chaplain was engaged with this man, the shelling outside intensified. More shell fragments than ever were striking the outside walls of our building, and I began to fear that those walls would eventually become so severely damaged that they would crumble, and we would lose our protection. Some shells occasionally fell so close that their explosions shook the foundation of the building and dislodged dust and dirt from our ceiling, which rained down on us. Eventually it became so intense that we could no longer move casualties in or out of the building, because it was impossible for anyone to pass safely through the hail of steel outside.

Then when the tumult all around us seemed to be at its worst, there was a pause, and the door burst open. A wide-eyed soldier ran in, excitedly yelling, "THE KRAUTS ARE IN THE DRAW RIGHT OUTSIDE! GET READY! THE AID STATION IS GOING TO BE CAPTURED."

Although in the past I had considered the possibility of being captured by the enemy a number of times, the suddenness of this perturbing announcement caught me by surprise. It was hard for me to believe that anything like this could be happening, but it became instantly imperative for me to consider all possible courses of action. If the enemy had broken through K Company just ahead on our left flank, we were next in line, and would certainly be overrun. It would be only a short time before we were all captured or killed.

We had previously given up our field radio to one of the line companies, and our field telephone was completely dead, probably because the line to our building had been completely cut by a shell explosion. We had no communication with the Battalion Command Post. I couldn't look for help or information there. Considering our entire situation, especially the shells still raining in all around us outside, and the room crammed full of wounded on litters inside, retreat to the rear was most certainly not possible. I quickly decided the obvious, that our course of action must be to stay within the shelter of the building regardless of the outcome of the fighting outside.

What I feared most was an enemy soldier kicking in the door and throwing grenades inside, or bursting into the room and spraying everywhere with a burp gun, so I asked one of the men to look outside and make sure that the large red cross which we had placed on the building near the door was still in place. I also made sure that every one of our medical people was wearing the red cross armband as well as his red cross helmet. I even considered hanging our large red cross flag on the wall opposite the door, but finally decided against it, because there was not enough light there for it to be readily seen. While they were helping us care for the wounded inside the aid station, the Graves Registration men did not carry their carbines, and I made sure that their weapons and the few others that were there in the room were put completely out of sight immediately. There were enough bloody bandages visible, and there was enough medical equipment in use, so that it would be difficult for anyone to mistake us for anything but a medical installation.

I also made a number of remarks directed at everyone present, saying in effect that no matter what happened we would continue operating as an aid station, that there were many worse things than being captured by the Germans, that we could do our job well no matter whose territory we were working in, and that we would continue to care for any and all wounded no matter what uniform they were wearing. This seemed to be effective in orienting everyone to a single plan of action, and things settled down promptly. Care of the wounded, which had been only momentarily interrupted, continued again.

No German soldier ever arrived at the door. In another half hour or so the shelling abated considerably, and the litter teams soon began to bring in more wounded. We began the evacuation of our casualties to the rear again, but there were so many that it was already daylight before we got them all out. The two cases, which had earlier given me so much concern, looked much better. Their bleeding appeared to be controlled, and their state of shock was steadily improving. They were not the first to leave the aid station, but as each one's condition stabilized he was carried back to a waiting vehicle by one of the litter teams, accompanied by some of the walking wounded we had accumulated.

Later that morning someone from the Battalion Command Post arrived with the word that a company of German mountain infantry had indeed reached the draw some fifty yards ahead of us, but had been almost annihilated by our artillery. What was left of it had been captured, including its captain. The counterattack, which turned out to be more massive than any other sustained by our division during the War, had been successfully repelled by our K Company and its supporting units. Later we learned that four companies of the famous German Mittenwald Division had carried out the attack, and had expected to surround the peak and regain Monte della Torraccia without much difficulty.

This enemy attack also produced our first wounded German prisoners. We treated and evacuated them in the same manner and through the same channels as we did our own wounded. Some were litter cases, but all were in good condition and I expected that all of them would survive. From the descriptions of the fighting which we had gotten from our men, I doubted that the Germans were able to evacuate many of their wounded from the field, and had to conclude that all of the enemy soldiers who had been more seriously wounded had died out there before our medics got to them.

The passage of wounded German soldiers through our aid station demonstrated to our men that a wounded German infantryman was not much different from one of ours. He too was visibly relieved when told that he would survive, and he too was glad to be alive and out of combat permanently.

After dawn the enemy shelling abated considerably and was no longer falling close to us. We continued to receive an occasional casualty, but little treatment was needed, and we were able to evacuate them promptly and without difficulty. It was now February 25, 1945, and no one in the Battalion had slept much for two nights. I had not slept at all for 48 hours, so after a K Ration breakfast I stretched out on the straw in the back of the room and slept for a little while.

At about noon we received some supplies by mule train, which came plodding up the trail carrying C and K Rations, water in five-gallon cans, and ammunition. This was the first time we saw mules since before we had left Camp Swift, and they were a most welcome sight coming up the trail with their packs bulging with needed materiel. Italian soldiers, wearing gray-green uniforms and Tyrolean hats with the long feather stuck in the band, were leading them. They were the Alpini, Italian Mountain Troops, and although Italy was no longer officially in the War, they were supporting the Italian Partisans and the Allied Forces against the Germans.

During the next several days we saw these mule trains often, as they continued to pass through our dooryard, bringing ammunition and supplies up to the front. We too were well supplied, and received plenty of C Rations, clean water, cigarettes by the case, and medical supplies. We had our two gasoline stoves brought up and also the large galvanized garbage cans, which we always had set up on them. We kept hot water for multiple purposes in one, but mostly dropped C Ration cans into it to be heated before we opened them. In the other we always kept brewed coffee, which seemed to be an incentive for officers and men from all over the area to drop in and chat when things were quiet. This coffee was certainly not a gourmet brew, but its qualities were persistent. We had sugar, but no cream, and used canned evaporated milk instead. It always amused me to dip a canteen cup full of this coffee out of the garbage can and add the evaporated milk, because the mixture invariably turned gray, or gray-green, instead of the normal tan coffee and cream color to which I had always been accustomed. But it was always hot, and it was wet, and the men generally drank it without complaint.

Our field telephone was soon in operation again, and the director of the Red Cross called me from Division Headquarters to compliment us for the job we had done and to ask if there was anything he could send up to us. I assured him that we were not in dire need of anything, but since we had left personal articles behind in favor of medical equipment and supplies, it would be nice for the men to have some soap, shaving cream and razor blades with which to clean themselves up a little. On one of the mule trains that afternoon a box arrived for us from the Red Cross, but it contained none of these items. There were a few cigarettes and some candy, but the bulk of the package consisted of paper hats, party favors and noisemakers of the type that were usually seen at a New Year's Eve party. It was good for something though. We all had a good laugh.

Later in the afternoon we received a few more casualties. One had occurred in very close proximity to the aid station and arrived inside within minutes. He was a lieutenant, a platoon leader, who had been struck in the right chest by what I was told had been a twenty-millimeter shell. He had a gaping chest wound and was already semi-conscious, in shock, and desperately short of breath. The hole in the chest was large enough so that I could see into the chest cavity and had an excellent view of the collapsed lung inside. It was bruised but didn't appear to be lacerated, and there was only a small amount of free blood visible.

After quickly tamponading the wound with a folded raincoat held in place by an elastic bandage as we had been taught to do, I started a unit of plasma and watched the tamponade closely. The patient's struggles to breathe were expelling air from his chest cavity past the compressed raincoat, which at the same time prevented air from returning into it through the wound. It was working effectively to re-expand the lung, and I was happy to note that the patient's color improved, while his respiratory rate decreased, and his struggles to breathe lessened considerably. A little later, when his pulse and blood pressure had returned to satisfactory levels, we evacuated him with plasma still running.

This man had been wounded almost on our doorstep, and was brought into the aid station immediately. His condition on arrival was most serious, and presented a difficult problem. We spent a considerable amount of time and effort in his resuscitation, and his condition was still precarious when we sent him to the rear. Had he not been brought into the aid station immediately after he was wounded, he would most certainly have died out in the field. I know that he survived, because several years after the War I heard about him. Barney Summers knew him quite well, and kept in touch with him. When Barney visited me some five or six years after the War he told me that this man was still hospitalized. He had barely survived the wound, and was still having a pretty miserable existence.

There is a lesson here, one that would be demonstrated to me repeatedly during the war and later on in my civilian hospital and emergency room practice. At the time I did not appreciate the principles involved, but because I saw cases like this over and over again during the whole of my medical career, I believe that they are valid. They apply to the case I have just described, and to many of the more serious cases which arise frequently in the medical field. Simply stated they are:

(1) In all serious injuries, in which the cause no longer exists or has been removed, and in which the victim has survived a **certain critical amount of elapsed time** before treatment begins, the rate of recovery to a **near normal condition** will be nearly 100 percent; and

(2) In these same kinds of injuries, the earlier **within that critical period of time** that definitive medical measures are begun, **the more resources will be wasted in futile efforts applied to cases in which a meaningful recovery was not possible from the beginning.**

Because in any given case we believe that we cannot predict the final outcome with certainty, much time, effort and money are regularly wasted in futile attempts to restore people who cannot recover no matter what treatment is rendered. Although our efforts usually fail in these cases, there are occasional survivors, always at a great expense, but the quality of life that is saved generally remains unbelievably poor, so in essence these cases are failures too. However, if elapsed time before treatment were to be considered in the life or death equation, nature itself would become an excellent indicator of the rate and quality of expected survival, and would make it possible to avoid a lot of futile treatment.

The truth of these statements was often illustrated in my personal experiences with combat casualties. Many of the men who were wounded in the field died. Some died instantly, but many did not. The vagaries of combat are such that company aid men cannot get to every wounded soldier the instant he is hurt, and even when one does arrive within minutes it usually takes an extended amount of time for a litter team to reach the scene, and carry him to the aid station. I don't know what the lag time was, between infliction of the wound and arrival at the aid station, but I feel sure that it averaged several hours. In the action we had just been through many of the wounded had lain in the field for several hours before being picked up, and then, because the carrying distances were long, it took another hour or two for the casualty to arrive at the aid station. In the entire War, over 98 percent of the casualties who reached an aid station alive, recovered to live fairly normal lives. This being true, it is obvious that time had performed a function, akin to a natural triage, and death had weeded out most of the casualties in which heroic but futile treatment might have otherwise been carried out.

These principles may also be illustrated in a more hypothetical way, by assuming that we had a magic way of transporting all of the wounded who were still alive to the aid station or the civilian emergency room within a minute or two after being injured. In such a scenario the majority of those who usually died in the field would, instead, make it in to the aid station still alive, and measures would be started which would result in more reaching the hospitals alive. Once there, heroic medical measures, very costly in time and materials, and requiring many times the medical manpower that we actually had available, could be applied to these cases, only to have most of them die anyway. A very few might survive for a time with a drastically impaired existence, but I believe that most of these marginal cases would fill out a shortened life span in a severely handicapped and miserable state.

In recent years our nation has become concerned about its high cost of medical care. Perhaps we as a people should be paying at least some attention to these principles.

The last counterattack of any size to come at us during the defense of della Torraccia was repelled on the afternoon of February 25th, but after that the enemy kept shelling our positions as if he had plenty of ammunition. From that time on while we remained in the line, we received only an occasional casualty. The bulk of our casualties had occurred during the first two days of heavy fighting, but I don't know exactly how many we treated. T/4 Harrison Swados, an aid man in L Company who was in the field during the entire battle, wrote a section in our 3rd Bn History in which he states that 85 litter casualties were carried off of the field in the attack on della Torraccia, and since this does not take into account the walking wounded, it would be reasonable to at least double this amount to estimate the total casualty count. Another one of the references states that K Company suffered a 12.5 percent casualty rate in repelling the main counterattack of the Mittenwald Division, and this would add about 25 more men put out of action. Adding a few more to the total to account for the losses in the other companies in the later defensive actions, a good estimate of the casualties suffered would be something above 200, or over 20 per cent of the battalion. Our medical detachment fared better: one company aid man wounded and evacuated in good condition, and another wounded and evacuated in serious condition.

We were now quite regularly seeing groups of German prisoners being marched past us to the rear, and occasionally one would be wounded. These were walking wounded, not in serious condition, and we did not evacuate them through medical channels. Instead I instructed the guards to drop them off at the collecting company on the way to the POW (prisoner of war) cages. All of them seemed to be relieved that they had been captured and were still alive. There would be many more in the days to come.

On February 26, 1945 the 2nd Battalion of the 86th moved up into the line to take over half of our defensive front. With such a defense in place we were sure that the enemy could not retake della Torraccia. He did continue to shell our positions however. Everyone had to stay pretty much under cover, and we remained in the farmhouse named Carge.

The next day I had my first close brush with death. It happened in the dooryard of the aid station at a time when things were quiet. I was standing there with a couple of men who had come for treatment of some minor problems, and there were several other men standing in the yard when an enemy mortar shell dropped in close to us. I was wearing my long Army coat and felt a shell fragment pass through the cloth near the hem on the right side, and when I looked and saw the ragged hole it had made I thought momentarily that I might have been hit, but there was no pain. When I looked at the calf of my leg there was not even a mark on it. Both of the men with whom I was standing were grazed by shell fragments, but fortunately did not sustain serious wounds. One had to be evacuated; the other suffered only a skin scrape, and returned to duty with a bandaid in place. We were all thankful that we weren't standing closer to where that shell had landed.

Soon after this incident another wounded soldier was brought in, who provided an excellent insight into the thinking of many of the men who had gone through the recent attack. I believe his story is typical of the state of mind of almost all wounded combat soldiers everywhere and at any time in history. I have forgotten this man's name and don't remember exactly when he arrived at the aid station, but I remember the man, the injury, and the circumstances of his treatment very well. He had been on a scouting patrol far to the front when he stepped on an antipersonnel mine of the type that the Germans called a Schuh mine. These mines had relatively low explosive power, could be made cheaply and easily in huge quantities, and were designed to permanently disable anyone unfortunate enough to step on one. They were generally buried just under the surface of the ground, and the injury they caused, when stepped upon, was most often loss of a foot, but sometimes there would be more or less serious injury higher up in the leg. Occasionally fragments reached the pelvis, and then there would be damage to the genitalia. It is not difficult to understand why these mines were feared.

This man had been first treated in the field by his company aid man, who had administered morphine and bandaged the stump of his leg. He could, of course, not walk, so was litter carried to the aid station. I had the litter team carry the stretcher directly into the operating area and place it on the supports provided. Although some time had passed since he had received the morphine, he was mentally alert and coherently described the circumstances surrounding his injury. He didn't complain of pain, and insisted upon seeing what I was going to do. Although he was a bit pale and a little shocky, his pulse and blood pressure remained quite normal, so I let him sit up and watch.

There was a large, very bloody bandage, the equivalent of several soldier's first aid packets, on the stump, and as I carefully removed it I could see that the foot was gone. All that remained were three or four small fragments of bone held together by some remaining shreds of ligaments. One of the fragments was still attached to the leg by the long tendon, which normally runs along the outside of the ankle. A long flap of skin, which had formerly covered the lateral side of the foot and ankle, remained attached at the lateral side of the leg, but had been completely separated from the tendon and bone fragments. It was very dirty and discolored, and was so ragged and tattered that I knew immediately it would be useless for anyone to try to use it as skin graft material. Above from where the ankle had been, both leg bones protruded an inch or two below beyond the battered soft tissues that remained. The main artery in the leg had been stretched downward and dangled freely between them, and whenever it was even slightly disturbed, more bleeding occurred from several tears in its wall.

Using a small amount of local anesthetic, I followed this dangling artery upward to a point where it appeared to be undamaged, and tied it off there, leaving the ligature ends very long. I also did not cut off the damaged portion of the artery, purposely, so that so that the next surgeon, who would operate in a hospital to construct a useful stump, would find it easily and tie it off permanently as he removed the rest of the dead and dying tissues. This single ligature controlled the bleeding very well.

Then I talked to the man about his injury. He was still sitting up and could see that his foot was gone. I explained that he would now be evacuated to a hospital, where one of the orthopedic surgeons would have to operate, probably under a general anesthetic, in order to build a good, strong stump to which an artificial foot and ankle could be attached. I also explained that, in order to do this, the remaining bones would need to be shortened and their ends smoothed, so that the bone ends could be covered with a thick pad of flesh, which would be needed for the artificial limb to fit comfortably and well. His would be an amputation below the knee, and with a good artificial foot and ankle he should be able to walk well enough that people need not know that he was an amputee. Then I told him I was going to remove the mangled portion of skin and the cluster of bone fragments, because I thought that they were beyond salvaging, and to incorporate all of that dirt and dead tissue against his wound inside the dressing, would only invite wound infection and later complications. I assured him that it wouldn't hurt, and to make doubly sure, I would use more local anesthetic.

Our patient, still sitting erect and watching the proceedings, agreed, so I went to work. After I had cut off the mangled skin and severed the long tendon, and while I was cleaning up the wound, applying more sulfa powder, and applying the dressing needed for transport, the man began to talk. I am not sure that after all of these years I can quote him exactly, but what he said went something like this:

"I'm lucky! I'm going home. The War's over for me, and I'm still alive! Losing my foot isn't too much of a price to pay. You guys are the unlucky ones. You have to go out there again. You have to go out there over and over again, but I'm going home. Even the guys who are dead are luckier than you are. They don't have to go out there anymore. But I'm the luckiest, because I'm still alive, and I'm going home!"

In another few minutes he was safely on his way to the collecting company. I don't know what happened to him after that, but I hope that my predictions for the outcome of his wound came true.

Of all of the casualties I treated during the War, this one was most vocal in expressing his feelings about being disabled and surviving. There were others occasionally who expressed similar feelings, and there were many who said nothing, but whose facial expression expressed it for them as soon as I told them that they were finished with the War and that I thought they would survive. These incidents demonstrated that the dread of going into infantry combat was so immense and so terrible that men were willing to trade almost any kind of wound for assurance that they would not have to return to it. It is remarkable that we saw hardly any self-inflicted wounds until the fighting in Europe had ended, and those that we saw then usually came about as a result of such foolishness as practicing "quick draws" with captured souvenir pistols.

As we continued to wait in our newly won positions, the brass higher up were planning our next move. We were sure it would involve continuing to attack, because the companies had almost immediately received replacements to bring them back to full strength.

These replacements were now quite noticeable. Most of our original infantrymen were six feet tall or taller, often making it necessary to carry them on our litters with their feet overhanging the end. Now there were a number of shorter men in the battalion who seemed conspicuous standing among their taller companions. However, they very quickly fit in well with their new units, and their height was not a problem. There was something about our officers and about the original 10th Mountain Division men that seemed to inspire confidence, and before long the newcomers were behaving just like the veterans.

The number of battalion staff meetings and briefings now increased, and all indications were that we were preparing for a new attack. There was much discussion about enemy mine fields and road conditions for the support units, which would be backing us up, and bringing in supplies. Plans were delayed several times because of these problems, and the next phase of our combat mission did not begin until March 3, 1945.

CHAPTER IX

THE SECOND ATTACK

We had barely settled into defensive positions around Monte della Torraccia when rumors began to circulate that our next mission would be to head for the city of *Bologna* and take it from the Germans. There were, however, more immediate matters and some serious problems to be faced before we could hope to achieve any such accomplishment. Two concerns uppermost in the minds of the staff were the problem of getting too far ahead of supply lines, and the dangers of the many enemy mine fields known to exist. Providing such things as road repairs and establishing future supply routes became high priorities, and the number of night patrols into enemy territory looking for information and prisoners to interrogate increased sharply.

After several postponements the second major offensive carried out by our division began early in the day on March 3, 1945. The 86th and 87th Regiments advanced abreast, and the 85th, which had suffered the most in carrying out the attack across the peaks of Belvedere and Gorgolesco, followed as division reserve. My battalion was not actually committed to the action until mid-afternoon.

We stayed at the farmhouse, Carge, all morning and waited for the word to move out and follow the troops. This move would also be made without vehicles, so the heavier items which had been brought up to us on the mules were sent back to the rear, and we distributed the rest of our equipment and supplies among the men, once again making each one responsible for as much as he could reasonably carry. We were prepared to take all of the medical essentials with us, but most of our personal and convenience items had to be returned to the rear.

We left Carge shortly after noon in the bright sunshine of a beautiful spring day. That old farmhouse had sheltered us for a full week, during which there had been some bad moments, and we now reluctantly left it behind.

Some one hundred yards into our march I looked back at it for the last time. Shell craters were scattered all around it in great numbers and several were within a few feet of its walls. It seemed almost miraculous that this beat up old building had protected us so well, and because I was most uneasy about the prospect of heading into another dangerous and disagreeable situation, it was difficult for me to leave this now familiar haven behind.

We walked slowly forward past rockslides and the many shell craters in the area where the enemy had, only a few days before, directed his strong counterattack at K Company. Then we passed through the area in which our men had made the assault upon the peak of della Torraccia. The dead of both sides had been cleared from the field, but the wreckage of the turf and the damage to the terrain caused by the battle reminded me of the recent carnage which had occurred there and added to my apprehension. As we continued we circled on the shoulder of the mountain and eventually reached its north-eastern slope. Here the regimental advance began with the 1st and 2nd Battalions advancing abreast. Our 3rd Battalion brought up the rear as the battalion reserve.

As we descended toward the valley beyond, artillery shells began falling near the troops ahead of us, and we had to stop on a sloping, grassy hillside. We had already been walking five yards apart, but now we scattered even wider, keeping as low a profile as possible and trying to conceal ourselves by lying in the grass. I was carrying medicines and plasma in my rucksack, and hand-carrying our gasoline lantern, guarding it against damage to the all-important, light-giving mantles. While I was lying there, clusters of spent bullets started to rain down upon me. These had most likely come from a machine gun far in the distance, because they landed with hardly any force at all, as if someone had thrown aloft a handful of pebbles. I had no difficulty scraping some of them out of the soft sod, and could see that they really were spent bullets. For a moment I thought they might make nice souvenirs, but, in the end, I didn't carry any of them away with me.

The situation ahead soon cleared without producing any casualties, and we continued into the valley where the entire battalion was advancing in a long, strung out column. There were occasional small actions along the route, off to one side or the other, to mop up small groups of enemy soldiers, which had been bypassed by the rapidly advancing troops ahead of us. Most of these confrontations were short and quickly settled. Prisoners were taken, sometimes without any exchange of shots, but more often after a noisy demonstration of the intense firepower our troops were capable of, after which the remaining enemy soldiers were usually quite willing to surrender. We soon saw large numbers of them being escorted to the rear by guards with rifles.

Most of this mopping up action was taking place near the head of the regimental column, and since we medics were marching near the rear with the reserve battalion, I didn't see much of it, nor do I remember treating any casualties from these relatively minor actions. However, it is possible that our battalion did have some casualties who were treated and evacuated through one of the other battalion aid stations.

Later that day our situation changed abruptly. At 3:30 p.m. we passed through the forward positions of the other two battalions while they were still engaging the enemy, and launched a major attack of our own upon the town of Campo del Sole, some hills to the West of it, and the territory to the North of it. These objectives were taken well before dark, and new defensive positions were quickly established in order to hold the ground that had been gained. During the first part of this action we moved our aid station into a suitable building, and started receiving wounded immediately. The fighting was intense, and produced serious casualties, but not in the numbers seen at della Torraccia. However, near the end of the day enough casualties occurred in a short period of time to once again require the use of litter teams called up from the collecting company in order to get them all out of the field before nightfall. Evacuation from the aid station to the rear was quick and easy, because we were able to use vehicles directly at the aid station to move our casualties back to the collecting company.

Several of the men from L Company who came through the aid station that afternoon had suffered particularly severe shell fragment wounds. These included huge, gaping flesh wounds and multiple open fractures. Later we learned that these wounds, and also several deaths, had been caused by short rounds from our own artillery. Comparing them to the wounds I was accustomed to seeing, which were caused by enemy shells, I concluded that our shell casings were thicker than theirs, and the heavier fragments caused larger and more serious wounds. Because that day all three of our battalions were fighting in close proximity of each other, we treated casualties from all three of them, and we also treated a number of Germans who had been wounded. Several of these Germans had been wounded by fragments from American hand grenades, and their wounds appeared to be larger and more traumatic than those inflicted by German grenades upon our men. From these observations I concluded that our grenades had heavier casings and were more powerful than the "Potato Masher," the German Grenade with the stick for a handle, which was being used against us. Realizing that these differences in weapons were significant, I was thankful that my ancestors had left Germany when they did, and that I was in the U.S. Army and not in the Wehrmacht.

Although I tried to treat all casualties equally, fairly, and based upon the immediate needs of each, I am sure that I was inclined toward treating our men first. In spite of this, I honestly believe that no wounded German soldier suffered excessively or died because his treatment was neglected or delayed while he was in our care or during his subsequent evacuation.

With the capture of the territory North of Campo del Sole the mission of our battalion was completed. Most of the other regimental objectives were also taken that same day, and the other two battalions took the rest of them the next morning. In this action Colonel Hampton was wounded and evacuated while the 1st Bn., which he commanded, completed its mission by taking the town of Sassamolare and the peak of Monte Grande D'Aiano. The regiment was now ordered to dig in and defend its new territory. The 87th, which had already taken Monte della Vedetta, Pietra Colora, Borre, Monte Acidola, and Monte della Croce, continued its attack for another day, and took the towns of Madna di Brasa and Castel D'Aiano, before it was ordered to dig in and hold. Meanwhile the 85th Regiment, which had been the Division Reserve, was committed on the right flank of the 87th, and continued to advance for still another day, taking Tora, Monte della Castellana, Monte della Spe, Monte Spicchione, Canolle and Mattiolo, before it was also ordered to dig in and hold.

As the result of all of these actions the 10th Mountain Division had taken a large, broad based peninsula of territory, which penetrated deep into the German lines. The 86th held the long left flank from Monteforte to Monte Grande D'Aiano; the 87th held the center on both sides and in front of the town of Castel D'Aiano, and the 85th held the right flank from Monte della Spe to Monte Castellana. The entire Division continued to prepare defenses, and we soon found ourselves in a state of static war consisting mainly of patrol activity and artillery exchanges. In the meantime our next moves were being planned.

After things quieted down we moved our aid station to a safer and more conveniently located building near Campo del Sole, and continued to receive casualties. At first they came as a result of enemy counterattacks, and later from patrol activity. Almost all of the wounds were caused by artillery and mortar shell fragments, and, although the casualties were not numerous, there were some almost every day. In a few days we started holding a daily sick call again, and I began to see and treat minor injuries and illnesses at the aid station once more.

While we were holding these positions, loudspeakers were brought up into the I Company area, and verbal propaganda was directed at the enemy across no-man's-land. I wasn't close to the speakers, and didn't pay a great deal of attention to the broadcasts, but I remember that the German language was spoken slowly and distinctly. I wondered if it was being broadcast live, or we were hearing a recording, but I knew that it was being heard by the enemy, because the response usually came quickly in the form of mortar and artillery shells aimed at the source of the sound.

During these same few days we were exposed to some new enemy shells, which had a very different sound than came from those to which we had become accustomed. Half scream and half whistle, it seemed that we could hear these shells coming from a lot farther away than we could hear the regular artillery shells. They always exploded high overhead with hardly any force at all, and only a feeble, popping sound, much like the sound of opening a bottle of champagne. Soon after the explosion hundreds of sheets of paper would come fluttering gently down to the ground, flooding the area with enemy propaganda leaflets.

It wasn't long before a number of these leaflets were brought into the aid station. There were some that tried to exploit the theme that soldiers' wives and sweethearts were being unfaithful. Some pointed out that there were "fat cats" at home who were profiteering and making millions at the expense of the soldiers who were dying at the front. Some encouraged our men to desert because the War was nearly over, and it would be foolish to die just before it ended. There was also one that presented some easy steps toward being taken prisoner, and described the pleasant life and conditions of ease in a typical German Prisoner of War camp. The ones that aroused my curiosity and interested me most pertained to the field of medicine. One of these was a leaflet that contained instructions on how to safely wound oneself in order to be evacuated, and it gave some ridiculous instructions, which, if followed, could easily have ultimately resulted in fatality. It did not mention the long and miserable complications or the crippling effects that some of these recommended wounds might produce. Another one contained instructions on how to produce a fake illness in order to be sent to a hospital, and this one also failed to mention any of the complications, which might result. One of them still stands out in my mind. It contained instructions on how to produce a "harmless" eye infection. In this scheme the soldier was instructed to place a little bit of smegma, the cheesy substance which accumulates under the foreskin, onto the inside of the lower eyelids, and to intermittently massage the eyeballs through the closed lids for several hours. This, the instructions went on to say, would result in very inflamed-looking but not painful eyes in about 24 hours, and would require evacuation to a hospital for treatment. Then it went on to say that these eyes would look much worse than they really were, because material from one's own body certainly would not cause any serious damage.

The second offensive of the division was now finished, and consolidation of the newly won territories was complete. Speculation was now stronger than ever that our next big move would be the breakout into the Po Valley and the capture of *Bologna*, but no one could really be sure what would come next.

CHAPTER X

I SPEAK GERMAN AGAIN

During the attack on Campo del Sole our troops captured large numbers of prisoners, and many were marched past our aid station toward the prisoner-of-war cages in the rear. Since the main medical support problem during the major attacks we had carried out so far had been the shortage of litter teams, and since there was here a large supply of able-bodied prisoners, I soon wondered if we could use some of them to make things easier for our men. It would mean that I would have to speak German to these prisoners, and I hesitated because I was suffering from a reluctance to use the German language, which I must explain.

My ancestral roots are entirely German. All of my great grandparents were born in Germany, and all of my grandparents were either born there, or emigrated to the United States as children. I was born into a close-knit German neighborhood in Detroit, where people knew each other well, belonged to the same organizations, and purposefully intermarried in order to preserve their German heritage.

My first language was German, the High German spoken in Thuringia and Saxony from where my people had come. When I was a child everyone I knew spoke German at home, and my grandparents insisted that always be spoken in their presence. In fact, until I was six or seven years old, whenever I addressed my grandfather in English, he would either not answer, or would answer gruffly in German, saying, "In my house German will be spoken!"

My parents moved out of the German community to another part of the city when I was about two years old, but continued to speak only German in our home, and when my sister was born, three years later, we even had a German speaking, live-in Baby sitter *(Kindermädchen)* for a time. At first I had no playmates who were not relatives of mine, and later as I grew older, I was very slow to make friends among the other children in the neighborhood because I was fearful, and the language difference made me bashful and shy. It was embarrassing not to understand all that was being said, and I always felt inferior during my casual contact with other children. There were also subtleties of neighborhood behavior that added to this feeling. For example, because they often overheard us speaking German, some of our neighbors of British descent commonly referred to us as "those foreigners."

At the age of five I started school, and this adventure began happily because my parents ceremoniously followed an old German custom of giving the new schoolchild a *Zuckertüte* (a paper bag containing sweets) as a present to celebrate the new beginning. Then they took me to the school, which was about a block and a half from our house, and duly enrolled me in kindergarten.

For several weeks I had been apprehensive about starting school, and I anticipated that it would not be pleasant. I had steeled myself to face the ordeal, but when my parents left me there alone, all of my resolve collapsed. I became fearful and embarrassed because it very quickly became apparent to me that I was "different" from my classmates. Always a shy, timid child, I was awed by my teachers and overwhelmed by the other children. They spoke only English, which I understood poorly, and they spoke it well. They were extremely confident, and I was filled with uncertainty and apprehension. Whenever I tried to speak English, I invariably mixed German words into what I was trying to say, and because my classmates often laughed at me for this, I soon stopped trying to talk. As the day progressed things continued to get worse. I was most unhappy. My first day in school became pure misery, and I was absolutely certain that I could never be at ease there.

The next morning I started the walk to school, but stopped in the only vacant lot on the way, where I played quietly by myself until I saw the other children leaving school to go home. Then I too went home, and acted as if I had been in school all morning. Since kindergarten lasted only a half-day, and since the vacant lot was partly wooded and contained some nice underbrush, which afforded good hiding places, this had not been difficult to do. It became my daily routine. Sometimes I was able to take a favorite toy along, and occasionally I was able to take my tricycle from the garage without it being noticed.

After about two weeks of this deception I awoke one morning to find a pouring rain falling outside. On this day my father took me to school in the family car, and seeing that I was reluctant to go inside, he accompanied me all of the way into the kindergarten classroom.

I remember the teacher smiling and saying, "Who is this little boy?"

"This is little Albert Meinke," said my father.

"Oh, yes," said the teacher, still smiling, "we had a child by that name on the first day of school, but he hasn't been here since."

The painful consequences of my truancy will not be detailed here. It is enough to say that for several weeks my father personally escorted me into the classroom, and after that I dutifully attended school by myself.

After a few weeks I was learning to understand English more easily, but I still could not speak it well. I continued to feel insecure and uneasy in school. Every day continued to be an ordeal, and I hated it. It was most embarrassing not to understand all that was said, but even worse was the ridicule, which came from my making stupid mistakes in front of the class, so I usually said nothing voluntarily and never volunteered for anything in school. I always held back, trying to be as inconspicuous as possible. I often tried to hide behind other children for fear of being called upon by the teacher. This reticence on my part lasted a long time, and as I grew older, I often tried to hide it under the guise of courtesy and politeness. Even to this day, unless I feel completely competent and well prepared, I become uneasy whenever I launch myself into any new situation.

I had been in school for more than a year before my parents realized that speaking nothing but German at home was causing a problem. In the fall, two or three weeks after I entered the first grade, it came as a severe shock to them to learn that I had been transferred into a special class for retarded children. At the same time a maternal cousin, three months older that I, found himself in a similar situation, and his mother was told by his teacher that her son was "quite slow to learn." He too had spoken only German at home before starting school.

These events were indeed a terrible blow to a family in which parents and grandparents continually extolled (in German of course) the virtues of courtesy, intelligence and ambition, and particularly emphasized that these qualities were the opposites of misbehavior, stupidity and laziness, human attributes which would under no circumstances be tolerated in our family.

It is to their credit that my elders perceived the problem to be one of language, and not mental retardation. In a short time English was spoken at home and also at the grandparents' houses whenever grandchildren were present. Subsequently all of the children in my generation did well in school, including my "slow to learn" cousin who earned a degree in engineering and had a long, successful career doing research for the U.S. Navy. All of my siblings and almost all of the many cousins I have on both sides of my family have college degrees, or have, or have had, successful careers.

After several weeks in the special class, I began speaking English much more freely, and returned to the regular classroom. I gained confidence rapidly. I a short time I no longer hated school, and before the end of the year I was doing very well. Late in the spring I was pleased to find myself near the head of the class, and the following year schoolwork became so easy for me that I was almost boring. It was no longer a challenge and I had no difficulty getting top grades without much effort on my part. This continued for years, until I entered medical school, and it was a fortunate circumstance, because it gave me time to pursue varied and necessary extracurricular activities.

My use of the German language had ceased somewhat abruptly after I had mastered it to the level of a seven-year-old child, and now, during World War II, I wasn't at all sure that I could speak to a German adult and make myself adequately understood. I faced the same situation now that I had faced many years before in kindergarten, except that now the languages were reversed. It might help that in college I had studied some German, because it was an easy way for me to obtain foreign language credit, but I wasn't sure about it. I had listened to radio broadcasts and recordings made by Hitler and other German political figures, and I knew that I couldn't understand this kind of German speech very well. I could hardly understand any of the German radio broadcasts, because the commentators seemed to use big words and speak too fast. I also knew that I couldn't understand scientific German without carefully studying it and laboriously translating it.

Up to now, when dealing with wounded prisoners, I had merely used a few German words and phrases, and never made any attempts at conversation. Now I gave the matter of my "hang-up" with the language a great deal of thought, and convinced myself that my fears were probably foolish and unfounded. In the end I made up my mind to tackle the language head-on, no matter how stupid my attempts to speak German might appear.

As groups of prisoners were being marched past our aid station, I began asking for volunteers to be litter bearers, and right from the beginning I was pleasantly surprised to find that they readily understood me. More important, whenever they spoke to me slowly I understood most of it very well. I'm not sure if it was because I seemed to speak German reasonably well, or my pronunciation was good, or they thought they might receive better treatment if they volunteered, but most of the prisoners seemed willing, and even anxious to serve. Later on it always surprised me a little that whenever I addressed a group of prisoners to call for volunteers, all of the group would usually step forward. Once the flow of prisoners to the rear had begun, there was always an ample number from which to choose. We made good use of these prisoner volunteers, and after we started using them, I don't believe that we ever again had to call for litter teams from the collecting company.

In choosing prisoner volunteers I tried to pick men who, although they were robust and strong, appeared meek and somewhat cowed by the circumstances surrounding their capture. Technically they were always under armed guard by one of the Graves Registration men, and whenever a prisoner team carried a casualty, a medic and the armed guard went along. The guards were not always graves registration men, for there never was any shortage of volunteers for this particular duty. Our men seemed to enjoy seeing the enemy work. It was extremely important to me that one of our medics be in attendance to see to it that no casualty was medically mishandled, but I doubted very much that the guard was really necessary, because these prisoners were not anxious to escape. They had had enough of war, and were thankful that they were alive and had been captured by Americans.

As time passed our Battalion continued to take more prisoners more easily on its combat patrols, and eventually this afforded me a number of opportunities to speak conversationally with some of them. The more I spoke, the more I remembered. Words, which I had not heard in years, came out of my mouth and sometimes startled me a little. I soon became confident with the language again.

In the beginning the prisoners were always stiff and formal, and I think that it was because they were all enlisted men, and had been trained to address officers that way. They knew that I was an officer, and in the German Army an enlisted man only spoke to an officer formally, and often with fear and trepidation. At first my attempts to strike up a conversation with a single prisoner invariably failed, but I soon discovered that it seemed easier for them if I spoke to them in small groups such as one of the litter teams we were using. My German was far from perfect, and I soon found that it helped the conversation along if I would frequently ask the Germans for help with the grammar. *"Wie soll ich es sagen?"* (How should I say it?) would often provoke a response, and once I could get one or two of them to offer a German word or a correction in grammar, and the help became spontaneous, I knew that I had established some degree of rapport. Later, after I had convinced the litter teams that I was merely the staff doctor (*der Stabsarzt*) and wasn't grilling them for military secrets, free and spontaneous conversation came much more easily.

Among the prisoners were youngsters, 15 and 16 year olds, who had been hastily pressed into service, marginally trained, and quickly sent to the front. There were also older men, who by our standards were too old for military service. The prisoners in these two groups were easiest for me to talk to, and they seemed more easily able to talk to me, especially the younger ones.

There were also some prisoners who had been in the German Army for a long time, even some who had been in the North African Campaign. These were the true Nazis, the diehards, the fanatics. It was impossible to start a conversation with any of them. The rest of the prisoners didn't seem to want to have anything to do with them, and more than one prisoner told me never to trust any of them. Whenever one occasionally volunteered for litter bearer duty, I rejected him, and promptly passed him on to the group of prisoners marching to the POW cages in the rear.

My conversations with prisoners never did turn up any information of military value, but it did give me a lot of insight into the workings of the German Army, and the morale of the German soldiers facing us all across the front. All of the prisoners I talked with were happy to have been captured without having been wounded, and were especially glad to have been captured by Americans. Almost all of them believed that Germany had already lost the War, and many were concerned about what would happen to them and their families at the very end. They feared reprisals by the Russians particularly, and it surprised me to learn that they were equally fearful of what the British and French might do to them. Many of them indicated that there were a lot of German soldiers facing us who were ready to surrender, but were kept from doing so for fear of reprisals to their families in Germany. Many admitted that they were generally afraid of their officers, and feared that the officers would shoot them in the back if they went toward our lines with their hands raised or carrying a white flag. They also said that there were still some fanatics, who were not officers, in front line units who were likely to do the same thing. Later on, in the Po Valley, we ran into one situation where exactly that did happen. German soldiers who were trying to surrender were shot from behind by other German soldiers.

During the few days after our second attack in which the Division was consolidating its newly won territory and preparing defenses, we had German prisoner litter teams with us all of the time, and, of course, we had to feed them. They hated the C Rations and K Rations that we gave them, and often expressed amazement that we ate them every day. The only complaint I ever heard from any prisoner about our treatment of them was about the bad food we Americans ate. The German soldier was quite accustomed to scrounging and living off the land, and even the forward infantry companies had field kitchens a mile or two behind the front where hot meals were prepared and brought forward to the foxholes. They also had such things as summer sausage, cheese, dried split pea soup, and dark, hard bread. Many of the German soldiers carried large sausage skins filled with lard with which they could cook on their own.

In time the prisoners taught us a few things about food, and I adopted some of their ways. Many of the fields all around us still had potatoes unharvested in them. We could easily tell where they were by the potatoes lying about on the edges of the shell craters. We just had to pick them up, or one man with his entrenching tool could dig up enough to feed all of us at the aid station. As long as we were in the Apennines there were potatoes still to be harvested in the ground. We ate them boiled, fried or roasted in the coals of an open fire, but most of us liked them best french fried in the lard which was readily available from the prisoners as they came through. My letters home also indicate that we ate pigeon and rabbit, and a number of times had steak grilled over an open fire in the fireplace in the kitchen of some farmhouse. What the letters failed to say, however, was that, although these steaks were extra choice, they were mule steaks.

The Division was using mules to supply the far forward areas, and during this time we had two Veterinary Corps Officers with us, Captain George A. Martin and Lieutenant Franklin D. Custer. Occasionally a mule would be killed in action or so badly wounded that it had to be "put down." Whenever that happened to a mule in otherwise good condition, someone would bring us steaks. We never asked any questions, and the fact that they tasted a bit like horsemeat didn't bother us. They were always a welcome relief from the canned meat and vegetable stew of the C Rations.

As time passed and I used the German language more and more, it began to feel quite natural to me. Before the fighting was over I found that I was even thinking in German again. At the end of the hostilities I found myself in the far North of Italy, and was able to visit Austria, and I was able to use the German language a lot. Today I am the only member of my extensive family in the United States that can hold a reasonable conversation in German, and I believe that I owe this ability to that period of time between the end of the War in Europe and our return to the United States, during which I was able to speak to German speaking people for several hours daily. For that I am grateful, and now I keep trying to use my first language as often as possible.

And in the late summer of 1945 when I first returned home, I was most happy to be able to say to my mother, *"Ich spreche wieder Deutsch."* "I am speaking German again."

CHAPTER XI

A WAITING PERIOD

My battalion had now participated in two major offensives. The first at Riva Ridge, Belvedere, Gorgolesco and della Torraccia had been bloody and prolonged. The second at Campo del Sole had been equally bloody but for us it had lasted only a few hours. By far the largest number of casualties had been sustained by the infantry, but enough replacements had already arrived so that the companies were at or above full strength again. This caused some concern, especially among the higher-ranking officers, that now there were enough newcomers in the ranks to impair unit fighting efficiency. Some said that additional training exercises were needed, and before long rumors were circulating that such exercises had been scheduled for all of the infantry units in the Division.

While we were holding the line just beyond Campo del Sole and after things had quieted down, I began to hear criticism of the fact that both times we had broken through the elaborate enemy defenses, our attacks had ceased. Most of this criticism came from junior officers, but there were also enlisted men who seemed to agree. I often heard expressions such as, "After we broke through there we could have gone on and taken *Bologna*!" "We could have gone all of the way to the Alps!" etc. There was definite resentment among the troops to the fact that we had twice attacked through fixed enemy defenses and breached them dramatically, only to stop and give him time to prepare new defenses through which we would have to do it all over again.

Now began another period of static war, which turned out to be a period of relative inactivity for the whole Division. Battalions were rotated through the front line, through rest areas, unit training areas, reserve areas, and back to the front. Less than half of the Infantry companies actually manned positions in the front line at any one time. The rest were either enjoying a rest period, were in training, or remained at the ready close to the front where they acted as reserves. We in the medical detachment were grateful for the respite. Casualties were few and we received them only when our battalion was actually manning the front, or was located very close to it in reserve. Our hardest job was moving from place to place, and we did this often. During this period the battalion moved into exactly the same positions more than once, and each time the men used the identical foxholes that they had occupied previously.

Although the front remained static, the fighting was now more violent than it had been when we first entered the front line in January. The enemy was always closer to us, and there was more direct and violent contact between the two sides. Enemy artillery was more active and more destructive. Each side was now trying to do as much damage as possible to the other, and as a result the number of casualties increased. On the other hand the Germans now seemed to be surrendering more readily. More and more prisoners were being captured by our patrols almost every day, and it was becoming more and more apparent that most of them thought that Germany had lost the War.

On March 8, 1945 we learned that we were to be relieved during the night, and would go to a rest area for a few days. This news was enthusiastically received. Everyone anticipated the welcome change. That afternoon we sent all of our prisoner volunteers to the POW cage, and packed our gear up well in advance of departure time.

Shortly after 2:00 a.m. on March 29th, in the darkness of the night, we were relieved by the men of the 2nd Battalion of the 87th. As they moved into our positions we cheerfully left them and marched the three miles downhill to waiting trucks, which took us to Campo Tizzoro. Although marching with full packs and riding in open trucks in the cold and the dark is not much fun, no complaints were heard, and once we had passed out of artillery range, everyone relaxed.

Campo Tizzoro was a small town located well behind the front. We arrived in darkness to find that everyone would stay either in a building or a tent, and have either a cot or a bed in which to sleep. We promptly installed the aid station on the second floor over some small shops in a run-down hotel on the main street, and soon afterward I turned in to sleep. When I awoke it was late in the morning. Field kitchens had been set up and food was being served from chow lines. We ate at tables once again. Somewhere near the center of town the engineers had set up enough showers so that everyone could have a hot shower, and there was clean clothing for everyone. I was still short of clothing since my footlocker had not yet turned up, and when I told the friendly supply sergeant my sad story, he cheerfully provided all I needed. From then on I had plenty to wear, and got along nicely by engaging native Italian women to do my laundry from time to time.

After eating breakfast, showering and donning some of my new clothing, I went to the local barbershop for my first civilian haircut in Italy. Up to now we in the Medical Detachment had given haircuts to each other, using the standard barber scissors and hand operated hair clippers that were in a barber kit that was included in our gear. There were no professional barbers among our men, and although I had had no previous experience, I found that I could give a pretty decent haircut, perhaps the best of anyone in the detachment. I remembered that Barney Summers had given me my previous haircut, and when he finished, he stepped back to look at his work, laughed heartily and said, "Meinke, you $#@<%$>% @*&&%%$%##@, if your wife could see you now, she'd shoot me!" Army lore has it that, in a situation like this, one could always find the best barber in the outfit by picking out the one with the worst haircut. Probably true, and perhaps the reason that my haircuts were in high demand.

When I entered the barbershop it reminded me very much of the barbershops at home. There were old magazines in the waiting area, hair clippings on the floor, and the smell of wet hair and hair tonic. A number of soldiers were waiting their turns and looking at the pictures in the magazines. The lone Italian barber was an "artist." He cut hair with grand flourishes, and every minute or two peered critically at the results of his efforts.

When my turn came I seated myself in the chair, and the barber suddenly became very talkative. He spoke in Italian, much too rapidly for me to understand any of it, but after much gesturing and some help from the gallery of soldiers still waiting for haircuts, it became clear to me that he wanted to know if he should leave some of my hair long in order to comb it up over my bald spot. This was a surprise. I didn't know that I had a bald spot, but with the aid of a couple of mirrors he showed it to me, and again I was surprised by the amount of almost bare skin that I saw. Could the hair have been rubbed off by the suspension straps of my helmet? After all, I had worn it day and night for weeks. I hoped that was it, but I knew better. This was the beginning of true male baldness, and later on, as the months and years slipped by, I wasn't surprised to see the thin spot slowly enlarge.

Somehow I got the barber to understand that I wanted the hair cut short all over. I don't think he approved, but he gave me an excellent haircut, replete with grand flourishes of the scissors and comb. At the end he applied some kind of hair tonic liberally, and when I paid him the five Lira for which he asked, and also a tip, I received a most gracious bow and a loud "Grazie

Tante." Actually I found this style of haircut so comfortable and easy to care for, that from then on I have never had any other kind, even after my Army days were over.

None of our soldiers showed up for sick call that afternoon, but I did see a few civilians. Movies were available in the evening for anyone who wanted to attend, but I didn't go. Instead I visited some of my friends at the collecting company and the medical battalion headquarters. It was a pleasure to engage in "medical talk" again.

What should have been the highlight of this rest period was a trip I made to Florence (*Firenze*), but I hardly even remember it, and would have forgotten it completely, had I not written about it in a letter to my wife. We traveled with my driver in a Jeep. Another officer came with us on the trip, but I don't remember now who he was. I remember seeing an American style traffic light there, which made me homesick, and I remember sitting among military officers of many nations at dinner in the Allied Forces Officers' Club. I remember that there were many shops open, and I did a lot of window-shopping. I even went into several shops hoping to find some gifts from Italy that I could send home, but I was deterred from buying by the exorbitant prices. They seemed preposterous to me until I remembered the peculiar currency exchange rules that had been imposed on Allied Military Personnel.

We were paid in "Army Lira" with a fixed value of one lira equal to one cent. On the black market the exchange rate was more than twenty lira for one cent, but none of us were paid in dollars and cents, so we never had any to trade. It was obvious to me that if I spent my army lira in Italy they would buy only one twentieth of what they were really worth. Only by buying money orders in dollar denominations and sending the money home, would I realize one cent for each army lira I received. Most of my salary was already going home as an allotment to my wife, but I also sent all of my extra cash home, including from time to time, my winnings from playing poker and bridge. The few trinkets that I eventually brought home with me were obtained through barter for such items as cigarettes, candy and soap.

There were other activities in which I participated during this rest period, not so much because I wanted to, but because I felt that it was expected of me. The officers' dances fell into this category, and I dutifully appeared, had a drink or two, and quickly withdrew, usually to write some letters before going to bed. I had never become very good at dancing, and it wasn't on my list of things to do for a good time. At one of the dances I met some doctors and nurses from the Michael Reese Hospital Unit, which had been overseas for a long time, and they seemed to be glad to talk to someone new.

They, too, were tired, and were more interested in swapping tales than danc-ing.

The Division Medical Battalion Headquarters and our Collecting Com-pany were nearby, so I had a chance to visit my good friends Dr. Pete Okumoto and Dr Wally Scheuerman who served in these units. Pete and I had gone through medical school, internship, and the training at Carlisle Barracks to-gether, and Wally was a medical fraternity brother of mine who had been a year ahead of me in medical school. I also had the opportunity to visit the hospital that was operating behind us and had been receiving our casualties. I especially wanted to look up some of the men who had come through our aid station, because I wanted to see for myself how they were being treated and how well they were recovering.

In one way my visit to the hospital was more enlightening than I had expected it to be. I don't remember exactly where the hospital was located, but it was close enough to the front so that exploding enemy artillery shells could be heard in the distance. My driver, Pfc. Charles Argyle and I drove there in a Jeep, and parked in a designated parking area that was guarded by U.S. soldiers. To enter the hospital we had to first walk along an alley that was about one city block long. The hospital buildings stood adjacent to the left side of this alley, and on the other side was a shallow ditch, on the other side of which was a long strip of vacant land. About half way along this alley three American officers were standing in a group, obviously discussing some-thing, and we had nearly reached them, when an incoming artillery round landed at least a mile and perhaps farther away. One of these officers imme-diately dove for the ditch and sprawled headlong into it. The other two, look-ing a bit sheepish, stood by. After we passed them Argyle and I agreed be-tween ourselves that the incoming round had fallen at least a mile away. Just then some soldiers emerged from the hospital, and as they walked past us we overheard this conversation.

"What the hell is that guy doing there in the ditch?"

"Oh, don't pay any attention. That's Major Whatsisname. He's the head psychiatrist here." The tone of voice carried more than just a hint of derision.

Once inside the hospital Argyle and I agreed upon a time and place to meet for the return trip, and went our separate ways. I met a number of doc-tors and had lunch with some of them. It was a pleasure to again talk about medicine with medical people.

After lunch I visited about two dozen patients from the 10th Mountain Division. Several of the wounded from my battalion were in various stages of recovery and were expecting to return to duty. They volunteered stories which were similar, and which disturbed me a lot. They went something like this:

"Sir, I wasn't scared when we went up to the front, and I wasn't particularly scared when we went into the attack, and I wasn't really scared when I got wounded, or when the medic fixed me up, but now, ever since that Major Whatsisname has been coming in every day to talk to me, I'm afraid to go back!"

After hearing this same thing for the third or fourth time I became really mad! During most of the return trip from the hospital I thought long and hard about the situation. I could recall that I had evacuated a number of men through Carge (my aid station at the time) with the diagnosis of "acute combat fatigue" or "combat exhaustion," but I couldn't think of any who had returned to duty. When we got back to our battalion area I asked some of our medics about theses cases, and also made some discreet inquiries among the line company officers. It seemed that almost none of these cases had returned to duty. Much later I was told by medical people stationed far to the rear that some of these men had been evacuated back to the States with major psychiatric diagnoses.

Combat Fatigue or Combat Exhaustion is an acute condition in which a soldier becomes temporarily useless and unable to function. Many things probably contribute to its cause, but the most important are lack of sleep, lack of food, excessive physical exertion and constant fear. These cases are always brought to the aid station by someone else, because they are unable to find it by themselves. They are incapable of obeying orders, act something like zombies, and some even resemble a catatonic state. The treatment is simple. They must be removed from the danger zone to allay their fear; they must be fed and allowed to sleep. Treated in this way, almost all of them get over the condition and are ready for action again in two or three days.

There must have been a reason for the failure of the men I had previously evacuated with combat exhaustion to return to duty, and after I witnessed the episode at the hospital entrance, I was more than ready to blame it on the psychiatrists. In those days I had a very low opinion of psychiatry. I had little use for it, and was sure that psychiatric treatment, poorly or erroneously applied, was of no benefit and could be harmful. I thought that most of the psychiatric treatment I had so far witnessed fell in the meddlesome or harmful category, and I believed that there were so few good psychiatrists in the United States that I could probably enumerate them all on my digits without removing my shoes.

After pondering the problem for a while, I arrived at what turned out to be a good solution. I felt sure that I was right about the treatment, because I had already kept some milder cases at the aid station as much as a whole day and overnight, then returned them to normal duty, with no difficulties or complications. It would make good sense to keep all of these cases under the protection of the aid station until they recovered, even if it took several days. There should be no need to evacuate any of them unless they actually turned psychotic.

So this is exactly what we did. Cases like these usually appeared only at intervals, when the stress of battle was at its greatest, and then there were often several together. If the aid station was relatively safe and located toward the rear when they were brought in, we kept them with us, but when we were attacking and on the move, we usually left them behind in a relatively safe place in the care of a couple of medics. Our litter bearers were made to order for this duty, for they had all completed the course at the Army Cooks' and Bakers' School. They weren't really missed up forward either, because we found it easy to replace them with German prisoner volunteers.

I didn't ask anyone's permission to do this, because I thought that if the practice were ever questioned, I could defend it on the basis that it was a medical judgment and that it was compatible with the Army's principle of getting men back to duty as quickly and as economically as possible. Now, in retrospect, I can say that the procedure was very successful. All of these cases returned to duty by at least the third day, and the psychiatrists didn't see any of them. I don't recall that any of them became psychotic or had to be evacuated.

There is also a sequel to this story. After the fighting in Europe had ceased, but before we left Italy, I received a nice letter from 5th Army Headquarters. It commended me because my unit, the 3rd Battalion of the 86th Mountain Infantry, had attained the best neuropsychiatric record in the entire 5th Army!

After three days of rest in Campo Tizzoro, our battalion became the division reserve, and we went back under the guns in the vicinity of Crocetta di Sotta. We rode in trucks to the village of Sassamolare, and waited there for nightfall. According to Lieutenant Brower's account of this move, we left the town well after dark on foot and in Jeeps. Toward the end of the march a wrong turn was taken, and the column went boldly out toward the German lines. Fortunately the mistake was discovered in time, steps were retraced, and we reached our destination without suffering any casualties. The Battalion Command Post was located in the tiny village of Gualandi, but our aid station remained a little farther back in a well-protected farmhouse.

Gualandi was typical of many Apennine villages. It was small and divided into two levels on the mountainside, Gualandi di Sotta and Gualandi di Sopra. Translated literally from the Italian, di sopra and di sotta mean upstairs and downstairs. These terms were descriptive and the names of other, similar villages in this part of Italy included them. In all of them so named, the mountainside was so steep that the upper level of the village was located almost vertically above the lower, and stairs were built upon or carved out of the rock between them.

Four days later we made another move, this time to relieve the 1st Battalion in their positions on Monte Grande D'Aiano. We were in the front line again. Although the line had remained static, the pace of warfare had increased some more, and enemy artillery fire was a constant threat to life and limb. We had gained the heights and were now looking down at them. They were expecting another attack at any time, and harassed us at every opportunity, desperately trying to delay it. No-mans-land had narrowed, and there was now a constant danger from snipers. Patrol activity by both sides was almost continuous. Probing attacks by small units of enemy soldiers were frequent, and our troops had to be ready to turn them back 24 hours a day. Isolated artillery shells would fall in near the aid station at unpredictable times, and concentrated enemy barrages would fall on some of the defensive terrain features on our side of the line from time to time. These activities produced casualties, but fortunately not many. However those that we did receive were difficult for me to justify, because we didn't seem to be gaining anything over the enemy and we weren't moving ahead. The War just didn't seem to be coming any closer to its all-important end. Almost all of the forward units, no matter whether they were in the line or stationed as reserves, were still in roadless territory and were supplied by mule train. That put them within mortar and artillery range of the enemy, so no one could relax. It was prudent to stay under protective cover and remain ever alert. From time to time we were treated to more propaganda leaflets, but the information in them was so obviously far from the truth as to be laughable. They had little or no influence on our men.

Our side also sent propaganda leaflets across to the enemy, and one such leaflet was in the form of a "Safe Conduct Pass" through our lines, issued to any German soldier who wanted to surrender. These seemed to be the most effective of any that we sent, because members of our intelligence unit, who did the first interrogation of prisoners at the front, told us a number of times that most of the Germans now being captured carried these passes in their wallets.

Our assignment on the front line lasted ten days this time, and as each day passed the enemy shelling seemed to increase. On March 25, 1945 K Company was the target of heavy concentrations almost the whole day, and suffered casualties, two killed and seven wounded. The following morning the shelling lessened considerably, and sometime in the middle of the day we learned that we would be relieved that night. We would be going far to the rear for training exercises.

As the front quieted down in the afternoon, Barney Summers asked for permission to go forward and see his brother-in-law, who was the first sergeant of I Company. Barney had introduced me to him when I first joined the battalion at Camp Swift. I still remember exactly what he looked like, but I am embarrassed to say that I don't exactly remember his name. After trying for a long time to recall it, the name Webb came to mind, and although I am not completely sure that is correct, I shall refer to him as Sergeant Webb. I got to know him quite well, because he often came to visit Barney at the aid station in the evenings. He was a quiet, confident, intelligent person, and I knew he had to be organized and efficient in order to run an infantry company as its first sergeant. Since we were all packed and ready for the move, I told Barney to go ahead. As was usual at this stage in all of our moves, we were earnestly hoping that there wouldn't be any more casualties before we left. While we waited a sack of mail arrived and was distributed. The men were beginning to read their letters. I had received a package, but before I could open it a call came in from the Battalion Command Post with the information that Sergeant Webb had just been killed. An enemy mortar shell had fallen directly into his foxhole. (*Author's note: After talking by phone to Barney Summers recently, I was happy to learn that I had the name right. His full name is Orville L. Webb. His body has been returned to the United States, and he is interred in the Arlington National Cemetery, near Washington, DC.*)

This sudden tragedy was keenly felt by all of us in the aid station. It also caused grief and sorrow among the men of I Company and many others in the battalion who knew him. Everyone seemed to have liked him very much, and the more time I had spent with him, the better I had liked him too. He was a fine person, and his death touched me all the more deeply because only a week previously, he, Barney and I had spent some time together celebrating the birth of his first child. Here was a very proud father, who had never seen his offspring, whose life had been snuffed out in an instant.

It was fortunate that Barney didn't return from the forward area right away, because it gave me time to think about what I might say to him. When he finally came back he looked terribly dejected and grief stricken, but he was able to talk about the tragedy. I didn't need to say anything; I just let him talk. He confirmed that his brother-in-law was dead, and, in terse sentences, related where and how it had happened. He said that he and his brother-in-law had discussed the possibility of something like this happening to one or the other of them, and he talked about the recent birth of the new baby. He indicated that he wished that instead of the baby's father, he could have been the one killed.

The time for our departure to the rear came soon, and since our vehicles had been loaded beforehand, we were ready to pull out. Barney's gear had been loaded by one of the men, so I motioned him into the Jeep, climbed in after him, and sat there next to him. Neither of us said a word throughout the whole trip, which was relatively long, because we went far south, all the way to Prunetta, where a regimental training area had been established.

At Prunetta the training sessions were structured and formal, and my part of the program consisted of lectures to groups of men on health subjects. I had done this before in connection with previous training programs, and it was not a difficult chore. One such lecture covered the purification of drinking water in the individual soldier's canteen, and the avoidance of native foods, which might be contaminated with infectious bacteria or harmful toxins. To consume native beef or native milk and dairy products, none of which were pasteurized, was banned, because of the possibility that these foods might contain the organisms of tuberculosis or brucellosis (undulant fever). At the time we had no cure for either disease. Untreated fresh salad greens and root vegetables were also banned, because they were often fertilized with human feces, which could carry parasitic and enteric diseases.

My lectures were always very informal. I encouraged questions from the men, because in my answers I could present some of my best sales pitches for following the rules. Detailed descriptions of tuberculous sputum and tuberculous joints, the abortions of undulant fever, the symptoms of severe enteric infections, the complications of gonorrhea and tertiary syphilis, the sequels of some of the parasitic diseases, emphasized by anecdotes about patients I had known, or heard about, or read about, did more to convince the men to obey the rules than anything else I could have said or done. The most popular lecture I gave was the one covering the venereal diseases. I usually gave it to a company of men at a time, but after the first few of these lectures there seemed to be extra people in attendance. These lectures were usually a part of a larger program, which began with the chaplain, who discussed the religious and moral implications of venereal disease. My turn came next, and I talked about the diseases themselves, their signs and symptoms, the prophylactic measures available and how to use them, and how, when and where to get them. Lastly the company commander spoke about "off limits areas" and disciplinary measures for violators. My part of the program was always the longest, and my audiences always seemed fascinated by the more graphic and detailed descriptions of the diseases. The men seemed to like the question and anecdote period at the end of my lecture so much that it often had to be cut off by the company commander, so he could get his few words in before the allotted time was up. The men usually summarized these venereal disease programs as follows:

The chaplain tells us to be good boys and not get it; the Doc tells us what it is, how to prevent it and what to do when we are exposed; then the company commander tells us where to go!

The training period at Prunetta lasted five days, and they were disagreeable days for the infantrymen. It rained much of the time and the ground was muddy. They slept in large pyramidal tents, which they were required to move during the worst of the weather, and there was an annoying problem getting the tent stakes to stay in place in the soft mud. There were drills, marches, inspections and weapons training exercises. The medics fared better, but I remember this period as being a very busy time, because a lot of the men had colds, and sick calls were long and tedious. We also saw and treated a lot of civilians.

When the training ended we became division reserve again and were sent to the same area near Crocetta di Sotta where we had been before. This time the highlight of our stay there was a speech by General Mark Clark, the Commander of the 5th Army. Before the general arrived the entire battalion gathered as an informal crowd within a field within sight of some of our mortar positions. Colonel Tomlinson, the regimental commander gave a short speech in which he didn't say much, but hinted that there were big things in the wind for our regiment, and that our 3rd Battalion would once again make a major thrust into the enemy lines. He finished just as General Clark arrived, and the General spoke immediately. I don't remember exactly what he said, but I remember that he gave a good speech. He was most complimentary to the entire 10th Mountain Division, and left no doubt in our minds that the division was slated for more "great and glorious accomplishments" soon. As soon as he had finished, he and his party left, but the battalion remained congregated to hear a few words from its commander, Colonel John Hay. I don't remember what he said to us either, but after he finished, I remember thinking that in appearance, in manner and in speech he was as good or better than the general. I thought that he was probably the best military leader we had seen that day, and was again truly thankful that I had chosen to serve with the 3rd Battalion.

For us in the medical detachment, being in the division reserve was not as bad as one might think. The whole battalion was usually far enough behind the front so that we didn't worry much about small arms fire, and our aid station was usually so well protected that, in contrast to the situation for the infantrymen, we didn't worry much about artillery. Troop training continued during these times, but on a much more informal basis. Groups of men were regularly withdrawn to a safe place for training sessions, and I remember occasionally giving medical lectures to some of them. We also occasionally held training sessions for our medics near the front. These were given by our own medical technicians and were much less extensive than what the infantrymen had to endure. I remember one soldier complaining that he had just been trained to fire a bazooka (a tube from which a rocket type missile was launched at the enemy) for the twelfth time, but generally there wasn't much grousing about this kind of training at the front. After all, a man's life might depend upon his buddy being able to fire his weapon automatically without thinking about it.

This time while the battalion was poised in reserve, we had the aid station on the main floor of a house which was very close to the one in which the battalion command post was located. Both were sheltered from enemy small arms fire, so the atmosphere surrounding us was relatively relaxed. Meals were more relaxed too. Instead of C Rations we were receiving new Ten in One Rations, made up of food packages designed to feed ten men at one time. They offered a greater variety of foods, and were much more popular than C Rations. In them were such things as canned bacon, butter, marmalade, canned chicken, etc. We set up an officers' mess where we ate meals prepared from these rations.

There were times when we were not very busy, and as was the custom at such times, several of the officers would get together and play poker. The room above the aid station was a good place for these games because it was more or less private, but still close to the phone in the room below. If necessary any of the participants in a game could be back in the battalion command post in less than a minute. I had often participated in these poker games, and usually came out a little bit ahead. I never lost much because before starting, I would always set a mental loss limit, and if I lost it, I would drop out of the game with the expectation that I would play again another time.

One afternoon I was among the officers playing poker in that room, and I was having phenomenally good luck. In a little over an hour I was over

$400 ahead, and I had just become aware of the amount when an enemy shell hit the building in the opposite corner from the room we were in. There was a loud explosion; I felt the floor shake, and in the far corner of the room I saw a part of the ceiling and some of the upper part of the wall fall in. No one was hurt, but this broke up the game instantly. Everyone scrambled down the stairs to better shelter below to wait out the artillery barrage, which followed. Later I went outside to look at the damage. From street level this building was only two stories tall, and the shell had hit the far corner of it at about the roofline. If it had been aimed a hair higher, or if the shell had traveled 15 or 20 feet farther, it would have come right through the flimsy roof into the room where we were, and we would probably all have been killed!

That was the last time I played poker in the Army, and, for that matter, it was the last time I ever played poker seriously. Yes, the shell hitting the building had scared me, but I was also frightened in a different sort of way by winning more than $400. In those days that was a lot of money, more than twice my monthly salary. So I sent it home and limited my gambling, from then on, to playing bridge for a tenth of a cent per point. Barney Summers and I usually played together, and issued a challenge to all comers. As a result we played often, and most of the time we won, sometimes as much as $10 in an evening. Late at night on April 4, 1945 we went back into the line, relieving the 2nd Battalion, which was holding the northernmost part of the front from Sasso Baldino to Monte Grande D'Aiano. Once again the action consisted of artillery and mortar fire exchanges and night patrols for information and prisoners. We stayed there until the night of April 10th, when we were relieved by the 10th Mountain Anti-Tank Battalion, and moved from there toward the line-of-departure for our next big push.

CHAPTER XII

TOILET FACILITIES

This chapter now interrupts the historical sequence in my stories. It is included here because by this time in the course of events I had seen almost all of the styles of toilets that there were in Italy. Many were amusing, and collectively they intrigued me. There were types and styles that I had never before seen, and which were radically different from those which I had known in the United States.

Naming this chapter wasn't easy. I seriously considered a large number of titles, and finally decided upon "THE COMPARATIVE ANATOMY OF TOILET FACILITIES," which is descriptive and has a nice ring to it. However, it would be too long to fit neatly at the top of a page or in an index, so I shortened it.

Perhaps squeamish or easily offended people shouldn't read this chapter at all. The subject matter certainly isn't appropriate at the dinner table, and having been made ever aware of this fact by my wife's eternal vigilance, I am always exceedingly careful to avoid bringing any part of it into a conversation at mealtime. However the topic seems to come up in casual conversation quite often, and frequently at dinner parties. Doctors' wives have a tendency to blame their husbands for bringing foul and nasty topics into the conversations, but most of such blame is actually undeserved. It is invariably someone else who asks the leading question which brings it to the table. Be that as it may, I have at times told the stories in this chapter in mixed company, and I don't think anyone was ever seriously offended. People generally seemed to like them, and many thought that some of the descriptions were funny.

Occasionally someone asks why I would want to include anything at all about toilets and waste disposal in my stories, and I feel obligated to explain that all good doctors are interested in sanitation because of its importance in the avoidance of pollution and the prevention of disease. Good sanitation practices were critical in wartime, and the study of such practices had been a large part of my Army training. My duties as a medical officer included inspection of mess facilities, the inspection of food and drinking water, and latrine inspections, and I always carried a responsibility to recommend measures to protect the men from avoidable disease. I addition. Italian plumbing amused and fascinated me because there was such a variety of it, and it was often so different from ours.

Until I entered the Army my life had been spent in Michigan, and my family and friends had indoor bathrooms with flush toilets, which operated on the same principles as those in use today. They flushed wastes away, through completely sealed soilpipes, into a sealed septic system or a city sewer. The toilet bowls all contained water, and had traps filled with water to block sewer gases from rising into the room. Our bathrooms did not stink or smell of sewage.

Outhouses presented a different situation. By the time the War began they had already been banned within most cities, but I was well acquainted with them because of my experiences at summer cottages and on a farm. They smelled, but most were not too objectionable. In most of them the floor and seat-bench were nearly airtight, and the seat holes had tight fitting lids. This did much to contain the odor.

Outhouses were set over holes in the ground to contain the wastes, and at the beginning of an outdoor cycle the holes were about six feet deep. In order to reduce the smell it was common practice to sprinkle lime, and occasionally a small amount of sand or earth, down into the pit from time to time. When the hole became too full, a new one was dug in a new spot. The outhouse was moved over it, and a new cycle was begun. The old hole was filled, often from a pile of earth that had been created when the hole was dug, with an excess of earth mounded high over it. In time this mound of earth would gradually disappear as the fecal material underneath it decayed.

In all of the Army barracks buildings I had seen, the toilets were no different than those we had at home, but out in the field the Army used the outhouse principle of disposal with something called a slit trench. I first heard about slit trenches when I was a medical student in R.O.T.C., but it wasn't until I went on a training bivouac during officers' training at Carlisle that I actually met one. It consisted of a trench about the width of a shovel and two to three feet deep. Its length was supposedly determined by the number of men who were expected to use it. Exact dimensions were prescribed in an Army manual. The sides were expected to be vertical, and the dirt removed from it had to be neatly piled alongside, about two feet away from it and parallel to it. When using it a man was expected to straddle the trench with one foot planted firmly on each side, and squat down to defecate. The toilet paper used was then to be dropped into it, and the man was expected to cover his deposit by adding some earth from the pile alongside. In combat it wouldn't do to have toilet paper flying in the wind all over the area because it could give the enemy information about out troop strength and concentration.

During combat, at least in the mountains of Northern Italy, slit trenches seldom met Army Manual standards. There were a number of reasons for this. We were in a part of the world where human wastes were treated casually, and were spread, together with animal manure, upon the fields each spring. None of the natives seemed to care what we did with it, and none of us in the forward combat areas seemed to care that the slit trenches didn't meet Army specifications. To the best of my knowledge nobody from the rear echelon ever came forward to inspect them.

The Army provided tan colored or olive drab toilet paper to every man. Everyone at or near the front was expected to use it, and generally did, but it was a rare thing for a soldier at the front to linger long enough to cover his deposit with dirt. It really didn't matter much that occasionally the wind would pick some of it up and blow it around the area, because it blended in so well with the dead leaves and other features of the landscape that it could not be easily recognized at a distance, and its presence couldn't actually provide the enemy with any information about troop strength or disposition. We didn't always fill in the trenches when we moved on either, especially later when we were attacking much of the time, but I am sure that this was no great problem. The dirt was right there, and anyone could easily refill one of them in a short time. My only concern was that, whenever we abandoned one, the waste was or could be buried deep enough to be walked upon without actually having any of it spurt up out of the ground.

Whenever any unit made a move in or near the combat zone, an early priority was to establish a latrine and dig the slit trenches. This duty did not normally fall upon the more intelligent and resourceful men in the unit, and often when the "volunteers" were not told exactly where to dig, slit trenches appeared in some unusual locations. During defensive periods when the front remained fixed and stable, headquarters and service units commonly stayed in small villages and towns, and established their latrines pretty much in the open, in abandoned vegetable gardens and vacant lots, wherever it was easiest to dig them. I heard a lot of complaints about this. To be squatting down over a slit trench in some village, and have a local signorina walk by, jauntily wave her hand and offer a cheery *"Buon Journo,"* had a most constipating effect. Indeed, I am sure that even the thought of something like this, actually did contribute to constipation in the ranks.

Outside of the towns the terrain and combat conditions were more important in deciding where to locate the latrine and dig the slit trench. On the mountain slopes there was often not enough soil over the rock to dig one, and lower down at the edges of the valleys the abundance of roots made digging difficult. It was much easier to dig out in the valleys in the small fields, which had been cultivated for many years, so this is where most of the trenches were dug. Such locations however had definite drawbacks. Being out in the open away from hillsides, they were often visible to the enemy, and tempted him into doing some long range sniping. In order to fire over the hills and avoid other obstructions to their line of fire, our artillery pieces often established themselves near the edges of these open locations, and the enemy invariably returned counterfire into the areas from which our artillery was firing. To hear a sniper's bullet sizzle past one's ear or to have artillery shells falling nearby while one was at the slit trench, also had a distinct constipating effect.

In rural areas human wastes were recycled by spreading them on the soil in the fields and vineyards. They were also carried out of the small towns and villages to be distributed in the same way. I didn't know how these wastes were handled in the larger cities, but I did know about the Cloaca Magna in Rome. From my studies of comparative anatomy, I knew, that in birds, the cloaca is a collecting organ at the distal end of the gastrointestinal tract in which not only the feces are held, but into which the urine also flows. Cloacal contents are expelled at intervals, and this admixture of feces and urine explains why birds never seem to be constipated. Magna is the Latin word for big, so Cloaca Magna meant to me, "large collecting organ for both urine and feces from which the mixture is eventually discharged." Many years after the War I flew over Rome, and had the opportunity to see the Cloaca Magna from above. When I saw the huge stream of sewage flowing out into the Tyrrhenian Sea, I could appreciate that it had been aptly named!

By the time I had returned from my trip to Florence, I believe I had seen almost all of the varieties of native Italian toilets that existed. In Chapter Five I have described the typical Italian farmhouse, and have described its toilet facilities in some detail. I won't repeat the description, but it belongs in this discussion here, as the starting point of the evolutionary line of toilets. It might be appropriate to review this description in Chapter Five at this time.

Although the marble slab with its four-inch hole was the standard for rural toilets, and I rarely saw anything else, there were a few farmhouses equipped with stools or toilet bowls of widely varied vintages. Eventually I had seen enough of them to realize that there had been a definite line of evolution from the primitive arrangement of the hole in the slab to the modern flush toilet, and that fixtures representing all of the stages of this evolution were still in use. Nevertheless, everywhere in the rural areas, no matter how old or how modern the fixture might be, it was always connected to the standard duct system which led to the manure pile on the ground floor of the house.

The crudest of these fixtures consisted of merely a large ceramic funnel, often with a crude attached toilet seat. The fixture was fastened to the floor and connected directly to the effluent soilpipe, which then became an extension of the funnel. There was no trap, and no provision for flushing. The sides of the bowl were always smeared with fecal material, which added its special aroma to the always present, odorous updrafts from below. I always assumed that in better times the bowl would be kept cleaner, perhaps by brushing and rinsing it with water from a pail, but during the War I never saw one of these that was clean.

Toilets that could be flushed were not common out in the country, and I saw them only on wealthy estates and in a very small number of farmhouses where I assumed only the wealthiest farmers lived. There were a few more in the villages and towns, and they seemed to be most numerous in the cities. Most were inoperable, because electricity was not available to pump the water needed. All could be flushed, however, after pouring an adequate quantity of water into the reservoir tank, or by directly and rapidly pouring enough water directly into the toilet bowl itself.

The simplest of the flush toilets consisted of a bowl, which funneled downward toward the rear and connected to a U shaped trap located under the floor. The bowl contained no water, but the fluid level in the trap was usually visible, and in these toilets one could easily see that the distance from the bowl to the trap varied from toilet to toilet. Because the bowl didn't contain water, its steeply sloping sides routinely became smeared with fecal matter. Some models tried to avoid this by incorporating a small ridge in the bowl which trapped about an inch of water, but this generally failed to completely prevent the problem, and flushing always required a powerful flow of water to keep the bowl reasonably clean. The powerful flush that was needed was often created by locating the reservoir high up, close to the ceiling, and having a large-bore pipe guide the water down into the bowl. A long chain fastened to the handle at the reservoir started the flushing action. Whenever the chain was pulled, water from the reservoir would come rushing into the bowl with such great force that there was often much splashing, so that whenever one of these toilets was in operating condition, one did not sit on it and pull the chain.

There appears to have been a definite and logical evolution from this early flush toilet to the modern ones we use today. This evolution involved the gradual rise of the trap upward from below floor level. Eventually it reached a position above the floor, and became incorporated into the bowl itself. The bowl became one arm of the U shaped trap and remained filled with water. Water in the bowl kept its sides from becoming badly soiled, because the waste matter floated almost weightless in it. Much less force was needed to clear the trap with such an arrangement, so ceiling reservoirs became obsolete, and tanks were mounted on the back of the bowl itself. In time, as the trap became incorporated higher and higher in the bowl, the outer shape of the modern stool changed from tall and thin to low and fat. In our "silent flush" toilets, it is the high level of water in the bowl, which is the same level as the water in the other, hidden arm of the trap, which allows the wastes to be flushed down the drain without much sound.

During the war I saw toilets representing almost all of the intermediate stages of this development, with widely varying levels of water in the traps and bowls, and years later when I was able to visit Europe, I saw that many of these intermediate stages were still in use not only in Italy, but in other countries as well.

People in the cities also seemed to regard sewage rather casually. Many neighborhoods reeked of it, because sewer lines were buried just under the street surface and were open at frequent intervals. Sometimes open ditches were being used as sewage conduits in congested urban areas, and I have already mentioned that it was quite common to see people, mostly men and boys, urinating or defecating right out in the open on the streets. In some places it was also common practice to pitch the contents of the overnight chamberpot out into the street through a second story window, and at certain hours of the morning it was wise to remain especially alert when walking down some of the narrow streets and alleys of the older sections of the cities.

Of all public toilets, the street corner booth was for me the most novel and amusing. I clearly remember the first time I saw one, a small booth standing in the middle of a wide sidewalk at a busy downtown street intersection. It was a little more than six feet long and about three feet wide, and it was divided in the middle by a partition rising up from the ground to a height of about four and a half feet. Its walls were thin partitions, which began a foot or so above the ground and rose to the same height. Solid entrance gates of

similar vertical dimensions shielded entrances at both ends, and anyone standing inside was fully visible above and below these barriers.

One time as I was observing one from a discreet distance and wondering
what it was, a middle-aged Italian man and woman came walking along the
street side by side. As they approached I noted that they were engaged in an
animated conversation. When they reached the corner they split up, went to
opposite ends of the booth and simultaneously entered. Their animated conversation continued across the partition. I wondered for a moment what they
were doing there, but I knew as soon as I saw the yellow stream of urine
disappearing into the pavement in front of the man' s feet. The woman's feet
were not visible because she was on the other side of the central partition, but
she did turn around so that her back was toward it, and seemed to sit or squat
down. All of this time she continued the conversation with her head turned
backward over her shoulder. She soon stood erect again, still talking, and the
couple emerged simultaneously from the booth. Still talking, they walked
side by side down the street beyond.

Another city toilet, which amused me very much, was an arrangement,
which I always think of as "The Pit." Although I had seen these toilets before, I remember them best in the men's room of one of the large railroad
stations. This was a spacious room with a high ceiling, glazed brick walls,
and ceramic tile on the floor. Factory style windows composed of multiple
small panes began some six feet above the floor and extended upward about
half of the way to the fourteen foot ceiling. They ran the full length of the
outside wall. Near this wall, facing toward the center of the room, were six of
these pits, spaced equidistantly in a row. No arrangements had been made for
individual privacy.

Each pit was square, about three feet across, had rounded corners, appeared to have been carved out of a single large block of stone and later set
into the floor. Each was shaped like a huge bowl with sides that sloped
smoothly down to a low spot in the middle near the back, where there was a
familiar-looking four inch drain hole. One might think of the whole thing as
a huge, square, eccentric funnel which had been set into the floor, which
drained downward to the rear, and connected with a soilpipe which drained
out under the outside wall of the building. Arising individually from the floor
of each pit and located forward of the drain hole were two massive pedestals,
which were shaped to look like large, raised shoe prints. Rising almost to the
level of the top of the bowl, they were over a foot high, and appeared to have
been carved out of the same block of stone from which the pit had been
created. These pedestals were so located that when a user stood on them, he

faced into the room, and when he then squatted down to defecate, he would come very close to hitting the drain hole.

Each pit had an overhead reservoir fastened to the ceiling, some fourteen feet above the floor. It provided the water for flushing. Coming through the large bore pipe from such a height, the water had a vigorous action, and often considerable splashing occurred. In public places such as this I could usually tell if the plumbing was in working order by observing the amount of wetness on the floor outside of the pits. Of all of the toilets in Italy, these seemed to amuse our men the most, for they would often joke about them, and admonish one another, "get off of those footprints before you pull the chain, unless you want your feet washed too!"

Italy also had a wide variety of urinals, ranging from highly decorative ceramic sculptures to plain pots and troughs, and it was in Italy that I was first introduced to an entire room that was nothing but a huge urinal. There were quite a few of those rooms in the cities. They had ceramic tile on the floor and half way or more up the walls. A tile trough, usually less than a foot wide and about three inches deep, ran along the base of the wall on three sides of the room. This trough was usually constructed with the same tiles as were used to make the floor, and was pitched to a low spot somewhere along its length, where the urine flowed either out through the wall, or down into a soil pipe of some kind. The technique here was to direct one's urinary stream to a low spot on the wall so that the urine could enter the trough silently, without turbulence and without splashing. Placing the stream directly into the trough always resulted in splashing to a degree that one's shoes and pant legs would become soiled.

I never did enter any private homes in the cities, nor did I go into any Ladies Rooms. If the sign on the door said *"Signore,"* or had a skirt logo on it I didn't enter. Therefore I cannot make any comments about the ladies' toilets in such places. The public toilets in the cities that I did enter all smelled as bad as their country cousins. In many the fixtures had no traps to block sewer gases from the room, and, indeed, one could often peer down into the soil pipes and see daylight, because the pipe merely ran out under the floor to an open sewer. Where traps did exist, they were often damaged, dry, or choked up with waste material, because they did not have enough water to operate properly.

My stories of toilets cannot be complete until I have told of an occurrence that happened within our regiment. My 3rd Battalion had just been rotated out of the front line to become the regimental reserve unit, and we set up our aid station in a farmhouse in a broad, shallow valley, just out of artillery range from the enemy. The regimental aid station was located on the ground floor of a super deluxe, four story farmhouse about two miles from us, and I visited there shortly after we arrived. The surgeons invited me up to the top floor where they had established their living quarters, and as we walked up I noted that there were no stair landings in this building. The stairs went straight up from one floor to the next in a single span, and the toilet rooms opened off of the hall next to the stairs on each floor. During my visit I used the toilet on the top floor, which had been reserved for officers. The room was neat and clean, larger than the average toilet room, and it had in it a modern flush toilet with a water level well up in the bowl. There was no objectionable odor. About a dozen five gallon water cans were lined up against one wall, obviously to be used for flushing. At the end of my visit, I returned to my own aid station. And gave no more thought to the regimental surgeon's toilet facilities.

Late that evening I joined a group of our men who had gone outside to enjoy the calm, peaceful serenity of this valley away from the front. The weather was unusually warm, and there was almost no wind. Sounds carried so well that we could hear occasional snatches of conversation from afar. An occasional enemy shell could be heard as it exploded in the far distance. All was quiet. The sky was clear and the valley was bathed in moonlight.

I had been outside but a short time, when, from across the valley in the direction of Regimental Headquarters, we heard a tremendous explosion. We all agreed immediately that we had never heard anything like it before, and we were completely at a loss to explain its origin. By this time we had been at the front long enough to recognize the sounds made by the various explosives that the enemy used against us, and this was something new and strange. Opinions were expressed as to its cause, including the possibility that the enemy had used one of its super powerful railroad guns, which were capable of firing large shells for distances in excess of twenty miles. I thought that someone or something had set off an unusually powerful antitank mine. We all hoped that no one had been hurt.

The next morning we learned what had caused the explosion. It had occurred at the Regimental Aid Station. I learned the details from several of my men who had talked to eyewitnesses from both inside and outside the building. The story as it was told to me follows:

It seems that some of the regimental officers had a little party earlier that evening, and when it ended one of the regimental surgeons returned from it in good control of his faculties, but feeling quite relaxed. As he climbed the stairs to his quarters he was smoking a cigarette, and when he reached the top floor the urge to urinate became overpowering. Instead of entering his room, he turned the other way, entered the toilet room, and relieved himself. Then, with lighted cigarette still dangling from his lips, he flushed the toilet bowl using one of the five-gallon cans in the room. What he didn't realize was that he had picked up a can of gasoline instead of one of the water cans. As soon as he saw that the bowl had flushed properly, he turned to leave the room, and upon reaching the door, decided that he no longer wanted the cigarette, which still dangled, from his lips. So, from the partially opened doorway, he flipped it across the room into the toilet bowl!

The resulting explosion was what we had heard the evening before. Gasoline had passed down the duct system all the way to the manure pile below, leaving the soil pipes filled with a highly explosive mixture of sewer gases, gasoline vapor and air. The explosion was so powerful that it blew away a wide vertical band of the outer wall of the building, from the top, all of the way to the ground. One of the witnesses who was outside said that he heard the explosion, and at the same time saw this portion of the building's outer wall fly outward. Then everything fell into the barnyard below, producing a large, instant heap of rubble. In a few seconds people appeared at almost all of the doors and windows in the building, and there was much shouting in Italian and waving of arms. An unbelievable number of people soon spewed forth from the doorway, still waving their arms, wringing their hands, and yelling. Fortunately there had been no one in any of the toilet rooms, and no one had been hurt.

When we discussed this incident among ourselves later, I ventured the opinion that this had been a poor way to treat one's hosts, and it would certainly not contribute to winning friends and favorably influencing the Italian people. Someone then told me that the American Military Government had been called to investigate, and in situations such as this, the American taxpayers would most likely pay damages to the owners of the building. I wonder if that actually happened.

CHAPTER XIII

BATTLEFIELD PROMOTION

During the period of relative quiet between major attacks in March and early April, a generous number of military leaves (of absence) were granted to men of the division. Florence and Montecatini were popular places to visit, but leaves to Rome were especially sought after, because Rome was far from the front and authorization for a stay covering several nights was required. Most of the Catholic men in the division were anxious to go because it would allow a visit to the Vatican and perhaps also to the Papal Palace. I too signed up for a leave in Rome, but in deference to them I allowed my application to be placed near the end of the waiting list.

I never did make it to Rome, but our regimental surgeon went for a few days sometime in the latter half of March when the front was reasonably quiet. Because my aid station was not far from Regimental Headquarters at the time, I was designated to fill in for him while he was gone. This meant that I had to split my time between two locations and hold a second sick call each day, but I wasn't overwhelmed with work.

Early one evening I happened to be at the Regimental Aid Station when a call came in from Headquarters. Colonel Robert L. Cook, the regimental executive officer, was on the line, and seemed surprised that Captain Randall, our regimental surgeon, wasn't there. After I told him who I was and explained why I was there, he stated the reason for his call. Our regimental commander, Colonel Clarence M. Tomlinson, was "under the weather." He had a little cold, and wasn't feeling at all well. They were out of booze, and he wondered if there was some medicinal whiskey available that he might have.

While Colonel Cook waited on the line, I searched the medicines and supplies there at the Regimental Aid Station, and found no whiskey. I reported this to him and said that, although I wasn't sure, there might possibly be some left at my 3rd Battalion Aid Station. If he would give me a little time, I would gladly go back there to check on it, and report back as soon as I could. He agreed. We ended our conversation, and my driver and I departed immediately in the Jeep to carry out this special mission.

Every medical unit in the Army was authorized to order and receive a monthly quota of whiskey, and no unit that I knew anything about ever ordered less than the maximum allowed. It was classified as a medicine, and was always included in an order with other medical supplies. The fact that it was ordered using its Latin name, *Spiritus Fruimenti*, fooled no one, and in spite of the fact that the indications for its use were at best nebulous and a matter of opinion, all of it was used up every month. I knew that it had been quite a while since we at the 3rd Battalion had ordered some, so I wasn't at all sure that I would find any.

As soon as we arrived, I made a quick search, and found that we had only one of the one-quart Army whiskey bottles left, and in it there remained only two or three ounces of whiskey. It would surely be a mistake to take this small amount to the Colonel. I racked my brain for another source, but I knew that there wasn't any more available in the entire area. Officers at the front could buy a fifth of whiskey every month through the PX (Post Exchange), but it had been several weeks since any of this had come through to us. Whenever any did arrive, the entire shipment never lasted more than a few days.

However, among our supplies were several quart bottles of ethyl alcohol, which we normally used for sterilizing instruments. This was pure ninety-five percent, 190 proof, grain alcohol, essentially the same thing as the "Grain Neutral Spirits" which the distilleries in the United States often included in large quantities in their whiskey blends.

I thought to myself, "Why not? Why not fix the Colonel up with something really good?"

One hundred and ninety proof alcohol, if swallowed would literally embalm the esophagus, so it had to be diluted. The formula for accomplishing this satisfactorily was not hard to figure out. I opened the whiskey bottle, with its pitiful inch of whiskey inside, and added 190 proof alcohol until it was not quite half full. Next I added enough clear water to nearly fill the bottle, and knew that the resulting mixture should be about 90 proof. However, the bottle was made of clear, uncolored glass, and when I looked at the mixture inside, I knew that it would never do. It was much too pale. It looked something like dilute urine. After thinking about this for a while, I had another inspiration. I put some granulated sugar into a clean tin can and heated it on our cook stove until it was well carmelized, almost to the point of charring. Then I added water to the can and stirred until the resulting solution became a deep, dark brown color. By adding it, a teaspoonful at a time, to the bottle, I soon attained a mixture that was the proper color for whiskey.

With a sense of triumph, and the bottle tucked under my arm, we hopped back into the Jeep for the short drive to Regimental Headquarters. When we arrived I knocked on the door of what had once been a lovely villa. A sergeant whom I didn't recognize, answered the door, and stood there expectantly. I told him my name, that I was the acting regimental surgeon, and was delivering the medicine that Colonel Cook had ordered for Colonel Tomlinson. He asked me to wait, left the door ajar, walked a short distance along a hallway toward the rear, and turned to the left to enter a room. I could hear muffled voices, and then, after a minute or so I heard Colonel Tomlinson say in a clear, loud voice, "Meinke? Meinke? Meinke? Who the hell is he." There followed some more muffled conversation. And in another minute the sergeant came back to the door and invited me in.

There were a number of officers in the room, but as I entered my attention focused immediately upon Colonel Tomlinson. Although I didn't know him well, I had seen him numerous times at a distance, and had attended staff meetings, which he had conducted. Viewed from this close up he still looked the part of a commanding officer. He was tall, erect and ramrod straight; he moved almost regally, without wasted motion. He definitely had a flair for command, and I had faith in his abilities, because John Hay, my battalion commander, had mentioned more than once that he was an excellent leader. As I have stated before, I had more faith in John Hay than I had in any other officer in the division.

Colonel Cook introduced me to the rest of the people in the room, but I don't remember now who the other officers were. Colonel Tomlinson didn't look very sick, but he might have had a cold, I handed him the bottle and as soon as he saw the label on it, his face lit up with a big grin. He unscrewed the cap immediately, and offered it to me, asking if I would like to have a snort. I refused as politely as I could, saying, "No thank you, Sir. I never drink anything at all when I'm on duty, and might have to take care of someone."

The Colonel then took a big breath, tipped the bottle to his lips, and swallowed a generous mouthful. In a few seconds his face turned livid. He shuddered, and his face became contorted. Then he exhaled vigorously, letting his breath out with a roar.

"Aggggggghhhhhh!!!!!!! Vile stuff!" he said.

Then he raised his eyebrows and one finger, and added, "BUT GOOOOOOD!!!"

He held the bottle up to admire it, and I breathed a sigh of relief, because I knew then that the Colonel thought he had a bottle of Army whiskey in his hand. I excused myself quickly and left.

Before the middle of the next month, on April 10, 1945, I received the order that I had been promoted, and was now a captain in the Army of the United States. Promotions had been discussed occasionally among the officers of my battalion, and I understood that regulations required me to remain a First Lieutenant for at least two and a half years before I would even become eligible to be promoted. I had only been in the Army for ten months, so this was totally unexpected and came as a complete surprise. I didn't even have insignia of my new rank put away somewhere, as was the custom for officers expecting promotion. At first I thought that a mistake had been made, but someone soon explained that I had received a battlefield promotion, in which case the "time in grade" requirement didn't apply.

I was pleased, mainly because the promotion meant a significant raise in pay, and I could start sending more money home to my wife for our future together. Whatever increase in military authority I might now have, wasn't important and didn't impress me much. However, everyone else in the Battalion appeared to be happy for me, and for several days I kept receiving congratulations. The company commanders, all infantry captains, seemed especially pleased that I had been elevated to their rank.

Because I didn't have any insignia of my new rank, Captain Frederic Dole, who commanded K Company, gave me a set of sterling silver captains' bars, which he said were "extras" that he carried. Nobody seemed to know where, in Italy, such insignia could be bought, so in my next letter home I asked my wife to buy several sets, and send them to me. We had been warned that small packages in the mail disappeared easily because they could be slipped unnoticed into an unscrupulous person's pocket, so I asked her to send them in a large box, and to fill the extra space up with cookies or other goodies. Her package arrived on June 23rd, well after the War in Europe had ended. Included in it were several sets of captains' bars. In the meantime I had received two from an officer who had been promoted, and bought two more from another officer. I still wore the bars that I had received from Captain Dole on my collar however, and planned to keep wearing them, especially if I had to go into combat in the Pacific. They had become my lucky bars, because both Dole and I were captains in the battalion who had come thorough much combat without being wounded.

The more I thought about my promotion, the more certain I became that the previous month's whiskey incident had something to do with it. Recommendation for the promotion must have gone up through command channels for approval, and since there had been no inkling that any such thing was brewing in the battalion, I had to believe that it had begun at Regimental Headquarters with Colonel Tomlinson. He hadn't even known who I was before I brought him the "whiskey," and at the time he seemed surprised that I, his acting regimental surgeon, was only a lieutenant. I don't think he knew then that all of his battalion surgeons were first lieutenants, and I think that when he discovered this, it bothered him as a matter of prestige. He was proud of his command, which now had proven itself in battle. He must surely have believed that his was one of the best regiments in existence, and it must have rankled him a little to learn that his battalion surgeons were all lieutenants at a time when, in most other divisions, these positions were held by captains. I believed that this was the explanation for my early promotion, and I became even more sure of it a short time later, when I learned that the other two battalion surgeons had also been promoted. I had merely been in the right unit, in the right place, at the right time, and had been able to produce a bottle of "whiskey" when it was needed.

When I had joined the division at Camp Swift the previous November, I was one of a group of medical officer who had been assigned to fill all of the remaining physician vacancies in the division. All of us were first lieutenants, and we had all been in the same training battalion at Carlisle. With the exception of my friend, Pete Okumoto, who was assigned to a collecting company, we all became battalion surgeons, and before the division returned to the United States the following August, we all had been promoted to the grade of captain.

Not long after my promotion, everyone in our battalion medical detachment received the COMBAT MEDICAL BADGE. This was something new. The badge showed an oval shaped wreath oriented horizontally upon which a litter, also oriented horizontally, was placed. Superimposed upon the litter, in the center of the badge was a Cadeuceus with the two snakes twined about a vertically oriented staff. Over the head of the staff was a block cross, similar in proportions to the standard red cross we were accustomed to seeing. Although this badge was not as wide as the COMBAT INFANTRY BADGE, which had a rifle superimposed over its wreath, the theme was similar. The award was a morale booster, and there is quite a story connected with it.

The Combat Infantry Badge had always been awarded to infantrymen who were engaged in combat, and the men who received it always wore it proudly. It also meant a slight increase in pay for them as long as they remained on combat status. In the earlier days of the War, medics, who were in combat with the Infantry, also received these badges, but later they were taken away from them. The reasons for this were not clear, and were never understood by the men at the front. This action caused a huge uproar and much consternation among the infantrymen, more so than the medics, because, during combat, medics working at the front were held in high esteem. Bill Mauldin satirizes the situation in his book, UP FRONT, in a cartoon on page 123 of the 1945 edition. It shows a dirty, unshaven, battered and tattered, steel helmeted medic confronting a clerk-type soldier sitting at a typewriter, wearing a garrison hat, and waving a pencil. The caption is: "Ya don't git combat pay 'cause ya don't fight."

This was the situation when we arrived in Italy, but the uproar over front line medics having to turn in their combat badges was still going on, and in the spring of 1945, the COMBAT MEDICAL BADGE was issued as the equivalent of the badges which had been taken away. The front line medic again had something that set him apart from his rear echelon counterparts, and he wore the badge proudly. I am not sure about it now, but I believe that combat pay was also restored.

CHAPTER XIV

BREAKOUT

The hiatus between the division's second and third major attacks lasted a little more than five weeks, and during about half of this time our 3rd Battalion was engaging the enemy somewhere on a defensive front. We spent most of the rest of the time only a short distance behind the line, as a part of the division reserve, and we were only away from the combat area for about a week, resting at Campo Tizzoro and training in Prunetta. During this entire time our higher staff officers spent a lot of time planning and preparing for the next major attack, which turned out to be the hectic, weeklong battle, which ended with the entire division astride Highway 9 in the Po Valley.

On April 6, 1945 we had been back in the line for only a day when I received word that the trip to Rome, for which I had signed up, had been permanently cancelled. A little later that same day another directive arrived which stated that no more leaves of any kind were to be granted. It appeared to me that our next action was imminent, and I became even more sure of it a few minutes later when one of the battalion staff officers came by and said,

"Doc, send your vehicles over to the motor pool at—, and **pick up your ten mules on the other side of that hill over there**."

This order came as a surprise. I knew that during the attack on della Torraccia we had been supplied by mule trains operated by Italian Alpini troops, and I knew that in March our off-road positions had been regularly supplied by a part of the division's Alpine Quartermaster Mule Pack Battalion, but I never expected to take charge of any of the beasts myself. Never in my life had I had any direct contact with mules, and having witnessed the horde of runaways at Camp Swift when I first arrived there, I wondered if I could steel myself and be able to handle this new situation. I thought about the situation for a few minutes, and remembered that mules were not completely strange to Barney Summers who hailed from Missouri and had encountered a few as he was growing up. Since he was our MAC (Medical Administrative Corps) officer, I could put him in charge of our transportation. So I turned the entire matter of the mules over to him, but nevertheless, I remained curious, and kept a close eye on the operation to see what was being done. I was leery that something would go wrong with those unpredictable mules.

None of our aid station personnel admitted to having had any training with Army mules, but there were a few men who had handled mules before. One was Pfc. Herbert Patton, who had grown up in Kentucky, and had handled mules there, so we put him in charge of the mule detail. It wasn't necessary to relieve him of any medical duties, because he was also our regular 3/4 ton truck driver, and he was without the truck whenever we operated in territory where we were using the mules. Another volunteer that I remember was Harold E. Rowland, from Little Rock, Arkansas. There were others, but I am not sure now who they were. These men were made totally responsible for the mules. They fed them, watered them, guarded them, were responsible for loading and unloading the packs used for transporting equipment and supplies, and they led them wherever they went. As long as these men acted as our mule detail, they were relieved of their regular litter bearer duties which were then taken over by German prisoner volunteers.

At about this time our two regimental veterinary officers became attached to our aid station, but we didn't see much of them. Mules were not brought in to the aid station for veterinary care, but were treated out in the field wherever they happened to be. These officers cared for all of the mules in the battalion, and the line companies used a lot more of them than we did.

At nightly battalion and occasional regimental staff meetings we learned about the general battle plan being developed for the anticipated attack. The main objectives this time were to again break through the enemy lines, break out of the Apennines into the Po Valley, and take the large city of *Bologna*. I soon discovered that I was not privy to as much information about this battle as I had been for the earlier ones, and realized that this was probably because most of our regiment was not scheduled to participate in the first day of the attack. In time I learned that my 3rd Battalion was not scheduled to begin its move until late on the second day, and I was again glad that I had chosen to serve the 3rd Battalion instead of one of the others. It was also somewhat reassuring to know that we would be attacking downhill, that the hills would not be as steep as before, and the valleys would be wider, shallower and more populated. This should make it easier for us to find suitable buildings for our aid station, and to evacuate casualties to the rear.

We were relieved from our defensive positions in the line on April 10,1945, and, using the mules for transport, the entire battalion moved in two stages to a designated final assembly area to prepare for the attack. We moved first to Riola, and moved again the next day to San Maria de Lebante. Just before we were finishing our first move toward the assembly area and were completing the setting up of our aid station in an unusually large barn, a regimental medical Jeep arrived and dropped off a medical officer with orders that he had been assigned to the Medical Detachment, 3rd Battalion, 86th Mountain Infantry. I was puzzled by this development because our table of organization definitely did not call for two medical officers. Nevertheless, I didn't question the orders. Actually I was glad to have the extra help.

First Lieutenant John Ninfo had entered the service from New York State. He was still relatively new in the Army, and this was his first day at the front. He had been inducted into the Army immediately after finishing his internship, and had gone through the same officer training at Carlisle Barracks that I had endured some seven months previously. Then he had been sent overseas for his first permanent assignment, and he had been in Italy only a few days when he arrived at our aid station. His ancestors had come to the United States from the Mediterranean Region of Europe, and he had married a girl of Italian ancestry whose maiden name was Marconi. He remained with our 3rd Battalion Medical Detachment for a while, and then served in the collecting company until the division was deactivated. After we returned from Europe to be stationed at Camp Carson, Colorado in September 1945, our wives came with us, and we rented apartments in the same building in Manitou Springs. The four of us got to know each other well. Sometimes we ate together in one apartment or another, and I remember that Margaret Ninfo had an outstanding original family recipe for Italian spaghetti sauce, which she cooked for us.

Soon after he left the service John entered a residency in obstetrics and gynecology at Flower Fifth Avenue Hospital in New York City, and while he was there my wife and I visited. During our stay John confided to me how he had felt on his first day at the front. For a long time he had been fearful about going into combat, and during the Jeep ride to the forward area he had worked himself into an advanced state of fright. However, when he walked into that big barn in which we were setting up the aid station, and met the grizzled old veteran in charge, and who seemed to know what he was doing, his fears vanished. He knew that everything was going to be all right. Now this was all very flattering, but I had to remind John that it was probably a good thing that he didn't know that the "grizzled old veteran" was himself a greenhorn who had only been in combat for about three months, had just been promoted to captain, and appeared old and grizzled only because he had not shaved or bathed in many days.

No sooner had we arrived in San Maria de Lebante when we learned that the attack, originally scheduled for that same morning, April 12, 1945, was delayed for 24 hours because of bad weather. The following day there was a second 24-hour postponement, and I assumed that it, too, was because of the weather. Our President, Franklin D. Roosevelt died on April 12th, but his death was not the reason for these delays. Rumors of the President's death had been rife for about twenty-four hours before official confirmation of this sad news reached us at the aid station on April 13th.

The several delays allowed time for numerous minor revisions in the battle plan, and finally the division attack began with the customary heavy artillery barrage early in the morning of April 14th. Soon our planes were doing a considerable amount of strafing and bombing. We could see and hear them diving to the attack. After a time we knew that the other two regiments had begun their advance because we could hear the rapid increase in intensity of small arms, machine gun and mortar fire. The progression of sounds reminded me very much of the initial phase of our early morning battalion attack on della Torraccia.

I remained with our aid station crew in the relative safety of our assembly area, and awaited reports of the progress of the attack. We were thus occupied all morning. By noon nothing that we were hearing out in front of us seemed to have changed, and we had received no word of the progress of the battle, so I walked over to the battalion command post to see if I could learn anything more.

The news was not good. Before they had been an hour into the attack, both leading battalions of the 85th had been stopped cold on the near edge of a large open valley known as the Pra del Bianco Bowl, because they encountered withering enemy fire from all kinds of weapons. (*Author's supplemental note: In this attack Lieutenant Robert Dole, a platoon leader in I Company of the 85th Mountain Infantry Regiment, who later became a well known United States Senator, and ran for the Presidency of our country, was severely wounded.*) The 87th which had been scheduled to advance along with the 85th on its right flank for a time, then veer off to the Northeast to attack the town of Torre Iussi, and Monte Pigna beyond it, had also been unable to cross the Pra del Bianco Bowl, and had not yet reached the area from which its main attack was to have started. In the meantime the 2nd Battalion of our regiment (the 86th) had started its mop-up operation toward Rocca Roffino, but almost immediately was pinned down by extremely accurate and heavy mortar fire from one of the hills, which should by that time have been taken by the 87th. The only reassuring thing in all of this information was the fact that there had been no new orders regarding the commitment of our battalion to the battle. We were still to be ready to move into the advance the next afternoon. As I left the battalion command post the atmosphere inside was grim, and reflected the anxieties of the officers who were trying to follow the course of the battle as it unfolded.

We sat around in our assembly area all afternoon, listening the sounds of battle coming from the North and the East. Early in the afternoon the noise intensified, as if a lot more artillery had been brought to bear on the trouble spot. Our planes continued to fly overhead on their bombing and strafing missions. The high-level din of combat continued on into the evening, but it was impossible to tell from the sounds how our troops were making out. From time to time someone from our Battalion Command Post came by to report that there had been some progress, but that it had been slow and diffi-cult.

That evening at the battalion staff meeting there was little new informa-tion. We were still in reserve and not scheduled to be committed until the following afternoon. No one seemed sorry about this, but we were all wor-ried, and some even wondered out loud if the main attack had been a failure. We really didn't know how much trouble the division had encountered that day, or exactly what progress had been made.

At our briefing the next morning we had much more information about the progress of the battle, and we learned that things had not been so bad the day before. Enemy defenses had been more elaborate and resistance more stubborn than expected, but by the end of the day all but one of the division objectives had been taken, and that one had fallen early the next morning. The attack was back on schedule, and we were definitely to be committed later in the day.

The battalion started its advance late in the afternoon on April 15th, and because the precautionary measure of keeping five yard interval between men was being observed, the column soon stretched out to a length of four or five miles. The medical detachment had once again been ordered to march near the rear, so it was almost dark before we even started. Our ten mules carried almost all of the aid station supplies and equipment, but each of us in the aid station crew hand carried some of the more delicate items in order to protect them from accidental damage. Each infantryman in the battalion car-ried extra ammunition, and K Rations to last three days. Men and mules were all heavily loaded as we carefully followed the route that our 2nd Battalion had taken the day before.

For several days we had been warned over and over again not to stray from the marked trail on this march, because we would be passing through an extensive mine field through which only a narrow passage would have been cleared. We were also warned repeatedly to be ever alert for booby traps in buildings, on abandoned equipment, and even on the bodies of dead soldiers.

We moved slowly forward. By the time we reached the yellow tapes staked out on the ground on both sides of the trail to mark where the ground had been cleared of mines, it was already dark. We began marching between the tapes and found that in places the path was so narrow that it would have been difficult for a truck or a tank to pass through without violating them. We soon reached and passed over a crude road, which the engineers had blasted out of the mountainside, allowing the rubble to fall down into the valley below. After that we were back between the tapes in the minefield once more. At times our column had to halt, because units up ahead were still fighting and trying to clear the Germans out of pockets of resistance. Rocca Roffeno and several surrounding villages, including some of the most rugged terrain in the Apennines, had been taken the evening before by our 2nd Battalion, and now it was engaged in some very heavy fighting ahead of us where it was attacking Monte Mantino.

To be sitting in the dark on the ground between the tapes in that mine-field, essentially alone because the man ahead and the man behind were at least five yards away, and to see the war going on all around, gave me an eerie feeling. Flares were being lofted into the sky intermittently, and continual heavy shelling was going on not far away. Occasionally a shell would land and detonate with what sounded like unusual vigor. I assumed that it happened that way because the shell had landed directly on a mine. This minefield was the most extensive and densest one that our division ever encountered. It was perhaps a mile and a half in depth, and because of the frequent and necessary stops, it took a long time for us to go through it. After we reached the other side, our advance continued in spurts of rapid movement between which there were long periods of waiting for whatever was going on up ahead to clear.

As we approached a small hamlet and were about to enter, word was passed back along the column to stay alert, because snipers were still active in the area. The village consisted of only about a dozen houses standing close together in a row along the uphill side of the narrow street. The buildings were two and three stories high, and their deep-set, upper windows seemed especially menacing as we advanced in the darkness. There were enough windows to shelter several snipers. On the opposite side of the street was a stone wall running the full length of the village. It was built of solid masonry, about seven feet high, and adorned here and there with sparse vines along the top. Our men instinctively stayed close in the shadow of the wall, and holding their weapons at the ready, watched the buildings intently as they passed through.

About two-thirds of the way through this little town I was momentarily startled to find the narrow street partially blocked by the body of one of our men lying crosswise in it with head toward the wall. I knew he was one of ours instantly, because I recognized the special jacket he was wearing, which had been designed for and issued to the mountain troops. It didn't take long for me to determine that there was no pulse and the body was getting cold, so I was there for only a minute. Because the street was so narrow, I had to leap over the body when I continued forward. Behind me someone else must have been startled to suddenly come upon the dead American, because I heard someone say in a loud stage whisper, "Move it! We can't afford to be trapped here!"

We advanced in this fashion until well after midnight, at which time we caught up with the whole battalion. Most of the troops were already dispersed in well-scattered foxholes on a large hillside. We were on the South slope of Monte Sette Croce near a place called Ca di Bello, and managed to install the aid station in a room on the ground floor of a small building located on an extremely bad rural road. We unloaded but didn't unpack, and we didn't receive nor did I hear of any casualties in our battalion that day.

Ahead of us the sounds of the fighting, which had continued until late in the evening, were now diminished, but the skies were still periodically lit up with flares and the flashes of artillery and mortar fire. To the Southeast, beyond our sector, we saw a particularly prolonged and heavy artillery display, and speculated that II Corps was probably beginning its attack. At the usual late-night battalion briefing I learned that the 2nd Battalion had taken Monte Mantino, now only a short distance ahead of us, and had dug in ready to defend it. We also had received orders. Early in the morning our battalion, followed by the 1st battalion would attack and take the lead for the day's fighting. After the briefing I managed to get about three hours of troubled sleep.

The next morning, April 16, 1945, things remained slow for us in spite of the fact that we had expected to go into the attack early. Our 2nd Battalion was still on and around Monte Mantino, but ahead of them the sounds of

battle has started up again in earnest. We were told that the 87th was behind
schedule in taking Monte Croce, Monte Mosco and the ridge between them,
but as soon as these areas were in division hands, our battalion would attack
Northward across this ridge to take Monte Moscoso and points farther North.

Because of this delay our advance through the 2nd Battalion was also
held up, and this allowed time for Colonel Hay to go forward with Colonel
Tomlinson and Major Pfaelzer of the regimental staff, to examine the terrain
and determine our route of advance in the forthcoming action.

When Colonel Hay returned he had quite a story to tell. The three of
them had driven forward, and then left their vehicle to go on foot to a vantage
point from which they could see the entire valley ahead. This spot turned out
to be too close to the enemy, because, as they stood there, a German machine
gun opened fire seriously wounding Colonel Tomlinson. The other two officers, still under fire, dragged him to safety. He was then quickly evacuated
from the field, and Lieutenant Colonel Robert L. Cook assumed command of
the regiment.

Colonel Hay also brought back some new and more accurate tactical
information, and briefed us once again on the battle situation as it pertained
to us. On the first day of the battle the 87th had begun by attacking to the
North, then it side-slipped the main assault by changing its direction of attack to the Northeast. Our Regiment's 2nd Battalion had started by attacking
to the East, then, after taking its objectives, changed direction to the Northeast and stayed on the right flank of the 87th until it veered off to attack, take
and hold Monte Mantino where it was now situated. This morning the 87th
had taken Monte Croce located to the Northwest of our 2nd Battalion, and
was now attacking along the ridge between Monte Croce and Monte Mosco,
and was expected to take and hold Monte Mosco soon. Once the capture of
this ridge was complete, the division's main direction of attack would change
to due North again, and our 3rd Battalion (86th) had been chosen initiate this
change. Closely followed by our 1st Battalion (86th) we would first pass through
part of the 2nd Battalion at Monte Mantino, then advance across the ridge
where the 87th was now fighting, and attack toward the more distant Monte
Moscoso. We would then become the spearhead of the division's drive toward the Po Valley.

From time to time groups of prisoners were still passing by us going to
the rear, and from them I recruited more litter bearers. I expected the front to
be extremely fluid and carrying distances to be long, and I wanted to be sure
that there would be enough men available to do the job.

Our advance began about noon, but we were soon held up again. It seemed that the 87th was having difficulty clearing that long ridge between the two mountains, which was to be our actual line of departure for our thrust to the North. After about an hour and a half spent marking time we were again briefed with the latest information about the cause of the delay. After an early morning artillery barrage, the day's fighting began with the 87th's attack on Monte Croce, but the mountain was so well defended that it was not secured until after 1:00 p.m. In the meantime, as the Germans withdrew, they withdrew along the high ground on the ridge toward Monte Mosco. They fought desperately to hold it, and it took until sometime after 2:00 p.m. for the 3rd Battalion of the 87th to reach Monte Mosco. Once there it took still more time to wrest it from the enemy and secure the area.

Our advance finally got under way at about 3:00 p.m. We passed quickly through our 2nd Battalion, across the newly captured ridge between the 2nd and 3rd Battalions of the 87th, and headed almost due North for Monte Moscoso with our 1st Battalion (86th) advancing almost abreast of us. We rushed full speed and practically unopposed through what appeared to be a huge hole in the German defenses which the two battalions of the 87th had created for us.

Before long, however, we encountered some enemy tanks for the first time. Some were knocked out with bazookas and anti tank grenades, but more often we called for and received air support by our fighter-bombers. (*Author's note: the Germans called these planes Jabos. Their full name was Jagdbombern.*) These strikes by the Air Force were very effective against tanks and road transport, and in this action they were critical, because in this portion of our advance we had neither armor nor artillery support. The roads behind us were impassable in places and there were severe traffic problems all over the region.

Our advance continued until late in the day, and mopping up operations continued on into the evening. The hills all around us reverberated with the explosive sounds of war. Flares lighting up parts of the landscape here and there were visible much of the time, and flashes of mortar and artillery shellfire were visible most of the time. Immediately behind us now was our 1st Battalion, also still engaged in mopping up, and we learned that our 2nd Battalion was following only about 1,000 yards behind them. On our right and behind us the 3rd Battalion of the 87th was busy repelling one desperate German counterattack after another. On our left the 2nd Battalion of the 87th had taken the town of Tole and was advancing toward Monte Ferra and the town of San Prospero. By the time our gains were buttoned up and defenses were established late that night, we knew that this had been a critical day in the attack. We had breached the enemy's main defense line, and he was beginning to use desperate measures to try to regain some of the critical territory he had lost. More important to me was the fact that now my battalion was the spearhead of a major offensive, and I must brace myself for increasing numbers of casualties. So far there had been remarkably few.

During our rapid advance that afternoon it had been difficult to keep the medical detachment together and we changed tactics so that we could stay closer to the line companies. We allowed our mule detail carrying the housekeeping equipment and extra medical supplied to lag behind, and catch up to us whenever we stopped for any long length of time and for the night. This made the medical part of the aid station more mobile and able to move more quickly. We were better able to keep our close contact with the Battalion Command Post. We also saved time and increased our mobility by treating more casualties right in the field where they had fallen, and moving them out to vehicle collecting points without actually running them through the aid station.

Late that afternoon as the whole battalion was advancing on foot, the entire staff of the aid station was keeping its normal combat position for moving forward, and was following closely behind M Company, our heavy weapons company. This should have put us behind our rapidly advancing Battalion Command Post and behind at least one of the forward companies, but this time it didn't work that way. M Company had somehow unknowingly passed between the two forward companies, and had reached a point well out ahead of them without being fired upon. We were right there too, and as soon as this situation was discovered we stopped and waited somewhat anxiously until the other line companies caught up and advanced to the fore once more.

From time to time during the advance, pockets of enemy resistance were encountered, and we had to stop and wait while the forward infantrymen cleared them out. We were usually close enough to these actions to watch the men of M Company place their mortars into position and fire them. Sometimes the terrain was such that I could witness the whole firefight, and I was constantly amazed at the intensity of the small arms firepower that our troops commanded. Always when I watched one of these "small" firefights, I would keep fingers crossed and pray that no one would be killed or badly hurt. Most of the actions that I saw, ended with a group of German surrendering, and by what seemed to have been a miracle, no one on either side wounded.

Once more our advance lasted until well into the evening, and after dark the mountainsides all around us were again lit up by the fireworks of combat. Skirmishes were going on in front of us, behind us and on both sides of us. In spite of all of the hectic combat activity, there had not been a great many casualties in the Battalion. I hoped fervently that this good fortune would continue.

Overnight on April 16-17, 1945 we stopped in a building which was near a road of much better quality than the one we had been on the night before, and during the night tanks of the 751st Tank Battalion overcame the traffic jams and landslides behind us, to arrive in our area in time to be included in our plans for the next morning's attack. It began very early, just at dawn, with Air Force fighter-bombers attacking and strafing long columns of German trucks and horse-drawn wagons, which were still out on the roads and fleeing toward the North. Our battalion column started forward at about 6:30 a.m., and encountered almost no opposition at first. The Germans had retreated most of the night, and many had been caught and killed on the roads by our planes early that morning. The air attacks had been devastating, and, as we advanced, we often saw many dead men and horses and a variety of ruined, burning German vehicles strewn along the roadside. At the head of our column the tanks and tank destroyers led the way, and from time to time some of the infantrymen rode on them. We were still acting as the spearhead for the regiment.

The medics had been ordered to travel behind a huge, noisy tank which literally blocked my view to the fore, but there came a time as we passed lengthwise through a wide, flat valley when I was able to see the column for a fairly long distance ahead. I noticed immediately that there were headquarters and company vehicles in the column, and then I realized that as far as I could see, forward and backward, ours were the only mules in the column. Meinke and his mules were following the exhaust of a noisy tank, and could keep up only because the infantry up ahead was still on foot!

Without a jeep it was impossible for me to catch up to the moving command post quickly, so it was some time before I eventually arrived there to register a complaint, and then I learned that all of the battalion mules, except ours, which had been forgotten, had been taken away the evening before. We soon had our vehicles again and the medics could all ride. However we also still had those mules, and it was another day or two before someone arrived to take them off of our hands. After that we never used mules again.

The battalion objective for that day was Monte Monascoso and the surrounding territory, and just as it looked as if we would take it without significant opposition, a whole company of German soldiers, who had hidden themselves in underbrush at a road junction near the base of the mountain, opened fire on I Company. They had waited until our tanks had passed well beyond them before revealing their presence. After a short but intense firefight, and with our tanks on the way back to the area, I Company's First Platoon took them all prisoner. Some of them later said that they had tried to surrender immediately, but were prevented from doing so at gunpoint by their non-commissioned officers. According to the commanding officer, who had been captured with them, this company had been hastily assembled and sent into the area during the night. They arrived sometime after 3:00 a.m., and did not know that we had occupied the hill in front of them the day before. They had not even had time to properly unpack before we arrived, and communications with their artillery and mortars had not yet been established. They had barely begun to dig their foxholes. It appeared that the speed of our advance had saved us from the severe enemy shelling that we would have received, if this company of Germans had had time to complete its communications network.

After this point in our advance there were enough satisfactory roads available so that we could carry litter casualties out of the field and bring them into the aid station on a jeep or in an ambulance. I don't remember how, but we acquired some more vehicles, and now had two jeeps and two ambulances as well as our 3/4-ton truck. For a while we also had a German ambulance, which K Company had captured, but we were unable to change the markings on the German vehicle and were therefore a little afraid that our troops would fire at it if we drove it around. We didn't keep it long, but turned it in to the motor pool, and sometime later I was told that it had been repainted and was being used to transport supplies.

The advance became so rapid that we now split the aid station, a section under each doctor, and moved forward by leapfrogging. We had to do this because it often became necessary to move forward, in order to keep up with the troops, well before all of the casualties in the aid station could be evacuated to the rear. It was no longer practical for all of us to move forward as a single unit. Therefore half of us remained behind to treat the remaining casualties and see to it that all were properly evacuated, while the other half moved ahead as a forward aid station to accept new ones. Sometimes the troops advanced so rapidly, that the need for the rear aid station to advance became urgent before all of its Casualties could be evacuated. When this occurred we brought the few remaining casualties along, and left them at the forward aid station, before continuing ahead to begin operations as the new forward aid station. With such a move completed, what had been the forward aid station became the rear one, and as soon as it had evacuated all casualties, it moved forward again, bypassed its sister unit, and once more became the forward aid station. Some of the men who were wounded during this time can honestly say that they were carried forward after they were hit, before they were sent to the rear.

Although we were using the roads again, casualties did not conveniently occur on them. Our infantry was still attacking across fields and through wooded areas, and men were being hit in places, which were well away from the roads. This created work for the litter teams, and we began using more and more German prisoners. German soldiers were surrendering by the hundreds daily, and there were still plenty of volunteers. At one time I had almost a hundred of them working for us, and we even managed to acquire a large German truck in which to transport some of them from time to time. A litter team consisted of four prisoners to do the carrying, one of our medics, and a Graves Registration man to act as a guard, and sometimes there was only one guard for several liner teams. Actually the guards were no longer needed, because none of these prisoners wanted to escape or do us any harm.

In the evening, when the battalion buttoned up in perimeter defenses for the night, we brought the two aid stations and all of our vehicles together. Shelling usually continued during the night, and occasionally produced casualties, and if there were still any being treated in the aid station in the morning, one section of the Aid Station moved out with the troops, while the other stayed behind until all had been properly evacuated. Then the leapfrogging began all over again.

One morning we set up a section of the aid station in a small village in a church basement, which had an outside entrance, so we didn't go through the church itself to get in and out. The line companies had already moved out, and our forward aid station section had moved out with them. Although these troops were advancing very rapidly again, battalion headquarters men, some reserve platoons, and some service personnel were still in the village. I was in charge of the aid station section that had stayed behind. We had finished the job of evacuating our casualties, and were prepared to move out to follow the action, when the Germans started to shell the village heavily. There were more casualties immediately. We were already out of the church basement and had our vehicles loaded, so instead of dragging them down into the basement again on this nice clear day, we cared for them out in the courtyard where there was more room to work. The courtyard was on the far side of the church, away from the enemy, and seemed quite safe, but in spite of this a mortar shell landed very close to us. I felt the blast and a sudden burning sensation in the calf of my right leg, and was sure I had been hit. I looked down, saw a ragged hole in my pant leg, and patted it with my hand, but there was no blood. I checked the casualties immediately. None of them had been hit, nor had anyone else in the area, so I went on with the business of treating and evacuating them. When I looked at my leg later, there was only a slightly reddened welt there. The skin had not been broken.

Our frequent moves sometimes produced a bit of excitement. While on the move we were particularly vulnerable, because we had to go out into the open, away from our usual protection. We made as much use of our vehicles as we could, but some of the distances had to be covered on foot while the vehicles could only take roundabout routes to arrive where we were going, and I had the ultimate responsibility to make sure that men and vehicles always came together at the end of each day.

One day during one of our leapfrog movements I was plodding along a narrow road with half of our aid station personnel and some litter teams. I didn't know exactly where we were, although the distinct sounds of battle up ahead told me where I had to go, and I knew that the other half of the aid station was somewhere up there. I felt sure that it was safer for us to be among our own troops, than to be isolated, so we continued toward the battle sounds as rapidly as we could. The road curved toward the right, around a hill on top of which stood a large stone house. As we approached it I made up my mind to investigate the house, and see what could be seen from up there.

A lone soldier carrying a rifle came around the curve toward us, and at first I paid little attention to him. As he came closer I looked again and suddenly realized that he was a German soldier. We were not armed of course, and were well marked as medics with our red crosses. Our party included some litter teams in German uniform, so it didn't surprise me that he did not shoot or threaten us with the rifle. When he got to within speaking distance of us, he announced in German who he was, and said that he wanted to surrender. He seemed relieved when I replied in German, and quickly told me that there were 15 more German soldiers in the house who would also surrender, but that the rest of his company was two or three hundred meters farther along the road, and contained some fanatics who would never surrender. I knew immediately that we were not traveling in the right direction, and was pondering what to do about the fifteen Germans in the house, when a group of armed British artillerymen appeared behind us. I hailed them, told them about the Germans in the house and gave them the information about the location of the German infantry company up ahead. In the next ten minutes I was able to arrange the surrender of all of the Germans in the house to the British. Then I retraced my steps down the hill and rejoined my men to seek another route to our Battalion Command Post.

On another occasion several of us were riding in the jeep along a country road with woods on the right and a pasture or meadow on the left. As we neared a crossroad, an enemy artillery shell landed not far from us in the meadow, and since this often signaled the arrival of more rounds, we left the jeep to lie in the only ditch available which was on the meadow side of the road. Another jeep, which was traveling at right angles to us on the crossroad ahead, stopped and parked on the edge of the road around the corner of the meadow from us. The four soldier occupants got out, and ran to take cover in the woods beyond. In less than a minute we heard more shells on the way. Several landed in the meadow and some in the woods, but none hit the road. There was a brief pause, and then I heard another incoming shell. This one had a peculiar sound, and I wondered momentarily if it was another leaflet carrying, propaganda shell. As I looked to my left, I was surprised that I could see it coming. It was rotating end over end, and landed short but still in the meadow. I saw it hit the ground, but it didn't explode. Instead it cartwheeled, bouncing at intervals for the full length of the meadow, and finally came to rest, without exploding, under the jeep which was parked on the crossroad ahead. More rounds came in after that, and we remained pinned down for about twenty minutes. Then, after a period of time during which all was quiet, we emerged, and the occupants of the other jeep also came out of the woods. We yelled at them, and they heard us, but I don't believe they quite understood what we were yelling because they continued to saunter toward their jeep. They had almost reached it when one of them apparently understood, stooped down, and looked underneath. In an instant all four soldiers scattered back into the woods. They soon emerged again, much farther away now, and one of them hurried up to the jeep, climbed into the driver's seat and slowly drove it forward a few feet. Then he gunned it, and sped up the road to pick up his buddies. They waved at us as they continued on their way.

Another incident involving enemy shelling occurred in a different meadow while I was advancing across it on foot with some of my men and couple of German litter teams. As we entered the open ground from a wooded area we could see two fallen enemy soldiers lying near the middle of the field. We were headed toward some farm buildings, and the bodies were well off to one side of our line of march. When we neared the center of the field, someone said that he saw one of the fallen enemy soldiers move, and I felt obligated to investigate. So I sent everyone on ahead, and took a prisoner litter team and a medical technician with me to take a look at them. The first one had been dead for some time; the second had probably survived his wounds for a time, but I checked carefully, and he was also dead. As I stood up beside the body, a mortar shell landed at the edge of the woods on our right, and one of the German litter bearers said to me in German, "We have to get out of here fast!" So we started trotting toward the farmhouse where by this time the rest of our group had already arrived. A second shell then fell at the edge of the woods on our left, and the German who had warned me to leave, now became more emphatic, urged us to run, and started to run as fast as he could toward the farmhouse. The rest of us followed at a sharply increased speed, and we had barely reached the safety of the building when a dozen or so mortar shells fell into the field where we had been. Some fell near the farmhouse, but we were safe inside.

When we left to continue the advance, I found that we had more German prisoners than we had started with, and after investigating I learned that a half dozen of them had survived our infantry attack and had lain scattered and hidden in the woods as our men passed through. Afterward they had hidden in the house, and when our medics arrived with their contingent of German litter bearers, these Germans mingled with them, and went unnoticed for a time. They all wanted to stay with us and would gladly do anything we asked, so I let them come along.

There was still a lot of daylight left when we halted our advance on April 17. We stopped in a woods at the edge of an unusually large, open, treeless basin, and the infantrymen began digging their foxholes for the night. Some 60 or 70 yards inside the woods I found a nice cottage, with thick stone walls, which would make an excellent aid station, and I planned to move in. Our vehicles, including the truckload of German prisoners, had just pulled into the yard, and our split aid station was back together for the night, when Colonel Hay called me up to the edge of the woods. He pointed to a farmhouse perhaps a thousand yards out in the valley, and said, "Doc, see that building out there?"

I admitted that I saw it

"Well," he continued, "I want you to set the aid station up out there tonight, and we'll attack past it first thing in the morning."

Then he pointed to the other side of the valley and added, be careful going out there, the Krauts are right over there in the woods."

I swallowed hard, and said the only thing I could, "Yes Sir."

We parted then, but I remained at the edge of the woods to consider this move. The valley was perhaps a mile and a half wide, and in it, as far as I could see, there was nowhere for anyone to hide or be shielded from enemy fire. It might be possible to sneak out after dark and make it to the house, but

it wasn't very likely that we could go unobserved and without drawing artillery or mortar fire. The day had been sunny and the sky was clear, and there
would surely be enough light during the night for us to be seen, but perhaps
not enough to be identified as medical personnel. If we were mistaken for an
infantry patrol, we would immediately attract all kinds of shellfire, and I felt
sure that there would be casualties among us.

The more I thought about making a move like this after dark, the less I
liked it. I had almost made up my mind to go back to Colonel Hay to see if he
would possibly change his order, and let us follow the troops in the morning,
but then I had an idea. If the enemy operated anything like we did, he was
over there digging his foxholes just as our men were doing here, and he would
not be nearly so ready to fire at us now, as he might be later in the night. We
had all of these German prisoners with us, and I didn't think that the Germans would fire at their own men. It would be safer for us to march out there
immediately, in daylight, in the open with our red cross banner flying, in two
lines, the prisoners toward the German side of the valley, and our men toward our side.

I explained the plan to our men, and understandably found that they had
little enthusiasm for marching that half-mile or more in the open ahead of our
troops. I didn't give the prisoners a chance to volunteer, but just told them
what to do. They willingly followed my orders and didn't complain. We loaded
up our rucksacks with supplies and food, took leave of our vehicles and drivers, and walked through the woods for some two or three hundred yards
parallel to the edge of the valley, so that when we emerged from the woods,
our line of march to the farmhouse would be at about a 45 degree angle to its
long axis. I deliberately chose this longer route to make sure that the left side
of our column was fully visible to the German side of the valley, and that the
right side was fully visible to our infantrymen.

So in daylight we started out of the woods toward our objective two by
two, German on the left, American on the right. I was in the lead with a
prisoner at my elbow. Someone near the head of the column carried the Red
Cross banner. I hadn't planned it that way, hut soon everyone was walking in
step, and there we were out in no mans land, marching as if we were on a
parade ground.

Not a shot was fired at us all of the way. I knew that there couldn't be
any American soldiers in the farmhouse, but as we neared it, I thought of the
possibility that there might be Germans waiting in ambush there. I asked the
German next to me if there could be any Germans there. He didn't think so,
but as a precaution I had the German side of our column move up by four or

five men in order to have a group of Germans at its head. This could be easily done because there were more of them in the column than there were Americans, and at the beginning of the march the last six or eight of the pairs were German. When we were still some distance from the house, I asked for a couple of German volunteers to go ahead and see if anyone was in it, and if they found any German soldiers to see if they would surrender. Two of them volunteered immediately, and as they started forward, I also asked them to check for booby traps. They ran ahead, and by the time our group reached die barnyard, they reported that the house was deserted.

As we entered I was glad to see that this was an unusually thick-walled, stone farmhouse, with plenty of room in the stable area, and extra rooms in which to operate. We were now out in plain sight between the two armies, and I was reasonably sure that the enemy must have seen us move. The fact that we had not been fired upon boded well, so I thought it would be a good idea to mark the building as a medical installation. Therefore, while we were setting up the aid station at ground level in the stable area, I sent two of the men to the top floor to stretch our large Red Cross banner over the outside wall between two of the windows.

I was concerned that enemy patrols might come by during the night, so this was one of the very few times that I felt the need for our own guards, and posted pairs, one American and one German at upstairs windows on all four sides of the building. The prisoners participated in this because it was my plan to not only challenge everyone approaching, but to also explain that we were a medical installation, and that they were welcome to come in without shooting. If a German patrol happened to come by, the Germans would be needed to do the talking. As things turned out, nobody showed up; we remained isolated out there the whole night long.

The shooting war began again in the morning. I had dozed and was awakened by shells falling all around. Two or three struck the building on the upper floor, but we were safe down below. Our infantrymen were advancing rapidly on both sides of us and there were casualties. The shelling lasted for several hours, but in spite of it we managed to get all of the wounded off the field and assembled in the aid station without suffering any casualties among our medics. Then, after the infantry had advanced well beyond us and things quieted down, we were able to evacuate all of them to the rear by jeep, and the cross-country leapfrog movements of the aid station sections began anew.

April 18 is remembered by the men of the 3rd Battalion because that day they ran into Checkpoint 50. For the uninitiated, a checkpoint is a spot on a military map which marks some prominent terrain feature, such as a knoll, a hill, a prominent building, a ridge, a river bend, etc. Checkpoints are identically numbered on all military maps used by the troops in a given area, and by using them as references, more rapid and accurate radio communication between units is made possible.

Our advance continued throughout the morning with our 3rd Battalion leading the regiment, and I Company out in front. Resistance was light, and a few prisoners were taken. Some were walking wounded, and were dropped off at the aid station as each group of prisoners passed by. One of these groups included a German medical officer, and I asked the German doctor if he would like to stay with us, or go back with the rest of the prisoners to the POW cage. He chose to stay, and immediately cooperated with me in the care of wounded prisoners. I was happy with this arrangement because I would now have another doctor with whom to talk, and I was even happier a little later, because we soon began receiving many more German wounded than Americans.

During the noon hour the town of Sulmonte fell to our troops, and the battalion advance continued toward Checkpoint 50, which was located several hundred yards North and West. The checkpoint was a hill with wide, sloping sides and a flat top which had several stone houses perched upon it, and except for a long, gently sloping ridge running toward the north, the valley floor all around it was flat, grass covered and virtually without any natural concealment.

That afternoon when the leading elements of I Company came over the ridge to approach it, they were fired upon by enemy machine guns. In another minute enemy mortars joined in, followed in a few more minutes by heavy artillery. A few minutes later when even larger artillery shells, estimated to be as much as 210 mm in size, fell into the area, it became clear that this was where the Germans were determined to stop our advance. Division Artillery was called for and concentrated its fire on Checkpoint 50.

Air Force fighter-bombers were called in, and they bombed and strafed the hilltop and its rear approaches. It seemed as if no living thing could survive such bombardment, but the enemy soldiers were extremely well dug in, and not only survived, but defended the hilltop to the bitter end with a fanaticism such as our troops had not before encountered.

Ultimately the hilltop had to be taken by direct assault. The heavy bombardment did allow our infantrymen to reach it, but not without casualties, and once on top our men had to ferret out the enemy soldiers, house-to-house, room-by-room, and dugout-by-dugout. In the end only a few were left to be taken prisoner, and it was not until the very end that any of them surrendered.

Heavy artillery continued to fall all around, but it was now all German.

It continued as Company L passed through to take the next two hills beyond Checkpoint 50. Miraculously there were only a few minor casualties during this part of the battle, and no loss of life. The enemy shelling continued until well into the night.

The whole regiment was temporarily held up by this battle for checkpoint 50, and since we were no longer moving forward our two aid station sections came together and established operations in a small stone building behind a ridge to the south of the action. I didn't directly observe any of the battle, but as we received casualties from it, and heard the comments and reports, a fairly accurate picture emerged. As was my custom I tried to monitor what was going on by listening on our field radio to the conversations between the Battalion Command Post, Regimental Headquarters and the companies in the field. I had already done this often enough to recognize code names and the code words that were regularly used. Although we carried the radio to reestablish contact with the battalion if we ever got lost, I had only once found it necessary to use our radio to broadcast, and that occurred in a Situation that had come about during our advance the day before. One of the company commanders had asked for instructions via radio regarding his next move, and Colonel Hay was sending them. Although I could hear both broadcasts clearly, it soon became obvious that they couldn't hear each other very well. This sometimes happened when there was a large hill between the two radios. I was able to break in, identify myself, and relay the messages in both directions.

I first became aware that the fighting at Checkpoint 50 had become intense early in the afternoon, and after that I listened to the radio frequently. We were getting I Company casualties, so I already knew that this company was bearing the brunt of the attack. Late in the afternoon, I overheard the I Company radio operator report the good news that they were on top of the hill, and that the objective had been taken. Then came the information that they had sustained more casualties than expected, and that the company was scattered. Only a few men were left at the top, and the company commander estimated that reinforcements would be needed to hold it through the night if the enemy should counterattack.

It would have been foolish to broadcast information about movement of troop units or their routes, because the Germans were probably monitoring our radio channels and would overhear it, but the terse reply came back instantly, "DIG IN TO DEFEND, AND WAIT FOR PINEAPPLE." This was an excellent response, perfectly understood by our men, but not likely to be understood by the Germans. K Company was the battalion's reserve company that day; K Company's commander was Captain Dole; and Dole was the name of a well-known American brand of canned pineapple, which was sold in grocery stores all over the United States. That night K Company, in full force, relieved I Company on the hilltop, and I company came down to spend the night behind L Company. Here was yet another small example of American resourcefulness in a difficult situation.

The captured German medical officer was in the aid station with us all afternoon that day, and I was glad to have him there. He was much older than I, perhaps in his mid-fifties. I don't remember his name. He spoke a little English, and it was obvious that I spoke German much better than he could speak English, so we spoke mainly in German. There were many times when I didn't understand some of the words he used, especially the technical terms, and whenever this happened a lengthy, roundabout discussion would follow until I finally understood. As my comprehension improved, so did my confidence in my ability to speak German, and I became much less self-conscious about using the language. I believe some of that confidence has stayed with me to this day.

He presented a bleak picture of medical practice in the German Army, where medical services had deteriorated from among the best in the world into conditions of desperation and severe shortages. He had been short of supplies and medicines for months. Bandages had been a serious problem, and when he had any, they were made of cheap paper. He had been short of antiseptics, soap, and narcotics. He had no antibiotics, although he knew that in the hospitals they were using neoprontosil, a red, dye-like powder that was the precursor of the sulfanilamide, with which we were regularly treating wounds at the front. He was interested in the fact that we already had, and were using several varieties of sulfonamides, and that in our hospitals we were regularly using the new wonder drug, penicillin, but he seemed skeptical when 1 told him what penicillin could do.

We also talked about medical education, and I learned that he had been trained in Vienna at the time when it was world-renowned as a medical center, and was, so to speak, the Mecca of Medicine. He said that in Vienna all patients who died in a hospital were subjected to an extensive autopsy, and he boasted that in 50 percent of these autopsies the clinical diagnosis had been correct. This prompted me to do a little bragging myself as I told him about my education. I explained that I was a year and a half out of medical school from the University of Michigan, and that in the senior year there all medical students were required to attend one hundred autopsies in person, and do the anatomic dissection for one of them. In only one or two of those that I had attended, had the clinical diagnosis been incorrect, and in only a very few others, although the main diagnosis had been correct, had other undiagnosed conditions been found, but always in their preclinical stages and usually only after microscopic examination of the tissues.

During all of the time that the German medical officer was with us, we were treating two or three wounded prisoners for every American. One of them who had been taken from Check Point 50 had been particularly severely wounded. He had multiple shell fragment wounds, an obvious fracture of his right leg and a probable fracture somewhere in the region of his right shoulder. When he was carried in, he was barely conscious, had an ashen complexion, profuse sweating, rapid pulse and low blood Pressure. He was obviously in shock, so I quickly reconstituted a unit of plasma and started to administer it intravenously through a large bore needle. The German Doctor was most curious about this, and asked what it was that I was administering. I told him, and when I explained how it was made, and the medical principles behind its use, he understood immediately, and said that he personally had never had anything like it to use at the front. With the plasma running I examined and rebandaged the wounds, and splinted the leg. The external bleeding was controlled. I could find no physical evidence of any internal bleeding except for that, which had occurred at the fracture sites, and when the prisoner's condition improved dramatically after only a small volume of the plasma had been administered, I was pretty certain that there was none. I knew that he was fully conscious again when he managed to scowl at me with a defiant expression on his face, and say, "Heil Hitler!" I also became aware that there was something definitely different about this particular prisoner, as compared to the rest of them. When I asked how he felt, and about the circumstances of his being wounded, he wouldn't answer, but just stared at the ceiling and glowered defiantly. He did let me inspect his splints and dressings at intervals, and raised no objection to the plasma administration or to the later addition of a bottle of normal saline to keep the intravenous line open. The other wounded Germans in the aid station and the volunteer litter bearers coming and going, seemed to shun him completely. It was normal for most prisoners to speak to each other freely and to their own wounded, and it was normal for wounded prisoners to speak to each other, albeit in quiet and subdued tones, but none seemed willing to speak to this man. Nor did he speak to anyone, and he didn't reply whenever I spoke to him. As his condition continued to improve the expression on his face showed increased defiance and eventually sheer animal hatred. The German medical officer didn't fare much better either, but when he "pulled rank," the man did give his name, rank and serial number.

After we had sent this man to the rear, my German colleague volun-teered a surprising amount of information about him, some of which came from our healthy prisoners, and some of which was common knowledge among the German troops. In the past he had been a member of Hitler's elite SS Troops, and had subsequently become a member of a famous German division, which had fought through the entire North African campaign, and had then fought the rear guard action in Sicily. He belonged to the famous 200th Regiment of the German 90th Panzer Grenadier Division, and was one of a few who had remained alive to be taken prisoner in the action on Check-point 50. This regiment had a reputation on both sides of the line for being efficient, well trained, extremely disciplined and ruthless. It had recently dwindled in size because no replacements had been available with which to compensate for the normal attrition of war, and because some of the men had been transferred to other units in order to try to instill some pride and "back-bone" into the groups of old men and boys that the Germans were now call-ing up to be soldiers. Originally the men in it had all been SS Troops or had come from Hitler Youth organizations. They and all others like them were feared and hated by the ordinary German soldier and by most German civil-ians. They were arrogant, fearless, ruthless, and treacherous fanatics, and would not hesitate to shoot anyone, even a soldier in a German uniform who looked like he might be trying to surrender. This man had been typical of the group. If we should have to handle any more of these fanatics, the Doctor warned, we should be sure to always search them for hidden weapons first, and carefully guard against the treachery they were capable of committing.

With Checkpoint 50 in our hands we moved the aid station forward again, and the German doctor now asked to go on to the rear. He knew that we had already been going constantly with little rest for three days, and said he was too old for that kind of activity, so I sent him back with the next group of prisoners passing through.

While there was still a lot of daylight left, we moved again and set up operations for the night in a stone cottage that stood all alone at the base of a cliff, which was perhaps one hundred feet high. I remember the house well. The kitchen was not very large, but had the usual open fireplace, and we soon had a nice fire going. Here the roads were good and we received and evacu-ated our casualties by jeep without any trouble. I remember that late that night someone brought in some mule steaks, and they were a delicious treat, broiled over the glowing coals in the fireplace.

The forward companies were well out ahead of us, and the men of the reserve company were digging in on the plateau at the top of the cliff, which stood only 15 or 20 feet behind our back door. To the right of us the plateau above us sloped down gradually to our level, and at the bottom, about 150 yards to our right, was a well defiladed, grassy bowl in which one of our field kitchens had been set up in order to give the troops a welcome hot meal. Several litter casualties arrived just before serving time, and while I was busy with them, one of my men took my mess kit and went through the chow line for me. An hour later, after I had eaten and my most seriously wounded patient, one with a severely compounded fracture of a femur, was coming out of shock, I stepped out of the back door with my mess kit in hand, intending to go to the field kitchen to wash it. As I stood there for a moment, a yellow stream, unmistakably urine, came down from above, missing me by only a foot or so. Because I was overtired and still tense from the difficulties of the day, this angered me more than it should have, and I was determined to put a stop to it and all similar nonsense in the future, so I made the end run along the base of the cliff, around past the field kitchen and up to the top. Some of the reserve company men were loafing about their foxholes there, and, in forceful terms, I demanded to know what had been going on. Finally, after some further questioning, one of the men, looking very sheepish, admitted that several of them had held a contest to see who could project his urinary stream the farthest, and he had won by going last, and projecting it over the edge of the cliff. He hadn't known that there was a building below. The men all apologized. They promised that it wouldn't happen again, and that was the end of it.

The next day, April 19, was much easier. The enemy had been routed, and was incapable of any organized resistance. We moved up to a new assembly area east of Checkpoint 50, and as we waited there to continue our attack toward the north, most of us suspected that this would be our last day in the Apennines. We were halfway up on a mountainside watching the activity in the valley below. The road running along the Lavino River, which flowed from Montepastore northeast to the Po Valley, was jammed. All kinds of military vehicles, including some heavy construction vehicles that I had never seen before, were traveling bumper-to-bumper toward the North. They stirred up a huge, long cloud of dust, which hung in the air high above the valley, and probably could be seen for miles. The enemy was apparently unable to interfere in any way with this massive troop movement, and the valley remained peaceful except for the heavy, muffled sounds of slowly moving traffic and the explosions of artillery fire far off in the distance.

What we were seeing on the road below was the 85th Mountain Infantry with its attached units moving from the left side of the division front to the right. Although the column as we saw it was traveling bumper-to-bumper at an easy pace, the head of this column was still meeting pockets of resistance, and wiping them out as they moved forward. The division was still advancing, two regiments abreast, the 87th on the left, and the 85th on the right. We, the 86th, had once more been designated division reserve, and were scheduled to follow along the road behind the 85th, once they had cleared the area. As the other two regiments advanced, they were to spread out a bit, and our regiment was to move up to an area behind and between them, and prepare to attack wherever it might be advantageous or necessary. This would once again place us almost exactly in the center of the division front.

Our turn on the road began at about 6 p.m. The weather had been unusually warm and dry for about a week, and the road was dusty. The men marched on foot, carrying their packs, but were not loaded down with extra ammunition this time because the battalion vehicles were with us. Our medical detachment even had extra vehicles. In addition to the jeep and our 3/4-ton truck, we had the two ambulances and a second jeep, and I believe that all of the medics except the company aid men, who marched with their platoons, were able to ride. We encountered no enemy shelling and the five-yard interval between men was ignored.

The men marched until dark, and then marched some more, stopping to rest for only five minutes each hour. The vehicles crawled along with them. Several times we all dismounted and everyone took cover in the ditches and fields while a plane flew over us in the dark. These planes didn't look like fighters and were probably our own observation planes, because they left us alone, but we "hit the dirt" anyway, because we couldn't take unnecessary chances. Sometimes we had to pull off of the road to allow a convoy of large trucks go by at a high rate of speed on its way to supply the troops up ahead, and then we would have to get off again when they returned, one and two at a time.

Shortly after midnight we reached our next assembly point. The weary troops turned off of the road into quickly designated company areas, dug well-dispersed foxholes and tried to get some sleep. We didn't unpack the aid station equipment, and I'm sure we holed up in some kind of building, but I don't remember now where it was or what it looked like.

As soon as things had settled down, another briefing session was called at the Battalion Command Post, and there I learned what was in store for us when the dawn arrived. The regiment would attack again at 8 a.m. to take the town of Ponte Ronca, then head northwest to cut Highway 9 in the Po Valley and take the town of Ponte Samoggia. Leading the attack would be our 3rd Battalion; the 1st Battalion would advance on our right, and the 2nd Battalion would march close behind to be committed as needed. The 85th Regiment would be advancing on the right flank, and the 87th Regiment would be advancing on the left, but much farther away. Should we suffer a flank attack on our left, our 2nd Battalion must be ready to meet it.

At 3 a.m. with less than three hours' rest, the battalion moved out again. The infantrymen were on foot, this time carrying full loads of ammunition. Everyone carried K Rations for several days. The march lasted another three hours or so, and sunrise was nearly upon us when we turned off of the main road and marched uphill toward the village of San Lorenzo to the line of departure for our morning attack. By the time we arrived it was light enough to see clearly, and although the dawn was hazy, we could see the flat horizon that was the floor of the Po Valley in the distance. We were on the brink of the breakout!

Our 3rd Battalion jumped off again at 8:30 a.m. There were still a lot of low hills and long ridges between us and the valley floor, and the battalion was mostly afoot with the vehicles following as closely behind as possible, using whatever roads and trails were available. Here and there the forward troops encountered pockets of resistance, and although these encounters would usually begin with a lot of shooting, there seemed to be little difficulty in persuading the Germans to surrender. Enemy artillery opened up about halfway through the morning, and continued incessantly for most of the day. A few enemy tanks were again encountered, and once more the Air Force was called upon to knock them out. We could see our planes bombing and strafing farther out in the valley too, and columns of smoke were rising here and there as a result of their efforts. We learned later that their targets included numerous enemy convoys of men and materiel, which were fleeing in front of our advance.

In his account of the action on the morning of April 20, David Brower states that just as we were descending the last ridge of the Apennines, two of our P-47 fighter planes, which had been flying sorties in the valley ahead of us, went down "just to the right of the battalion." I remember both of them well. Our aid station was on the move at the time, and we were following the infantry on foot. Our vehicles were following behind us as best they could, and trying to stay close in order to evacuate the few casualties we were receiving directly from the field. We were headed north along a wooded ridge near its top, and up ahead and in the valley beyond the ridge to our right, we could hear occasional intense bursts of small arms fire as groups of enemy soldiers were being flushed out. The Germans were surrendering readily in large numbers as soon as our men displayed the awesome concentrations of small arms fire that they could produce. Usually none of our men were hurt in these skirmishes. Our casualties were few, and were caused mainly by artillery and mortar shells, which now seemed to be coming from many different directions, including some from our rear.

As we moved slowly through the woods along the western slope of the ridge, what sounded to me like an artillery piece began firing on the other side of it. I paid little attention to it until all of a sudden the P-47s came swooping down out of the sky to strafe something in that area. I don't remember exactly how many there were, but they came diving down at a steep angle, one at a time, firing as they came, then pulled up, gained altitude, made a wide circle and repeated the attack. It seemed as if they were only a hundred feet or so above the crest of the ridge we were on when they were at the low point in their dive. The firing on the other side of the ridge continued, and since I only had to go a few yards to reach the top, I decided to climb up to see if I could see what was happening.

Staying low to avoid showing my silhouette on the skyline, I peered over the crest of the ridge, and there, perhaps a hundred feet below and a hundred yards away, parked next to a stone building, was a huge enemy tank. It looked bigger than any of ours, and was intermittently firing its long gun at something toward our rear. As I watched, the P-47s broke off their attack and left, probably to refuel and rearm. However, while I was still watching a few minutes later, a single plane came roaring down out of the sky at a very steep angle, with all guns blazing. It was headed directly at the tank, and the pilot didn't pull out of the dive! I watched as the plane continued with undiminished speed, and crashed dead center on the turret of the tank. There was a big explosion, and a huge ball of fire engulfed the area, but not much debris flew from it. I knew that it was impossible for the pilot to have survived, and I was sure that the occupants of the tank were now cooking inside because the whole area was burning with great intensity, so I didn't go down the hill for a closer look.

The pilot of the second plane fared better. We were still advancing along the top of the same ridge, and I first spotted the plane when it was still quite a distance away, because it was trailing smoke. It came flying up the valley toward us at a very low altitude, and just before it came abreast of us the pilot flipped it upside down, dropped out, and opened his chute. The plane continued on and crashed somewhere out of sight behind us just after the pilot landed on a patch of grass in front of a building on the other side of the road in the valley immediately below us. It looked to me as if he had bailed out only about three or four hundred feet above the valley floor, and it seemed as if the chute had hardly opened before he hit the ground.

I raced down the hill with one of the medical technicians and got to him immediately. Both legs were broken, but that seemed to be the extent of his injuries. At first I wondered if the tail of the plane had struck them as he dropped out of it, but quickly realized that this wasn't likely, because at that time his forward velocity and the plane's forward velocity were about the same. Even if the tail had struck him, the difference in velocities would have been so small that serious injury would be improbable. The fractures were painful so I injected the contents of a morphine styrette into his arm immediately, and in a short time we had the legs securely splinted. The medic with me started to fill out the usual casualty tag, which was routinely attached to all casualties in order to let the next doctor in the evacuation chain know what had been done, and when asked his name, I was startled to hear the pilot reply, "Roy Hazen." I was surprised a second time when I heard him say that he was from Detroit.

While I was attending the Detroit Public Schools I had been casually acquainted with a fellow by that name, and I remembered playing for a while on the same neighborhood pickup baseball team with him. He had been a year or two behind me in high school, and again later at Albion College, but I had not seen him in over five years, and I wasn't exactly sure that I could remember what he looked like. By this time the morphine was taking effect and our patient was becoming groggy. Our litter jeep arrived, and since there was still shooting going on all around, this was not a good time for casual conversation. Therefore we loaded him promptly and sent him to the rear.

For many years after this incident I wondered whether or not this pilot was the Roy Hazen I had known. I recently learned that he was not because I have found my old acquaintance still living in southeastern Michigan, and discovered that he had also become a doctor, and that he was still in medical school while I was in Italy.

By noon that day (April 20) we were in the last of the foothills of the Apennines, and an hour later all three battalions of the 86th were on the valley floor. Now there was a slight delay while tanks, tank destroyers and reconnaissance jeeps outfitted with heavy 50 caliber machine guns came out of the hills to lead our advance in the flatlands. The lead infantrymen rode these vehicles and others, and it soon became a pattern to advance a kilometer or so at a time, from one road intersection to the next, dismount and engage the Germans who were trying to impede us until they either surrendered or were killed. There also were many forays laterally into the fields and farm-houses to clean out small pockets of resistance. Many enemy soldiers were bypassed, but they generally posed no problem. Once they realized that they had been isolated from their main forces, they surrendered readily, and as columns of prisoners were being marched to the rear, their numbers continu-ally grew, as more and more thoroughly defeated and disconsolate enemy soldiers came out of the houses and hedges to join them, waving anything they had that was white.

By mid-afternoon the 1st Battalion had reached and straddled Highway 9 a few miles northwest of Bologna, cutting off the enemy's main escape and supply route for his forces on the eastern half of the front. Our 3rd Battalion took the town of Ponte Samoggia early that evening, and before nightfall the entire division was astride Highway 9, and preparing perimeter defenses.

A long and confusing battle was over. The 10th Mountain Division had spearheaded the drive, and was the first division to break out of the Apen-nines into the Po Valley. My battalion had been the point of the spearhead for most of the last four days of the battle. The entire six-day period had been one of unusual activity and confusion, made worse for most of us because we didn't have a completely clear picture of the whole action. My own confu-sion was augmented by chronic fatigue, because during the entire six days it was never possible for any of us to sleep for a decent length of time, and whenever there was time for sleep, it was impossible to sleep in any degree of comfort, because one had to first find a suitably protected shelter some-where, or dig a foxhole out in the open in which to make his bed. Officers generally got less sleep than the men, because during the so-called quiet pe-riods, they frequently had to confer at the various levels of command in order to continually coordinate each step of the advance. Medics, particularly those working in the aid station, also got little sleep because much combat action occurred late in the day, and much of the time casualties were treated and evacuated well on into the night hours.

I admit that I was confused during most of this battle. I hardly knew what day it was, nor did I care, and I was often not certain about exactly where I was. However I always saw to it that our battalion aid station stayed close to M Company, and I usually knew the location of the Battalion Com-mand Post, and I could therefore estimate the relative positions of the line companies. Among many other things, the living from hour to hour, the ac-tivities blending from one day into the next, the uncertainty about my loca-tion at times, and the anxiety about the outcome of my efforts contributed to a considerable confusion concerning parts and details of this period, which I ultimately took home with me.

During the battle my mind was continually filled with the urgent problems of the hour, and at the time I did not expect ever to he writing about what was happening. Therefore, in order to write this story of the breakout with any order or sense to it, I had to spend a lot of time doing research, and in doing it I was pleased to find only minor discrepancies of time, rather than dates or places. The material in my bibliography corresponds well with the events I remembered, and with the material in the letters I wrote home. To the best of my knowledge everything I have written here is true. All of the events I have presented actually happened.

CHAPTER XV

TASK FORCE DUFF

The weather was unusually warm on the afternoon of April 20th when the battalion emerged from the foothills of the Apennines onto the floor of the Po Valley, and some of the men shed shirts and undershirts for a few hours. Although the nature of the fighting didn't change much, combat in the flatland was a new experience. I felt naked and exposed there, and many of the men admitted to having similar feelings. Gone were the ravines and gullies, and the protecting hills to which we had become accustomed. Decent and safe hiding places were few and hard to find.

The infantry companies did not exactly follow the roads, but often attacked from farmhouse to farmhouse across fields and through woodlots, and didn't appear to be having much difficulty getting the Germans who remained in them to surrender. The aid station and Battalion Command Post followed as closely as possible in vehicles, using whatever farm lanes, open fields and roads were available. Out in front of us the P-47s appeared to be having a field day of bombing and strafing, and we hoped that they were knocking out the enemy tanks that we suspected were there. Here and there in the distance columns of smoke were rising where fires had started, and in several places we saw the unmistakable, dense, black smoke of burning petroleum products.

The forward companies encountered very little small arms fire, and at the rear of the battalion there was practically none. However enemy artillery was still active and dangerous, and it seemed to be shelling the roads and approaches to the villages. Because we were moving ahead so rapidly, the bulk of the shells passed over the leading companies, and tended to land among the troops closer to the rear.

Whenever a barrage began, we all jumped out of our vehicles and "hit the ditch," or whatever small depression was handy. These were usually ex-

tremely shallow ditches in an otherwise flat land, and I can still remember
the feeling of utter helplessness, whenever I found myself lying on my belly
in one of them with shells falling all around. Under these circumstances I
couldn't fight, and I had to suppress the almost overwhelming urge for flight,
because standing up in such a situation would probably have been fatal.

As we advanced in the valley, deliriously happy Italians of both sexes
and all ages lined the roads at each farm and at most road intersections. They
cheered and waved. They offered us bread, sausage, and wine, and some of
the women and children threw flowers. When they saw our red crosses, there
were repeated shouts of *"Croce Rosa, Croce Rosa!"* and before long I found
myself holding short medical consultations and treating Italian civilians again.
One farmer gave me several bottles of wine in old, dusty, dark glass bottles,
and we opened one. It contained some excellent sparkling burgundy, so I
slipped the rest of the bottles into my rucksack in the back of the jeep for
drinking at a later time.

These offerings of food and wine made me wonder, because I thought
that the Germans had foraged so thoroughly that there was little left for the
Italians, but Consiglio told me that most of the farmers had been able to
successfully hide more from the Germans than the Germans suspected. Enemy soldiers had also told them that the Americans were short of food, and
often went hungry, so now these people were generously sharing what they
had with us.

Late in the afternoon we reached a main road, and headed northwest on
it. We were on Highway 9, and were following it toward Ponte Samoggia.
The skies were clear and almost cloudless, and our planes were still busy
attacking targets well ahead of us. It appeared that they had so disrupted and
disorganized the retreating enemy that he could no longer use his artillery
effectively, and the firing had all but stopped. The infantrymen, who had
until now walked all of the way, became scroungers, and commandeered all
kinds of vehicles. More and more of them appeared in the column as we
progressed. There were horses and wagons, motor scooters, bicycles, private
automobiles and trucks, and a number of small three-wheeled cars, which
often pulled trailers loaded with our men and their equipment. There were
even some enemy vehicles in our column, with their iron crosses hastily
smeared over. These vehicles had apparently been abandoned for lack of
fuel, but they ran very well on our gasoline.

The forward companies reached Ponte Samoggia at about dusk, and we
had to wait while they captured the town, but when the skirmish was over
they had taken its main bridge still intact, an accomplishment which, I be-

lieve, immediately changed the division battle plan. We followed Battalion Headquarters into town and set up our aid station in a building.

Late that night, April 20-21, in a room dimly lit with candles, the evening staff meeting was held. The regimental and all three battalion staffs were present as well as a number of company commanders. When I arrived I saw that this was going to be a much bigger meeting than usual. A major new operation was in development. A task force was being organized to thrust deep into enemy territory and try to capture the bridge across the Panaro River at Bomporto, some 30 miles north of us, before the enemy could destroy it. I don't remember that we called it TASK FORCE DUFF at the time, but General Robinson Duff, the division executive officer and second in command, had been selected to lead it, and this task force has been known by that name ever since. I can't even remember if General Duff attended the meeting, but he probably was there.

The task force had already been completely planned and our meeting was mainly for the purpose of giving out specific assignments and coordinating operations between its various components. It was to be completely motorized and start for Bomporto at daybreak. To get there it would have to travel the entire distance through enemy territory, completely surrounded, without flank protection, and with an excellent possibility that it would be cut off from our main forces if the enemy opposed it at all. Once the bridge was captured intact, the task force was to defend it and keep it from being destroyed, until our main forces could fight their way up to it.

As the meeting continued, I stayed on the periphery and listened to all of the instructions, but didn't concentrate or pay particular attention to the unit designations of the components of the task force. The Division History states that it was made up of the 2nd Battalion of the 86th Mountain Infantry, Company D of the 751st Tank Battalion, one platoon of the 701st Tank Destroyer Battalion, Company B of the 126th Engineer Battalion and the 91st Armored Reconnaissance Squad, but I remember it a little differently. Only two infantry companies from the 2nd Battalion were included, and as I remember it, they were the only infantry in the task force. Even though I didn't pay much attention to unit designations, I did try to appreciate the numbers of tanks, tank destroyers and armored vehicles involved, and I remember thinking that, considering the task that had been assigned, this was not a very large force.

My complacency was suddenly shattered and the briefing suddenly caught my complete, undivided attention when the medical support for the task force was discussed, and Colonel Hay told me that I had "volunteered" to head the medical contingent. He assured me that I didn't have great cause for worry, because our 3rd Battalion would be coming forward behind us as fast as it possibly could.

The rest of my orders and instructions followed quickly. I would have 14 ambulances with drivers, with which to set up shuttle system for evacuating casualties to the rear. Most of time they would be traveling unprotected through unsecured areas, but would most likely be allowed to pass unmolested, because the farther north we had come the more the Germans had respected the Red Cross. In addition I would have a medical Jeep and a 3/4 ton truck to carry supplies and equipment. I would have some of the 2nd Battalion Medical Detachment enlisted men with me, and the company aid men would travel with their companies.

This staff meeting lasted a long time, and when it was finished, the entire task force plan had been decided. The ambulances and supplies would be coming up from the rear, so I personally didn't have much to do in preparation for the departure. I wondered why I had been picked for this assignment, and whether or not someone in the higher echelon had had this in mind when a week earlier the additional doctor had been assigned to our 3rd Battalion Medical Detachment. I tried to sleep, but anxiety and the anticipation of the events likely to occur during the upcoming trek bothered me, and tired as I was, I slept only fitfully for the rest of the night.

The task force departed from the vicinity of Ponte Samoggia just after dawn, and I soon found myself riding in the jeep somewhere in the rear half of the column. Immediately ahead were two supply trucks, a truckload of infantrymen and then a tank. Immediately behind was the medical supply truck, an ambulance several headquarters vehicles and then another tank. The rest of the ambulances were to follow and establish themselves at pickup points along the route in order to form a shuttle service. As a loaded ambulance passed each pickup point on its way to the rear, the ambulance stationed there would move up one point. As a result, whenever I dispatched a loaded ambulance to the rear the next one had only a short distance to come to pick up the next casualties.

At first there was no enemy opposition, and the task force was able to move ahead rapidly. No one walked so the speed of the column was faster than the approximately 3 miles per hour sustained by infantrymen on foot. The column wasn't very long, because at every crossroads I could see the reconnaisance jeeps speed down the side roads to the right and left, looking for signs of enemy soldiers. We passed by wrecked enemy convoys several times, and I noted that this was not new carnage. The fires had burned themselves out, and the carcasses of dead horses and oxen were bloated, as were the corpses of many, many dead German soldiers. This had been the work of our Air Force two or three days before, and I noted that our planes were still at it up ahead. After we had passed several road crossings, German artillery opened up, not at us, but toward Ponte Samoggia, which was by now well behind us.

Now we ran into enemy opposition in the form of roadblocks at most of the road intersections, and occasionally small arms fire came from some of the farmhouses. We were delayed at almost every crossroad as the Germans tried to slow our advance. In some places it took quite a long time to overrun the enemy strongpoint, but more often there was only a short firefight before we could advance beyond it. Although for most of the day enemy artillery was active all across the front, their shells landed behind us. I don't recall that very much fell near us, nor do I recall much mortar fire. I believe that we were moving ahead so fast, and German communications were so wrecked that the enemy didn't know where we were.

It became standard procedure to capture a group of enemy soldiers at an intersection, speed to the next one, and do it all over again. I was close enough to the head of the column to see the infantry squads unload, deploy into the fields on both flanks and advance to the objective with the lead tanks. A few shots from the 75 mm guns on the tanks and some machine gun fire usually persuaded the Germans to surrender. Then the reconnaissance jeeps would go out in both directions to return in a few minutes, and the column would continue the advance.

Prisoners began to accumulate, and there were so many that they were sent to the rear in marching columns without guards. The rest of the division was following behind us on foot, and would pick them up. Casualties were amazingly light and most of them were German. None were seriously wounded. We treated all alike, and evacuated them to the rear as soon as there was an ambulance full. Among the Germans, some of the walking wounded who weren't disabled, wanted to stay with their comrades, and I let them march to the rear with the other prisoners.

Crowds of jubilant Italians again lined the road, shouting, *"Viva! Salute! Salve! Bravi! Liberatore."* and other things, while dancing in their yards, waving at us, offering eggs, bread, cheese and wine, and throwing flowers at us. The small villages on our route seemed to offer the most enemy opposition, and whenever we approached one, the Italians would all disappear. Then, after the village had been taken and all enemy soldiers had been killed or captured, the crowd would gather again, cheering more enthusiastically than ever, as the rear of our column passed through. In a number of places the natives told us that we were close behind the fleeing enemy, and I believe that this information was relayed to the Air Force, because our planes again became very active in the skies ahead.

Late in the morning we had just passed through a town, and were delayed by a firefight, which was going on at the head of the column, when a German artillery piece opened up, firing toward the town we had just left. Several enemy artillery pieces had already been captured and disabled, but this one had apparently been missed. It was located about 200 yards to our left, and was well hidden with camouflage materials. Some of the men from the trucks in front of us and a couple of medics went out and persuaded the gun crew to surrender without firing another shot. Two German artillery officers and two privates had been manning the gun, and they were sent trudging toward the rear with the next group of prisoners to come along.

At about noon we were held up by a longer-than-usual firefight up ahead, and while it was going on, I remember sitting in the warm sunshine on a low stone wall, eating lunch consisting of K-Rations supplemented with Italian bread and red wine. As the afternoon progressed enemy opposition became much less, and we advanced faster. There were almost no casualties, and this resulted in a longer distance in the gap between the ambulance accompanying me, and the one at the most advanced pickup point behind us.

Sometime around 4 p.m. the head of the column reached the bridge at Bomporto, and took it intact after a short but intense firefight. Explosive charges to destroy the bridge had been placed and wired, but the enemy was apparently surprised by our unexpected arrival, and did not set them off. The leading elements of the column were soon across the bridge and into the town proper, but now there was a delay while the engineers removed the charges before the rest of the column crossed.

While this was going on we set up an aid station in a building at the roadside, and began receiving wounded, mostly German, from the battle for the bridge. There were also some of our men who had become ill, and it wasn't long before I had an ambulance full of casualties to send to the rear. At dusk a sergeant from one of the 2nd Battalion companies came in accompanied by one of his buddies. He looked seriously ill, with face flushed, and he had a fever of over 105 degrees F. After examining him I was pretty sure that he had pneumonia, and when I told him that he would be evacuated he protested that he didn't want to leave his unit. I had to explain his problem in detail, and his buddy had to insist that he go, before the sergeant agreed. I gave him a loading dose of sulfadiazine and some aspirin for the fever, and tried to make him as comfortable as possible on a pallet on the floor, where he soon fell asleep. Several other soldiers came in now with colds and other minor complaints. None wanted to be evacuated, so I treated symptoms and let them return to duty. Three more walking wounded who were not seriously injured but needed formal surgical repair of their wounds came in, and I had them ready for evacuation by the time the next shuttle ambulance arrived. I was then able to evacuate all of the casualties we had left.

The task force had accomplished its mission. It had captured the bridge intact, and the town of Bomporto was in our hands. The rest of the regiment began to arrive much sooner than it had been thought possible, and the 2nd Battalion medics who had been working with me rejoined their detachment as it came past. I rejoined my own unit, which crossed the bridge into the town together with the 3rd Battalion Command Post. While defenses were being prepared for the night, the Regimental Command Post also moved into the town. The whole regiment had reached this objective in record time.

As soon as we arrived in Bomporto, Consiglio made arrangements with the proprietor of a cobbler shop for us to stay there, and we set up the aid station in the large front room, which contained shoe repair equipment and shelves containing customers' shoes. The proprietor was an older man, very patriotic and very emotional. He was so happy to be liberated, that from time to time as he talked about it, he shed real tears. He brought out small Italian and American flags and displayed them in his shop window, and after we were completely set up, he plied us with fried eggs and bread. There were no casualties in the aid station that evening, but civilians soon began to ask for medical help, and for a time I once again had a brisk practice.

Another regimental briefing session was held that evening. I had assumed that the mission of the task force had been completed with the capture of the bridge at Bomporto, but now I learned that not only had the mission been extended to include reaching the Po River as fast as possible, but the size of the task force had also been increased to include the whole division. Because, on this first day, the entire regiment had not only been able to quickly mop up after the task force, but was also able to reach Bomporto so quickly, and because the other two regiments had also been able to move up so quickly that they were now close by and covering both of our flanks, enemy attack upon our rear was improbable. Although flank attacks were anticipated by the other regiments, such attacks could be countered with units reserved for that purpose. It was hoped that the enemy was now so disorganized that he could no longer mount any real resistance, and that our forward progress would be swift.

The increase in the size of the task force created a transport problem.

There were only enough trucks available to carry one battalion of infantry at a time, so an elaborate plan was devised to leapfrog the battalions forward. The advance or attacking battalion would ride, and go forward as rapidly as possible, while the other two battalions would follow on foot and engage in mopping-up activities using only their intrinsic organizational and supply vehicles. At intervals, depending upon the resistance met, the forward battalion would give up the personnel trucks, which would return to pick up one of the rear battalions, and then come forward again, pass through the battalion it had dropped off, and spearhead the rapid advance once more.

No one in the 2nd Battalion slept that night because that battalion started out immediately at about 10 p.m. (April 21). They followed the road north toward the city of San Benedetto Po, which was very close to the Po River. Part of their mission was to establish strongpoints at all of the bridges along the route, so that the Germans couldn't destroy them. At about 4 a.m. (April 22) the 2nd Battalion gave up the trucks, which then came back to pick up our 3rd Battalion. Together with our intrinsic vehicles plus some extra supply and ammunition trucks, we formed in a column, which left on the road to San Benedetto about fifteen minutes later. As we passed through the 2nd Battalion we picked up tanks, tank destroyers, self-propelled guns, heavy artillery, signal corps people, engineers and reconnaissance units, all of which had their own transportation. This made a much longer column, and appeared to me to be a much more formidable force than the one I had been in the day before. About an hour out from our passage through the 2nd Battalion there was a delay because a bridge was out. After some scouting about, an alternate route was found with its bridge still intact, and after using the detour we were soon back on the road to San Benedetto again.

We had traveled only a short distance farther when our column was attacked by four German tanks accompanied by infantry. This occurred well up ahead of me so I didn't actually see the action, but it was a serious situation. The German tanks had long barreled 88 mm cannons, compared to ours which had shorter 75 mm guns, and this gave them significantly more range and firepower than our tanks. The German tanks also had thicker armor plate than ours, which made it harder to knock them out. The ensuing fight resulted in two of the German tanks being destroyed and left burning, while the other two retreated. Most of the enemy infantry was either killed or captured, and eventually our column moved forward again.

Mid-morning found us still advancing in the vanguard of the division task force. Cheering and gesticulating Italians again lined the roads, demonstrating their happiness at being freed from the Germans, and again plying us with eggs, bread, cheese and wine. They also supplied us with the information that a large group of Germans had just passed through, and that the "Fascisti" were aiding them. Some of the Fascists were even said to be wearing German or Partisan uniforms, and fighting alongside the Germans.

Our combat procedure was the same as it had been the day before. There would be a short fire fight at a crossroad at the head of the column, and when it subsided the reconnaissance vehicles would go out to the right and left, and another group of prisoners would start walking without guards, to the rear.

Throughout the day portions of our column were stopped when German vehicles and columns of vehicles came up to us, not realizing we were American until too late. These were mainly rear echelon troops, which had been bypassed and were trying to get back North of the Po River before we cut them off, and they surrendered easily. Most of the German soldiers we now encountered surrendered meekly, and it seemed as if there were always hundreds of them marching in long lines, unguarded, to our rear. Most were happy to become prisoners of the Americans, rather than the British or Russians, and many expressed a fear of reprisals from the Italian Partisans that were now active in large numbers behind their lines. Later that afternoon, because of the Partisan activity, German officers were allowed to keep sidearms, and later we even saw columns of prisoners, guarded by their own German soldiers carrying rifles, marching in orderly columns to our rear.

The column made excellent time when we were moving, but there were frequent stops, not only to fight, but for such things as deciding which fork in the road to take. Reconnoitering became necessary because the division had advanced so rapidly that we had gone off of the maps that were available to us, and we often questioned the natives in order to avoid wrong turns. Whenever a stop was made, the distance between vehicles would shorten until each one came to a full stop only a few feet behind the one ahead. We normally stayed in the vehicles, unless we received the signal from up front that there would be time to dismount for a while. Whenever we dismounted, happy Italians would surround us, and occasionally German soldiers came out of the houses to give themselves up.

During one stop that afternoon, I noticed that before we had time to dismount an unusually large number of Italians had surrounded our vehicles, but suddenly they vanished. Just as I wondered what had happened to them, I heard firing and saw an enemy armored car, poorly camouflaged with a few branches, speeding toward us from our left, with machine guns blazing. Just ahead of my jeep was a supply truck, then some truckloads of infantrymen from M Company. There was instant scrambling as everyone left the vehicles in a hurry. I hopped out of the jeep, vaulted over a low stone wall, crouched behind it, and peered forward in time to see one of our tanks, which was standing slightly ahead of the M Company trucks, rotating its 75 mm gun barrel around past its rear to point toward the oncoming enemy vehicle which was still coming at us at a high rate of speed and still firing its guns. When it reached a point about 150 yards away, our tank fired and scored a direct hit. I saw bodies fly up out of the vehicle. A second shot came within seconds, and the enemy armored car, now completely stopped, went up in flames.

The danger was now over, and men arose from the ditches up and down the column. I ran forward to survey the carnage caused by the German machine guns, and was amazed to find that no one had been hurt. A bullet had grazed one man's finger, and I gave him a supply of band-aids. The incident had produced no American or Italian casualties.

Before long, however, we suffered an attack in which we were not so lucky. A flight of our P-38 fighters passed overhead, and in spite of the fact that all of our vehicles carried panels on top to identify them as American, they turned one at a time to dive upon and strafe our column. During this advance we had often passed wreckage and carnage caused by such action, and I am sure that most of us were terrified to have our own planes attack our column. The main point of the attack was some distance ahead of where I was, but everyone in my vicinity departed the vehicles and ran as fast away from them laterally as they could. Yellow smoke was the signal to our aircraft that we were friendly, and yellow smoke grenades were set off immediately. Soon large amounts of thick, yellow smoke were rising from many points along the column, but the planes didn't break off the attack until after three of them had strafed the column. Some of our men were killed, but I don't remember exactly how many, and I didn't stop to count because there were also a number of seriously wounded men needing attention.

The stop and go advance continued all afternoon without encountering any serious enemy opposition. We were mainly bypassing enemy units and collecting prisoners by the dozens. The Germans were more eager than ever to surrender, and many admitted that they feared the Italian Partisans who were becoming more and more active behind their lines.

At dusk our time to ride ended, and I watched the personnel trucks return toward the rear. The infantrymen set out on foot once more. This didn't change the transport for us in the medical detachment, because we had our organizational vehicles and ambulances to ride, but forward progress would now be much slower. As the last of the trucks were leaving there was a sudden outburst of intense firing a short way ahead of us and to the right of the column. I thought at first we were being attacked by a large force of Germans with tanks and artillery, but the uproar ended too quickly for this to be so. We continued to advance, and as we passed the next crossroad I saw a number of burning enemy trucks that had apparently been carrying ammunition when they were spotted and destroyed by one of our tank destroyers.

The advance on foot continued on into the evening, and although we progressed much more slowly now, we were clearing the enemy from his positions much more thoroughly. Larger numbers of prisoners were willingly giving themselves up. The 1st Battalion arrived well after dark in the trucks we had sent back, and passed through us to take the lead in the advance. The rural roadway was narrow with hardly any shoulder on which to stop while the big trucks passed, and in most places the ditches were deep and filled with water, so we could not drive off into the fields. Somehow we managed to let the 1st Battalion pass through, but after that things didn't improve much. We still had task force armor and reconnaissance vehicles with us, and the tactical situation required that some of them move up and down the column frequently. There were also vehicles coming and going as liaison between the rear and the 1st Battalion ahead. The ambulance shuttle was still working, and occasionally an ambulance would pass by. On one stretch of road, which ran along the edge of a canal, the shoulder was so narrow that it was hard to find enough room to pull off to allow a tank to pass. Wherever there was even a marginal amount of space on the shoulder the vehicles would pull off in a crowded bumper-to-bumper line, with vehicles so close together that getting back on the road became difficult.

While we were on this stretch of road, a small enemy plane flew very low over us. Everything in the column stopped and everybody took to what little cover there was. Our men had orders not to fire at planes, and no one did. The plane circled and flew back across the column again, about 100 feet above the second vehicle on the road ahead of my jeep, and I clearly saw the iron crosses on the wings. Someone in the vicinity identified it as a Stuka, and as it disappeared into the night I remember thinking that it appeared small and had a weak engine sound compared to our P-47s and P-38s.

Sometime after midnight we stopped for the rest of the night in a small town, and established the Battalion Command Post and the aid station in some buildings. We didn't unpack any of our equipment because we had no casualties at the time. The infantrymen were dispersed in a defense perimeter around us, getting whatever sleep they could in foxholes.

That night the information we received at the battalion briefing was very tentative and sketchy. The only communication we had with anyone was by radio and that was often none too good. We had no maps, but estimated that we were about ten miles from the Po River and the one bridge over it that our Air Force had not destroyed. Enemy troops by the thousands were heading toward it to cross the river and avoid being cut off. Earlier in the evening somewhere ahead of us the 1st Battalion had been engaged by a large enemy force, including tanks and bazookas, which had destroyed a number of their vehicles, and the battle was still going on.   We had bypassed this action and were again in the lead, but the 2nd Battalion was now coming up in trucks once more, and we would follow it toward the bridge at daylight. We could see that ahead of us in the direction of San Benedetto there was a lot of activity. Much of it looked like ammunition dumps being blown up, and we speculated as to whether the Germans were doing it in preparation for clearing out of the territory south of the river, or whether the Partisans were freely executing their sabotage plans. Our situation remained tense for the rest of the night, and most of us slept only fitfully.

At daylight on April 23 we began to advance again. The 2nd Battalion was now ahead of us but was apparently having a problem in starting their advance, so we turned West toward another main highway in order to bypass them. On the way we came across several abandoned enemy artillery pieces, and made sure that they were permanently put out of action by welding the breeches closed with thermite bombs, as we had done to all of the big guns we had earlier found or captured. Then we came upon a really "Big Bertha," a huge, long-barreled gun mounted on a platform as big as a railroad flatcar, with many axles and rubber tired wheels. Our column had stopped for a while, and my jeep was at the edge of the field in which the gun stood. Several Italians were standing around looking at it, and some of our engineers went out to make sure that the gun was incapable of being fired. I also walked over to it with some of my men to get a closer look. This was a huge gun, and guesses as to the size of the bore were anywhere from 280 to 360 mm. Only the 16-inch guns on the largest of battleships were bigger (400 mm). The barrel was level with the ground and aimed toward the road at about a 45-degree angle. One of the Italians in the group around it now told us the story of this gun, and one of our soldiers interpreted. First he pointed out the row of tall umbrella pine trees bordering the road in the area where the gun was aimed about a quarter of a mile away, and he emphasized that one of the trees in the row was missing. Then he said that the Germans had abandoned the gun fully loaded and ready to fire. Later when a group of Italians were curiously inspecting the gun, one of them did something to it, and it went off. The shell hit the trunk of the missing tree a few meters above the ground and exploded, destroying much of the tree trunk, and toppling its umbrella top to the ground. A little while later when we went by that stump, I noticed that its end had been reduced to shreds like toothpicks, the adjacent tree trunks were gouged and badly damaged, and the earth all around was torn up. I believed the story.

When we reached the main road we turned north on it, and thought that we once again were leading the regiment's advance. We were now on a wide road with much wider shoulders than we had ever been on before. The terrible destruction that our Air Force had inflicted upon the German convoys the previous day was awesome, and was evident everywhere along the route. An unbelievable number of wrecked and burned enemy vehicles lay strewn about on both sides. Smoke still rose from the wreckage in places. Some vehicles had a dead and badly burned driver at the wheel, and some contained other corpses. Dozens of dead German soldiers were scattered about, and many of them were severely torn up or badly burned. Sometimes there were only pieces of bodies recognizable to mark what had once been human beings. Most conspicuous of all were the dead horses, and there were so many that it was hard to believe that there were any left at all on the Italian farms.

We also found German vehicles intact, abandoned because they had run out of fuel. Some had just been left at the roadside, but many had been pushed off into barns and sheds, or into the fields where attempts had been made to camouflage them with branches or straw. At one point we came upon a German motor pool full of vehicles, including a dozen or so large vans, like the moving vans we used at home to move furniture, and in that motor pool I noted that some of the German trucks had American tires on their wheels. I distinctly remember seeing the brand name "Firestone," and I believe that there were also tires made by Goodyear on some of those enemy vehicles. This reminded me of the 92nd Division fiasco of the Christmas past, and I surmised that the enemy might have gotten these tires as a result of it.

Although at this time we were not officially the mechanized battalion, we had commandeered or captured enough motorized vehicles so that everyone rode. There were plenty of captured enemy trucks available, but these were dangerous because sometimes our men would fire upon them, so few were used, and those that were included in our caravan had the German crosses carefully covered up. The vehicles our men used were many and varied. Civilian trucks and trailers were popular, and at every opportunity our men upgraded their transport. There seemed to be no dearth of talent in the ranks when it came to jump starting a car or truck.

We now entered a more industrialized area, and the road was lined with what appeared to be small factories, warehouses, and shipping yards. One building that we entered was a German supply depot containing mostly food items, blankets, and a few articles of clothing. I was mainly interested in the food, and took some chocolate bars and some bars of dehydrated split pea soup with me. The chocolate was of extra fine quality, and the pea soup tasted remarkably like that which my mother and grandmother had made at home.

A little bit farther along, we entered another warehouse and found it piled high with cases, some containing bottles of an excellent French champagne, and some containing bottles of cognac. Several of us immediately had the same idea, and with the battalion commander's permission a "work detail" was recruited to return to the German motor pool, commandeer several of the moving vans, load them with as much of this good stuff as possible, and follow us for the rest of the War. This worked out perfectly as planned, and for a while, after the fighting was over, every man in the battalion received a bottle of one kind or the other every other day. Once the moving vans were safely loaded and back in our midst, we were generous about telling people from other units where we had found the stuff, even giving specific directions on how to get there. In the same yard, not far away there was a similar building which we had investigated, and found it to be filled with peculiarly shaped "dishpans" which no one recognized until I pointed out that they were douche bowls. Several times in the next few days I heard that the building containing the beverages had been cleaned out completely, but the douche bowls still remained.

In addition to the many abandoned enemy trucks and cars we were now finding a lot of self-propelled artillery pieces with empty fuel tanks. These were usually hidden in sheds and barns, or camouflaged in the fields. After the first few were discovered they were searched for diligently, because we didn't want any bypassed Germans turning them upon us later from our rear. The engineers were kept busy putting them permanently out of action with thermite bombs.

We marched into San Benedetto Po in the early afternoon, only to march right out again and bivouac in a hayfield on the outskirts of the town. There the companies established defensive positions designed to repel any attack coming from the South, and this seemed very odd at the time.

We now learned that Colonel John Hay had been moved up to become the regimental executive officer, and Major William Drake assumed command of the 3rd Battalion. The change didn't disturb me at all. I had great confidence in both of these men, and was sure that the battalion would be well led by Major Drake. I was also quite happy about Colonel Hay's transfer to Regimental Headquarters, and felt that it would strengthen the regimental command considerably.

CHAPTER XVI

ACROSS THE PO

When we entered San Benedetto Po shortly after noon on April 23, we were surprised to find the Regimental Command Post already established there. We thought that we would be the first to arrive, because we thought that the 1st Battalion had been delayed by the severe battle in which it had engaged during the previous night, and that the 2nd Battalion had also been delayed because some of the troop transport trucks had been shot up in the same battle. The order to leave the town immediately and establish defenses facing the South also confused us, and it wasn't until later in the afternoon that the situation became clear. We had not arrived first at the head of the task force after all, because when we had stopped for the night (April 22-23), the 85th and 87th Regiments had continued, and had arrived at the Po River well ahead of us. Regimental Headquarters and our 2nd Battalion, riding in the trucks, had also arrived ahead of us, and by the time we finally marched into town and became a part of the division reserve, the 87th was already beginning to cross the river.

We had no sooner finished setting up our defenses, when we received word to be prepared to move out on two hours' notice to make the river crossing. That evening we were relieved from our defensive positions by the 10th Antitank Battalion, and carrying our equipment in the expectation of crossing in assault boats, we began the march to the river in the dark at 9:00 p.m.

It must be remembered that nowhere in the overall planning for the Allied Forces in Italy and nowhere in its training was it anticipated that the 10th Mountain Division would ever make an assault across a major river. Crossing the Po was to have occurred well to the East in the British Eighth Army sector. The initial breakout into the Po Valley had been planned to occur there, but when the 10th Mountain Division was first to break into the Po

Valley and had established itself in its entirety around Ponte Samoggia, it was also destined to become the first across the Po. In the original plan our division was to have crossed much later under more peaceful conditions, to help police northwest Italy after the end of the War. No bridging equipment or special river crossing personnel had even been assigned to IV Corps, let alone our division, and what there was of such equipment in Italy was stored somewhere far to the east and well behind us.

It was fortunate that when we first broke out of the Apennines and began to advance across the Po Valley, someone higher up the command had had the foresight to order up some assault boats and paddles to be delivered to the town of Anzola, where 50 of them were turned over to our division late in the evening on April 22. As soon as these boats reached the riverbank a little after 8:00 a.m. on April 23, the decision to cross was made, and the companies of the 87th started across shortly after noon. They had already established a beachhead, and the 85th was in the process of crossing the river by the time we were relieved by the antitank men.

We marched to an assembly area where we waited for quite a while. Enemy shells were falling into the areas all around us, but none came close enough to cause any great alarm. While we waited, some enemy bombers flew over and dropped a few bombs some distance behind us. Before long we continued on foot and headed for the river. The infantrymen were again heavily loaded, but carried only weapons and ammunition, and the medics carried only medical supplies and aid station equipment. Strict blackout conditions were observed. The march was interrupted frequently for various reasons, and several times we had to stop take cover because enemy shells dropped in close to our column.

At about 3 a.m. (April 24) we reached some woods near the river, and I could see that there was only a road and a narrow strip of brushy terrain between us and the riverbank. There weren't enough boats to take the whole battalion across at one time, so the crossing was made in waves of several boats crossing at the same time. The medics, and I with them, went in the last wave, and after we were across, one of the other battalions of the 86th began making its crossing.

We waited quietly in the woods while the boats were making the early trips. It was dark and damp there, and the night had turned cold. The men were only lightly clothed, because it had been hot in the valley for several days, and many shivered as they waited. Enemy shells passed overhead occasionally, but landed well behind us.

Finally word came for our group to approach the boats, and we crossed the road to the riverbank. There, in the bright moonlight, I had my first and only close look at one of these craft. It was an ugly sheet metal scow that didn't look very manageable or sturdy, but it was deep and had plenty of freeboard. Each boat held twelve men, and three engineers with paddles provided the power. We climbed aboard rapidly and kneeled, six on each side with our packs and gear piled between us in the middle. Two engineers paddled at the rear, and one was stationed at the prow.

Boats were loaded quickly, and a group of them, mine included, was shoved out onto the river. There was plenty of moonlight, and as we crossed, I could see the other boats and the men in them very clearly. I was certain that we could be easily seen from either shore. We heard small arms fire to the north and West of us. Artillery was falling in the same general area, and also behind us on the south side of the river, but no shot of any kind was fired at us while we were on the water. I was thankful that we were going into the rear of an established beachhead, instead of making a fresh, direct assault into enemy territory.

The river at this point appeared to be a little more than 200 Yards wide, and it took some ten to fifteen minutes to paddle across. Its surface was smooth, but there was a current, and we drifted downstream as we crossed. Dawn was just breaking in the east as I stepped out of the boat onto a sandbank on the other side, and as I strapped my rucksack to my back and picked up a bag of equipment and my first aid kit, I thought about the engineers and their return trip. Even though the boat would be completely empty it would probably take them longer to go back, because they would have to paddle some distance upstream.

We didn't linger on the shore, but quickly joined the forming battalion column and marched for several miles to another assembly area near the town of Governolo on the banks of the Mincio River where we dug foxholes and set up defensive perimeters once more. The Mincio is a tributary of the Po, which flows from Mantua *(Mantova)* almost parallel to the Po at this point, and empties into it a few miles downstream. We would have to cross it to continue our advance toward the north. Although the bridges had all been bombed out, this river wasn't as wide as the Po, and the engineers quickly ran a pontoon bridge across near one of them, which was sturdy enough to carry all of the traffic needed. The 2nd Battalion, and then the 1st followed closely behind us, and before noon the whole regiment was together again, awaiting the new orders, which were not long in coming. We had crossed the Po River without suffering any casualties, and for that I was thankful.

CHAPTER XVII

TASK FORCE DARBY - VERONA

Later in the morning, not long after we had crossed the Po River, orders for our next assignment arrived. Our regiment (the 86th Mountain Infantry) had been chosen to become yet another task force, complete with tanks, tank destroyers, self-propelled artillery, reconnaissance vehicles, engineers, etc., to advance northward, bypass Mantua *(Mantova)*, and proceed as rapidly as possible along Highway 62 to capture the historic city of *Verona*. It was important to take this city quickly to seal off the main escape route for all of the Germans who had been bypassed in the recent actions, and also to trap most of the enemy units located all over northwest Italy. Their main escape route ran from Verona up through the Brenner Pass, and there was only one lesser pass, quite a distance west of Brenner, which might also be used. Once Verona was in our hands, the back of the enemy forces in Italy would be broken, and it would be very difficult for the German Armies to escape into Austria.

General Duff had been wounded and evacuated the day before as his task force had approached San Benedetto, and the division artillery commander, General Ruffner, then led Task Force Duff to its successful completion. General Duff's sudden departure left the division staff without an executive officer, and within hours Colonel William 0. Darby was named in his place. Colonel Darby was already famous as the commander of Darby's Rangers, a unit which had seen action in North Africa, and had gained a reputation as one of the toughest, most efficient fighting forces in the American Army. His first assignment in this new position was to lead the task force to take Verona.

Task Force Darby immediately faced a major problem. Jeeps and some of the lighter vehicles were able to get across the Po River soon after the beachhead was established, but the heavier trucks, self-propelled howitzers, and especially the tanks we needed were another matter. The engineers were still at work on the bridge, and our advance toward Verona had to be delayed until the heavy vehicles could come across. We therefore remained in place near Governolo during the night, and expected to start out early the next morning. However, when dawn came there was another delay because the bridge still wasn't ready. Finally, at about midday (April 25), by working continually around the clock, the engineers had it finished well enough for heavy vehicles to cross, and at 2:30 p.m. we received the word that our armor was on its way. In the meantime, early that morning, the 1st Battalion of the 85th had advanced northward some 40 miles out of the beachhead, and captured the airfield at Villafranca.

We left our assembly area at 4:30 p.m., and following the same route toward the airfield, arrived somewhere near it just before dusk. There was now another delay, and we waited at the roadside for the armor and other units to come up and integrate themselves into our column. Although we came very close to it, I never did see the airfield itself.

When the heavy vehicles finally arrived, Task Force Darby was complete, and got under way without further delay at about 9 p.m. Everyone rode in some kind of a vehicle. Nobody walked. There were more tanks, tank destroyers, self-propelled howitzers and other heavy vehicles in this column than I had seen in Task Force Duff, and there also seemed to be more trucks, including a number of captured enemy trucks which had been completely repainted in order to cover up the iron crosses. They had also been stenciled with the white star insignia of the Allied Forces in order to identify them as friendly to us. Engineer units with bridging equipment, including long spans of what appeared to be Bailey bridge sections, were also present in the column.

There was almost no opposition to our advance, and the few times that infantry was needed, the men left their trucks, quickly did the needed mopping up, and climbed aboard the vehicles again. The enemy had apparently not had time to destroy the roadway and bridges, and whatever minor repairs were needed from time to time were quickly accomplished by the engineer outfits with us. Prisoner of war cages were set up every 10 miles along the way, and ambulance stations as well as casualty pickup points were located along the route near them, but casualties were so few and so minor that they were not really needed. Ambulances, which were also included within the column, were sufficient to directly evacuate the few casualties that occurred.

The routine followed during this advance was like that of the previous task forces. The head of the column entered every crossroads cautiously, and stopped a little beyond it. Then reconnaissance vehicles went out in three directions to probe for enemy positions. Usually none were found because the Germans had apparently retreated well ahead of us. The column then sped to the next road intersection, and repeated the process. The head of the column was too far ahead for me to see this happening, but I knew it was going on, and from time to time, whenever we crossed a particularly wide, main road, there were our tanks or tank destroyers, stationed at a distance, one on each side, to guard against a flank attack. In the darkness we passed through villages that seemed deserted, and the few Italians we did see all gave us the same message, *"Tedeschi tutto via."* "The Germans are all gone."

Around 2 a.m., while we were stopped at the roadside, my section of the column was attacked by an enemy plane. Most of us were already out of the vehicles stretching our legs, when we heard the plane, flying low and coming in from our left. No one paid particular attention to it until someone yelled, "Hey, that's not ours!" By this time the plane had started to dive at us, and I just had time to drop to the ground near the shoulder of the road next to my jeep. The plane roared down with machine guns chattering. It seemed to be diving straight at me, and then I saw the row of dancing sparks made by steel, or steel jacketed machine gun bullets striking the pavement between my jeep and the tank, which stood about 30 feet in front of it. As the plane pulled out of its dive and passed overhead I rolled over just in time to see the iron crosses on its wings. We had strict orders not to fire at any planes, and no one did. The plane circled at a low altitude over the area to our right, crossed back over the column again, and flew off to the northwest. I called out to see if anyone had been hurt, and was glad to find that no one had been hit.

There were several strange things about this aerial attack that puzzled me. No one had recognized the type of plane. To me it seemed unusually small and flimsy compared to our fighters. The machine gun fire, which had bounced off of the pavement only a few feet from me seemed to lack the power and authority of that which I had recently witnessed coming from our planes. These observations made me wonder if this perhaps had been a Fascist pilot in an Italian plane. Another thing, which puzzled me, is the fact that one of our planes would have strafed the column lengthwise, not at right angles. Perhaps the pilot didn't know that we were Americans, and deliberately missed to see if we would fire back at him. When no one did, he may have concluded that we were a German column. We shall never know.

We continued to travel along Highway 62 in this manner all night, and reached the outskirts of Verona at dawn. Our introduction to the city was spectacular and memorable, and is well described in David R. Brower's account of our entrance into the city in "Remount Blue," the history of our 3rd

Battalion. I quote directly from it:

"….., the 3rd Battalion continued through the night in rapid pursuit, and approached the outskirts of Verona at 0600 (6 am.) on the 26th. At that hour Verona's several bridges were blown by the fleeing Germans, in an explosion so great that shock waves could be seen to spread in swiftly expanding concentric circles in the cirrus clouds, after which a column of dust and smoke mushroomed into the sky.

As we reached the marshalling yard we came upon a macabre sight. At a main intersection a number of Kraut trucks were strewn about in disorder. One truck, loaded with ammunition and pyrotechnics, was burning furiously with a beautiful display of signal flares and colored smokes. On the road around the truck were bodies; some were badly dismembered, others were charred and motionless, and a few were still moaning and writhing. One German officer, blinded at least by blood, lay in the rubble with his hands over a sucking wound in his chest. Sullen German aid men—at least they wore the red cross—wouldn't touch him until ordered to do so by Captain Meincke, the battalion surgeon, when he came upon the scene, and launched into an effective German tirade."

I remember the massive explosion and the cloud of dust and smoke which rose into the sky when the bridges were blown up. I was far enough back in the column to get a panoramic view of it, and although at the time the general public had not yet seen pictures of the mushroom cloud of an atomic bomb explosion, I know now that this is what it looked like.

We arrived at the river a short time later, and the bridges had indeed been blown, but the one to which our route took us still had a narrow bit of the roadbed left intact. None of our vehicles could cross it to enter the inner city, but men on foot could walk across unimpeded. As we in the medical detachment crossed, foot soldiers of the 2nd Battalion and most of those of our 3rd Battalion were already in the city, mopping up and taking prisoners.

A lot of rubble, several wrecked enemy vehicles, and the burning German truck were within sight of the bridge, and the scene was just as Lieutenant Brower described it. First I checked the dozen or so bodies which were lying about. The dismembered ones were most certainly dead. Some of the other charred and blackened bodies still showed an occasional gasp or a bit of agonal movement, but I was sure that there was no one salvageable or able to survive in this group. Treatment of any kind was not indicated, because it was quite apparent that all were too far gone to be having any pain or suffering. Next I turned my attention to the German officer with the open chest wound, who had by this time managed to crawl away from the mass of dead bodies. I had the German medics pick him up, and told them where to move him, so that I could examine him more easily. The medics themselves still appeared to be dazed, and while I was telling them what to do, I had to repeat myself several times. These instructions were probably what Lieutenant Brower interpreted as an "effective German tirade," although they weren't meant to be anything of the kind.

The German officer had a large, open hole in the right side of his chest, and was very short of breath. I could see lung tissue inside. The lung didn't appear to be to be lacerated and there was hardly any blood visible in the chest cavity, so I immediately applied the standard dressing for pneumothorax and made sure that its one-way valve action was working properly. I was quickly reassured that the treatment was effective, because the man's respiratory rate improved promptly. Although there was black soot all over his face, hands and uniform, he seemed to have been burned hardly at all, and I felt that he could survive.

Just as I was about to tell the two German medics how to evacuate their wounded officer, one of the charred bodies lying near the burning truck startled us. It rose to its feet and walked slowly toward me, looking like a blackened ghoul arising from the rubble in a horror movie. I quickly stepped over to meet the man, and spoke to him, but I don't think he heard me. I gently led him over to a nearby wall, sat him down so he leaned against it, and took a closer look. Most of the flesh was burned away on both hands, and a lot of exposed and charred bone was visible. His head and neck had been burned black; his eyelids had been almost burned away, and the corneas at the front of the eyeballs had been coagulated white by the heat. He couldn't close his eyes, and this gave his face an eerie, ghoulish expression. When I exposed his torso and arms, wherever it wasn't charred the skin appeared to be cooked all the way through. The burns were all third degree, and involved practically his whole body surface. I was sure that survival was impossible. I also knew that third degree burns are painless, because the nerve endings which pick up pain sensation in the skin are dead, but I asked loudly and repeatedly if he had any pain. There never was any reply. The man was still breathing shallowly, and although there must have been a pulse, I couldn't find it. He still moved his limbs occasionally, but never made a sound. Once when I thought I detected a bit of a facial grimace, I did wonder if he were having some pain, so I emptied the contents of a morphine styrette as deep as I could into his arm, and left him sitting there.

I turned my attention back to the wounded officer again, and found him in a much improved condition, so I told the German medics to carry him on their litter, across the bridge, and along the road over which we had come. If they saw other prisoners being marched to the rear, they could ask for help with the carrying. They were to take their patient to the first of our ambulances that they saw, to be evacuated, and they might possibly be allowed to go with him if they volunteered. Then I watched them carry their burden across the damaged bridge and on down the road, and that was the last I ever saw of them.

I turned again to the burned German soldier that I had left propped against the wall, and found that in those few minutes he had died. I left him sitting there, with the charred skeletons of his hands in his lap, and the opaque, whitened corneae of his eyes staring straight ahead, but seeing nothing.

We went on into the old walled city and set up the aid station in an empty store. The whole city seemed to be in an uproar with deliriously happy Italians singing and dancing in the streets, and the mopping up operations were almost a lark. The Italians seemed eager to tell where any remaining Germans were hiding, and to expose those who tried to escape by changing into civilian clothes. Local Partisans were rounding up known Fascists and carting them off to jail.

The 1st Battalion didn't come into the city. Instead, with the aid of the engineers and their bridging equipment, they crossed the Adige River with tanks, tank destroyers and self-propelled artillery, and continued to advance, this time to the northwest, to the town of Bussolengo.

By noon things had pretty well settled down inside Verona. We received word that we might stay there for a few days, and this made everyone happy, because we had now been on the move for some twelve days and nights during which no one ever got a full night's sleep. The Italians were generous about offering rooms and beds in their homes, and I think that by mid-afternoon every man in the battalion had made arrangements for a bed in which to sleep that night.

Our men in the medical detachment had carried medical supplies and equipment in their rucksacks, and we now had no rations. When I checked at Battalion Headquarters about getting some, I learned that a Regimental Supply Depot was being set up about a block away, so three of us set out on foot to find it. As we walked down the street, a large, three-wheeled motor scooter, driven by one of our soldiers and pulling a flatbed trailer loaded with cases of rations, passed us. None of our vehicles could cross the river yet, but our supply people had already commandeered vehicles within the city to transport materiel. We followed the load of rations down the street to the Regimental Supply Depot, and found that already an impressive number of supplies had been stocked. Near the center of the room were two piles side by side, one of C Rations and one of K Rations, and when I presented my request the supply sergeant pointed to them, and told us to help ourselves.

I had met this supply sergeant several times before, and recognized him, but I don't remember his name. The first time was at Camp Swift, where he had already developed a reputation for running a very efficient operation. Now, I could tell that something was bothering him, and he was mad.

Some headquarters men followed us into the warehouse, and also sensed that something was wrong. When one of them asked what was the matter, the story came out:

Shortly before we arrived, a major and a lieutenant from the American Military Government had come into the depot to get some rations, and the sergeant had treated them just as he had treated us, by telling them to help themselves. The major looked at the pile of K Rations, then at the pile of C Rations. Then he raised his nose into the air, and said something to the effect that he and his people couldn't eat that swill. They were accustomed to dining formally, on things like fried chicken and roast beef. I don't exactly remember what the outcome of the encounter was, but the supply sergeant was obviously still holding his pent-up ire in check.

My sympathies were with the sergeant. These Military Government people seemed to have no idea of the supply problems inherent in a military campaign such as the one that we had just finished. With supply runs of up to a hundred miles, much of it through enemy territory, and hundreds of items needed, I often wondered how the supplies kept up with us. During my entire combat experience, I don't remember a single time when what we needed was not available. If it wasn't available instantly, it always became so in a remarkably short time. In my opinion the division's supply personnel come high on the list of unsung heroes.

We carried both C and K Rations back to the aid station, ate lunch, and settled in to stay for a while. That afternoon I held a formal sick call for the first time in many days, and afterward things had settled down well enough so that I also treated a few civilians.

At about 5 p.m. the city went wild. Church bells rang, cannons and other weapons were fired into the air, and music played everywhere through loudspeakers, while mobs of people cheered and danced in the streets. It was the biggest mob demonstration we had seen so far. Soldiers and civilians alike were celebrating in the streets, singing, and yelling, "The War is over! *Basta!*

Tedeschi kaput." I cautioned our men to stay inside, because this looked to me like a good time for someone to get hurt, and I contacted Battalion Head-quarters for confirmation that the war had truly ended. No official word had been received there about an end to the War.

Actually the War was not over, but the situation didn't became clear until we learned that the Mayor of Verona had made a speech to a huge crowd of people assembled in a large city square. What he had said was that Verona had been liberated, and that as far as Verona was concerned, the War was over. This brought our ecstatic soldiers back to reality, and their celebrations ceased. However, the local populace continued to celebrate on into the evening.

At 6 p.m. we received the distressing news that we had to leave Verona immediately. When the order came to me I was told that we were being kicked out by the American Military Government, and I couldn't help but wonder what our supply sergeant thought about that. I was also told that we were being replaced in Verona by the 85th, and I wondered about this too, because I thought it was sheer foolishness to be switching the locations of the regi-ments for what I perceived to be no apparent reasonable purpose. It wasn't until several days later that I realized that the 85th referred to was the 85th Division, and not our 85th Mountain Infantry Regiment.

So we reluctantly packed everything up again. At about 9 p.m. we marched out over the same partially blown bridge that we had used to come into the city. The trucks were waiting for us, and so were our medical vehi-cles. It was already dark, and it was raining hard. After some delay the col-umn started to move, and it was the beginning of a terrible trip. Everyone was tired. The road was congested and muddy, and the column made fre-quent stops. The drivers of the personnel trucks had hardly slept at all for days, because they were continually making shuttle runs such as this one, and were transporting one troop unit after another in quick succession. The drivers of the five or six trucks directly behind us fell asleep almost every time we stopped, and most of the time I had to walk up and down the column to wake them up when we started up again. This went on until about 4 a.m., when we turned off into a huge field near a small village. The infantrymen then dug foxholes in the rain in which to try to sleep, but the medics were more fortunate, because we were able to set up in a dry barn.

Task Force Darby had been completely successful, but now, for the men who had done the job, it came to a totally miserable and uncomfortable end in that rainswept field near Bussolengo.

CHAPTER XVIII

LAGO DI GARDA

Every man in it was exhausted when the battalion finally settled down in the cold rain near Bussolengo. The barn in which we set up the aid station kept us dry, but the infantrymen stayed out in the field in their foxholes and slept as best they could.

I slept soundly until nearly 4 p.m. (April 27), and then was able to walk into the nearby village, where I was fortunate enough to get a much-needed shave and haircut in the local barbershop. I returned in time to attend the evening briefing and learn about our next mission.

We were to begin leapfrogging the regiments, in order to always keep fresh troops at the head of the advance, and the 87th had already started this action. It had gone west to the shore of Lake Garda, turned north along the shore, and had already advanced well beyond San Zeno before encountering enemy resistance. The 85th was now in the process of passing through the 87th and would continue the advance for eight hours, after which our regiment would pass through both of them and carry on for the following eight hours. After that the rear regiment would pass through to the front every eight hours. The plan gave each regiment eight hours in combat, and sixteen in which to rest each day. We were ordered to be ready to move out later that night, whenever the trucks came for us.

We left just before midnight, and followed the route that the other two regiments had earlier taken up the east shore of Lake Garda. We passed through the 87th, and stopped among the rear elements of the 85th, where the infantrymen detrucked and continued forward on foot. We soon passed beyond the forward elements of the 85th at the small village of Navene just as dawn was breaking (April 28). Our regiment (the 86th) was now once again leading the Division advance. The 2nd Battalion was in the lead with our 3rd Battalion following closely behind it.

The advance continued for a little more than a mile, and then ran into a situation that stopped it cold. Here the sheer rock face of Monte Baldo came down several hundred feet almost perpendicularly into the waters of Lake Garda, and the road, which paralleled the shoreline, passed through a tunnel running through a part of the mountain. The Germans had blown up the entrance of this tunnel, effectively sealing it off with tons of rock and debris, and, as soon as our troops appeared, they began to shell the road leading to it from the other side of the lake. The men had to take cover and dig in as best they could to protect themselves. Now our 3rd Battalion, following closely, was ordered to disperse laterally on the steep mountainside toward the East and take advantage of whatever cover was there. This cleared the road for more rapid movement to and from the far forward area.

Our 3rd Battalion Command Post now established itself in a villa on the shore at Malcesine, about a mile and a half south of Navene, and although we didn't unpack any of our vehicles, we used a part of the building as the aid station. I remember the villa well. It was neat, clean, and expensively furnished, with pictures still hanging on the walls. The day was overcast and windy, but the view from it was spectacular, and now for the first time it was light enough for me to get a good view of the lake. We had not seen the wide southern part of it because we had gone past it in the dark, but here at the north end the lake was indeed beautiful, and the visible countryside was extremely mountainous. Lake Garda appeared to be about a mile and a half wide here, and was bordered on both sides by high, snow capped mountains, whose sides sloped very steeply to the water's edge and gave the impression that they continued to slope steeply beneath its surface.

As soon as our battalion had moved off of the road, artillery moved up past us to fire at enemy gun emplacements on the opposite shore, and this soon resulted in a significant lessening of the shelling that the 2nd Battalion was receiving up ahead. However the prospects for getting to the north end of the lake looked hopeless, especially since we knew that beyond this first tunnel the road ahead ran through five more of them, all of which would be easy for the enemy to defend or blow up. A flanking movement over the mountains to the east might be possible, but such a move would require mountain climbing equipment that we now didn't have, and would take a long time during which our men would be completely exposed to the enemy shooting from the other side of the lake. On those mountainsides they would stand out like targets in a shooting gallery.

Fortunately, our overall plan of attack included the possibility of surprising the Germans with an amphibious attack across Lake Garda, and a fleet of amphibious trucks known as DUKWs, or "DUCKS" for short, had been kept close behind the regiments. They were now very close because they had already been used as land vehicles in the leapfrog advancements of the regiments. Shortly after noon, as soon as we saw the empty DUCKS go forward past us at Malcesine, I knew that we would be committed to an amphibious operation. The nature of the enemy shelling changed a short time later, and I was sure that the 2nd Battalion had taken to the water. It not only increased tremendously, but we were hearing and seeing antiaircraft fire with air bursts occurring at low levels out over the waters of the lake. Our Air Force already knew that the Germans had a lot of anti-aircraft guns at the north end of Lake Garda, and we were now being made aware of their presence.

During the amphibious assault by the 2nd Battalion word came for us to move up, and we advanced slowly, on foot. When we arrived at the embarkation point from which the DUKWs were leaving intermittently to bypass the sealed-up tunnel, we learned that, in spite of the antiaircraft fire, the 2nd Battalion had successfully bypassed the first two tunnels and had already taken the third, with few casualties. I was told at the time that there had been none, but this information didn't turn out to be quite true. As soon as the last of the 2nd Battalion completed the amphibious move, our 3rd Battalion began its move across the water.

My turn to climb aboard one of the DUCKS came toward the end of the movement, and I felt encouraged because I had not yet heard that any casualties had occurred. The only sheltered place for loading was more than a mile from the first tunnel in a small cove near Navene. The DUKWs had square prows, and were not built for speed. I guessed that in choppy water they could safely make a speed of about 6 miles per hour, and calculated in my head that we would be on the water about ten minutes before we reached the first tunnel. I didn't know how far beyond that we had to go.

The group I was in, 24 men, walked down the slope toward Our DUKW and started to board as soon as it reached the shore. It had always been my habit to hang back and see that everyone else got safely aboard, or through whatever else the exercise might be, and this time I also planned to be the last to board and take my place at the back of the row of men along one side or the other of the craft. As I reached the DUCK, the soldier marching abreast of me hesitated, and I was just about to say, "After you," when I thought, "Oh what the Hell!" and hopped aboard, taking my place as the second to last one in the row of twelve men, on the left side. We had been instructed to remove everything from our persons, which might weight us down or prevent us from swimming, and put it into our rucksacks or include it somewhere else in our gear. We now placed all of our gear along the center of the cockpit, and kneeled along the gunwale.

After clearing the protective cove, the driver headed about a hundred yards out into the lake before he turned north to travel parallel to the shore. He explained that this was necessary because earlier, when they had gone closer in, the enemy had shelled the cliffs above and caused a lot of falling rock that endangered the craft. I put my hand down into the water. It was ice cold, and I wondered how long a swimmer could survive in it. I was a good swimmer and had even won a few ribbons for participation in fifty and one hundred yard freestyle races in school. If I wasn't wounded, didn't hesitate, and went all out, I thought that could make it to the shore before significant hypothermia could occur. Other DUKWs, well spread apart, were bobbing on the water ahead of us and behind us.

Because the mountain slopes all around were tall and steep, the German artillery pieces and 88 mm antiaircraft guns in the area could only be located well above the water level of the lake, and fortunately for us, the barrels of these guns apparently couldn't be depressed below the horizontal or at least not far enough below it for them to be fired directly at us. This was reassuring, but now as we traveled northward I was introduced for the first time to airbursts exploding overhead, and it was frightening. Just as the bombardment began, the first of the tunnels up ahead came into view, and it seemed farther away than I had estimated. I dreaded going over that open water at a snail's pace for that mile or more with those antiaircraft shells exploding just over our heads. Whenever one exploded, black puffs of smoke appeared in the air, and a hail of fragments whizzed down to strike the water, causing multiple splashes of various sizes. They weren't exploding very high above us either, perhaps only fifty or a hundred yards.

About half way along in the course of our ride, we were suddenly diverted from anxiously watching the airbursts above by one of the men on the right side of our craft, who pointed across the lake and yelled, "Oh my God! There's a big door opening up in the cliff over there, and they're rolling a big gun out! God, it's huge! See it! See it there, half way up the mountain!" I didn't see it, although I looked in that general direction, but some of the other men now said that they too saw it. For a moment I was scared, but then reason took over. If the enemy couldn't depress this gun barrel any more than they could the others, it couldn't be any real threat to us no matter how big it was. I was more afraid of the airbursts from the enemy 88s, and was thankful that they had now let up a little. I looked toward the near shore and saw that

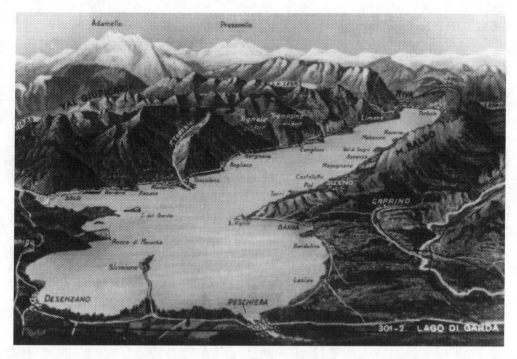

THE TOPOGRAPHY SURROUNDING LAKE GARDA
The tunnels that were bypassed by amphibious assault were carved out of solid rock in the precipitous side of Monte Baldo between Navene and Torbole.

we were about as far as we were going to get from it, and as I eyed this expanse of water, I wondered if I could make it now if we sank. I thought I could probably do it; at least I hoped so.

In time we came abreast of the first tunnel, which was completely blocked with rocks and debris, and I could see huge gaps in the road between it and the second tunnel, where two bridges had been reduced to piles of rubble. Once past this first tunnel our course took us closer to the shore, and it soon appeared that we were going to land between the second and third tunnels. With only about another 200 yards to go, I estimated that we had been on the water about fifteen minutes. Now the enemy antiaircraft guns really opened up again with great intensity. The sky above was continually filled with explosions and hundreds of those black puffs of smoke. Shell fragments were raining down all around us, and several times during the last two or three minutes I saw showers of fragments hit the water only a few feet away. At last we reached the shore and landed in a small cove where there was a little bit of beach. The men quickly picked up their gear, vaulted over the side, and scrambled hurriedly up the steep slope to the other side of the road where there was some cover. I had picked up my rucksack and my first aid kit, and had started for the front of the craft, when I looked back and noticed that the man behind me hadn't moved. He remained crouched on his knees with his head bent forward. I went back to him and found that he was dead! He had taken a shell fragment in the middle of his back. I didn't take time to determine if there were any other wounds, but just made certain that he was really dead, and that there was nothing I could do for him. Then I told the driver to take him back and turn him over to the Graves Registration detail, and I too vaulted out of the DUKW and scrambled up the slope to the other side of the road.

As I sat there in the shelter of a big rock, I realized that I had just had another close call with death. Ninety-nine percent of the time, under similar circumstances, I would have been the last man in that row. I couldn't understand what had happened to alter my pattern of being polite, of standing aside for someone else to pass, as I had done all of my life, and wondered if there had perhaps been something supernatural connected with my stepping in ahead of the man who had been killed. I felt a bit guilty, but nevertheless was very glad to be still alive.

While we were making the amphibious pass around the first two tunnels, the 2nd Battalion had continued the attack, and by the time I landed, had cleared out tunnels number 3 and number 4. As the leading elements began to attack tunnel number 5 they found that the road in front of it had been blown, so they established defensive positions for the night at that point. My medics and I stayed hidden among the rocks on the hillside between tunnel number 2 and number 3, while enemy shells from the other side of the lake continued to pass overhead, and explode on the mountainside behind us. In the morning (April 29) our 3rd Battalion was scheduled to pass through the 2nd Battalion, attack tunnel number 5, and continue the advance beyond it. I received orders to have my medics ready at 6 a.m. to follow the action.

The rest of the afternoon and evening became another period of misery. It was raining and had turned cold. We spent some time huddled behind the boulders for protection against the enemy artillery and also a lot of 20-millimeter rounds he was firing at us from across the lake. Later that evening we passed through tunnel number 3 and stayed in a shallow ravine that was not much more than a big ditch. Between tunnel number 3 and tunnel number 4 there was almost a mile of road, and the rocky, brush covered slope here was not as steep as the slope along the road behind us had been. The entire battalion spread out in this area for the night, and I spent this miserable time with my aid station crew in that rocky ditch. Light rain continued. Most of us

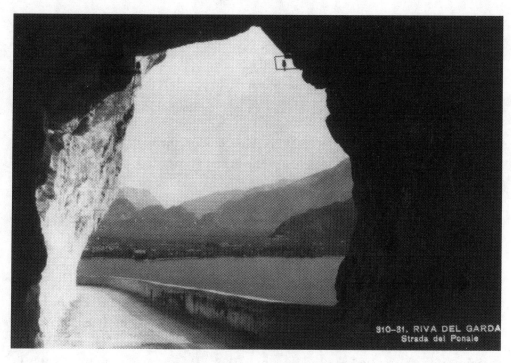

A TUNNEL ALONG THE SHORE OF LAKE GARDA
The towns of Riva and Torbole are seen in the distance. Arco is farther away at the other end of the valley.

It was in a tunnel like this one that two companies of American soldiers were making preparations for their next advance when an enemy 88 mm shell entered the forward end of the tunnel and exploded inside. It took a long time to treat and evacuate the numerous casualties caused by this single shell.

were too miserable to sleep. However, the enemy shelling eventually stopped, and for that I was glad.

The rain finally stopped at about 3 a.m. (April 29), and as things began to dry off a bit, I fell asleep. When I awoke my muscles were stiff and I had numerous sore spots where rocks had pressed hard against my body. I had been so tired that I had slept for a long time without changing position. I looked about and saw that the ditch was empty except for the half dozen of my medics who were with me and who appeared to be still asleep. It was full daylight, and the sun was shining. I looked at my watch, and saw that it was almost ten o'clock. I had goofed! My battalion had attacked at dawn. We were supposed to have been close behind them, and here we were, still in that ditch.

I woke everybody up immediately, and briefed the men on the situation.

We had to move as fast as possible to catch up with our battalion, and if they were hungry they could eat their dog biscuits on the march. We started off immediately, but I don't think anybody ate.

We had to go more than half of a mile to reach tunnel number 4, and as we hurried along the enemy started shelling in earnest once again. Most of it was coming in well ahead of us and didn't slow us down. We passed through groups of 2nd Battalion men, and had just passed through tunnel number 4, when word came that all medics were urgently needed in the next tunnel ahead, which was now only a short distance away. I started off at a trot with the rest of the medics following. We ran right into the tunnel, and continued toward the forward end. The scene that greeted us there looked as if it should have been in a nightmare or a horror movie.

This had been the site where the day before a contingent of German soldiers had met disaster when the explosives they were placing to blow up the tunnel had gone off prematurely and killed a lot of them. Rock and rubble, including body parts of these Germans still littered the far entrance of the tunnel, and was perhaps three or four feet deep. Now a German 88 mm antiaircraft airburst had exploded some 30 or 40 feet inside the tunnel while more than two companies of our men were in it. There must have been over a hundred of them lying sprawled, one on top of another on the tunnel floor. This tunnel wasn't very long, and about halfway through I began stepping over the bodies of the fallen. Many were still, but a lot of them were moving and moaning. It was hard to know where to begin. I did notice, however, that there was not a lot of blood in evidence, and I hoped that most of them were suffering only from concussion, and not from serious shell fragment wounds.

Then I noticed a Red Cross helmet on one of the men lying nearby. I had passed him, but now I turned back, and as I kneeled down beside him, I recognized him immediately. He was one of my M Company aid men, T/5 Charles T. Ladd, from Massachusetts. His face was pallid, his pupils were already dilated, and he was taking his last three or four gasping breaths. In less than a minute he was dead. I saw no obvious wounds, but I couldn't take time to look very long or very hard, because there were so many others still living that needed attention. Later I concluded that he had been hit somewhere in the back by a large shell fragment, that a major blood vessel such as the aorta had been torn, and that he had died of massive internal bleeding. There was nothing I could have done.

As I turned to the next man it suddenly struck me that Charley Ladd had been an aid man with M Company, our heavy weapons company, and this was the company behind which the medical detachment routinely took its place during any forward movement. This time we weren't there, because we had overslept in a ditch at the side of the road. I WAS SUPPOSED TO HAVE BEEN IN THAT TUNNEL WHEN THE SHELL WENT OFF, but I wasn't! If we hadn't been so dead tired; if we hadn't fouled up and overslept; if we hadn't been late in catching up with the battalion, I too could now be wounded or dead!

Second Battalion medics and litter teams were also present to help, and we began to sort out this medical mess as rapidly as we could. We set up a work area at the rear end of the tunnel, and processed casualties there. The Regimental History states that there had been five killed, one of whom was Captain Lawrence Ely, the commander of the 2nd Battalion's H Company, and 50 wounded; the Battalion History has it seven dead and 44 wounded. I wasn't counting, but at the time it seemed like more.

Because we were still isolated on a long, narrow beachhead, evacuation of the wounded had to be by water. The 2nd Battalion Medics established a collecting point near tunnel number 3, where we had landed the day before, and as soon as we had established a triage procedure, we started sending the wounded there. I learned later that German artillery had brought more guns to bear on this area, and had really zeroed in on the water route. The slow moving DUKWs were just that, sitting ducks for enemy artillery, so our engineers brought up some faster assault boats, equipped them with outboard motors, and used them for this ferry service. Whenever a boatload of ammunition or supplies arrived, two litter wounded could make the return trip in these much faster craft.

Among the wounded that morning were Major William Drake, the commander of the 3rd Battalion, and Major John Seamans, who was then commanding the 2nd Battalion. Captain Everett Bailey took Command of the 3rd, and Captain Jack Carpenter the 2nd. I knew both men, had confidence in them, and was sure that both battalions would continue to do well under their direction.

Both of the wounded battalion commanders were among the walking wounded. I don't specifically remember Major Drake's wounds. They were relatively minor, but serious enough to need definitive surgical repair, so I sent him back to the casualty pickup point early, along with the first of the litter wounded.

Major Seamans had a shoulder wound. He stood off to one side, and waited for a long time before he let me redress it, saying that the other wounded men needed me more. Finally, when there was no one else in need of attention in our immediate area, he let me look. It was a nasty-looking but not serious wound which involved some of the shoulder girdle muscles, and it too needed surgical repair. I told him to go back with the next group of wounded to leave, but he refused, and stayed with us, mingling with and encouraging the wounded men. He finally left with the last group to go. I remember watching him leave, proud and erect, with his right arm in a sling and a bloody bandage on his shoulder, and I thought to myself that here was an officer who truly cared for his men, and appreciated their sacrifices. After that I never saw him again or heard anything more about him.

We had arrived at tunnel number 5 within minutes after the shell exploded, and it took more than two hours to organize the wounded and get those that needed to be evacuated for treatment out of the area. As I had suspected, many suffered only blast injury but only a few of these seemed to be serious. Those who had not been unconscious recovered in a matter of minutes, and I am sure that some of these didn't bother to seek medical care. I observed the rest for a while, and again encountered the phenomenon of men, even under such terrible circumstances as these, not wanting to be evacuated. They absolutely did not want to let their comrades-in-arms down, and they didn't ever want to be assigned to another unit. I let most of them return to duty, but did do a lot of quick and repeated neurological examinations in order to at least try to be sure I wasn't sending someone back into combat who was incapable of functioning properly.

As the last of the tunnel casualties started for the rear, one of the battalion officers briefed me on the combat situation. The battalion had attacked on schedule that morning (April 29), and had captured last two tunnels without much difficulty. It was now deployed in front of tunnel number 6, and attacking the town of Torbole. Before dawn the 1st Battalion had gone eastward into the mountains near tunnel number 3, then turned northward through the rugged terrain, and had gone to within a half mile of their objective, the town of Nago, located about a mile northeast of Torbole. There they met stiff opposition, and couldn't advance any farther. At these two towns the Germans were at last making a strong stand with all of the resources they had, and it was becoming very tough for the battalions to gain any ground.

Now I was abruptly introduced to yet another crisis. There were inside the tunnel near its rear entrance, several small rooms, which had been hollowed out of the solid rock and fitted with heavy doors. An officer—I don't remember which one—came up to me and asked if I would take a look at Colonel Cook, the regimental commander, who was now in one of them. He told me that Colonel Cook was acting strangely, seemed incoherent at times, and had issued some orders that didn't make sense. As we walked together to

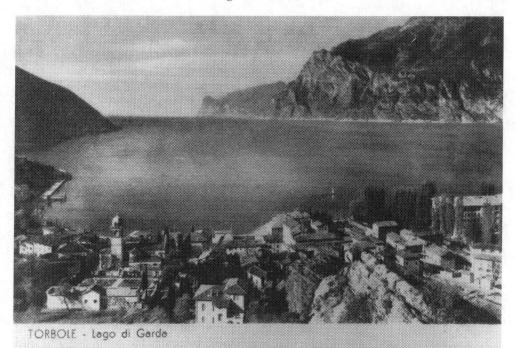

TORBOLE - Lago di Garda

TORBOLE AND THE NORTH END OF LAKE GARDA VIEWED FROM THE HEIGHTS NORTH AND EAST OF TOWN
The roads on both sides of the lake pass through tunnels. The ones that caused our troops so much trouble are located in the mountain coming down to the waters edge on the left.

see the colonel I kept thinking that the regiment didn't need this, with another battle just about to begin.

When I arrived inside the windowless, candlelit room, there were several other officers present. I don't remember who they were now, but they corroborated the story I had just heard. Colonel Cook just sat there, motionless, his face drawn and expressionless. He exhibited typical symptoms of combat fatigue, but it appeared that he had not yet succumbed completely. I was able to question him, but answers were slow in coming. Yes, he had not slept in over 48 hours. No, he didn't feel sick. No, he had no pain. No, he had not been injured. Yes, he didn't know what day this was. The Colonel was very obviously in no condition to lead.

Now I worried because I wasn't sure how much authority I had in this situation. It had been no problem in the past for me to diagnose combat fatigue, and evacuate a man or hold him for treatment. For quite a while now we had not been evacuating these cases, but keeping them quiet somewhere toward the rear, and returning them to duty when they recovered. But this was the regimental commander. Did I have the authority to order him to do this, or must I declare him incompetent, and evacuate him to the mercy of the psychiatrists? I knew that Colonel Cook was a career officer who had gone through West Point, and I was sure that he didn't want "Evacuated because of Combat Exhaustion" to appear on his military record.

Some of the other officers present now joined the halting conversation, and after a while the colonel agreed that he was "overtired" and "not thinking clearly." I persuaded him to give up command to John Hay, who was then the executive officer of the regiment. He also agreed to go to the rear under some pretext, and hole up somewhere for eight or ten hours of sleep. Then, if there still was a problem, we could decide upon something else. To the best of my knowledge, this is exactly what he did, and since that time I have never ever heard another word about this incident from anyone, anywhere.

That afternoon and all night I stayed near the rear of tunnel number 5 with my aid station crew, listening to the sounds of the battles for Nago and Torbole. I was glad that John Hay was leading the Regiment, for I had confidence in him. This turned out to be the last big battle of the war for us, and before it was over Colonel Cook was back in command. Later, when I read about this action in the regimental and division histories, the following passages provoked a knowing smile. I quote:

From the Division History: "(30 April 1945) At 300050B (12:50 a.m.) the Germans launched determined counter-attacks on both towns (Torbole and Nago). The attack was made by armor and supporting infantry. At 0125B (1:25 a.m.) the commanding general ordered that the troops should withdraw to the hills to the east of the towns if necessary. The commander of the 86th Mountain Infantry, Lt. Colonel Cook, was of the opinion that the troops would be able to hold the town and requested permission to remain in the town fighting a delaying withdrawal if it became necessary. The general approved."

From the Regimental History: "At 0055 (12:55 a.m.) the Germans launched determined counter attacks on both positions (Nago and Torbole). The attacks were made by armor and supporting infantry. At 0125 (1:25 am.) General Hays ordered Colonel Cook to pull his troops out of Torbole into the high ground to the east. Colonel Cook and Colonel Hay were of the opinion that the battalions could hold their ground. They suggested a delay in withdrawal, and General Hays approved."

Our 3rd Battalion troops had all but completely taken the town of Torbole when the Germans began these counterattacks, which were led by the dreaded

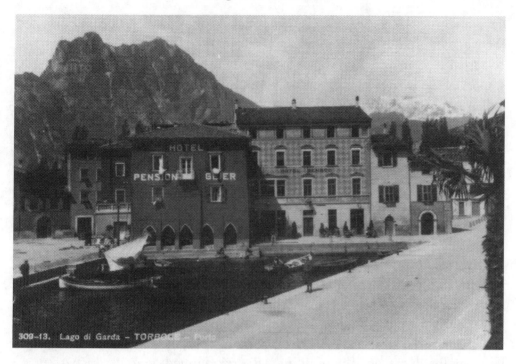

THE ROAD TO RIVA AS IT PASSES BETWEEN THE WATERFRONT AND THE VILLAGE SQUABE IN TORBOLE
The square is just to the right of the roadway shown in the picture.
This is the place where Colonel Darby and Sergeant Evans were standing when they were killed by a German artillery shell on April 30, 1945, just two days before the hostilities ended.

and powerful Tiger Tanks. They had pushed our men back out of at least half of the town when the bazooka teams of the 2nd Battalion were sent forward to help, and apparently turned the tide. The battle continued in the north half of the town for several hours, then abated.

When daylight arrived (April 30) the Germans had retreated. Patrols were sent out and found that the bridge between Torbole and Riva had been blown, but an alternate route was found with a bridge over the Sarca River still intact. When the lead patrol reached Riva early that afternoon there were still Germans there, who looked as if they were ready to fight, but when the entire 2nd Battalion appeared, they fled to the North without firing a shot. By noon the 1st Battalion had taken the town of Nago, and now Regimental Headquarters and the 3rd Battalion Command Post moved into Torbole.

We walked through tunnel number 5, past the bodies of our dead which had been neatly laid aside and discreetly covered, but decaying pieces of dead enemy soldiers were still evident where they had earlier met disaster. We walked through tunnel number 6, and emerged from it onto a long, curved sweep of road in a relatively flat area along the shore. I remember having to step over the bodies of three dead German soldiers lying in the road about half way to the town and noticing that although they were wearing the German Army uniform, two of them were mere boys. I thought that they could not have been more than 15 years old. When we reached the town square I saw that many of the buildings had been damaged but were still standing.

The southwest side of the square was on the water's edge and was composed entirely of wharf and small dock facilities. The other three sides were made up of multistoried buildings, and the word "ALBERGO" painted on several of them indicated that in better times they had been resort hotels. We established our 3rd Battalion Aid Station on the ground floor of one of them, and the regimental and battalion command posts moved into another. Enemy shells were still occasionally coming in from the North and Northwest, but most of them were falling harmlessly into the water, and only rarely did one land behind the town. The road from the south passed through the square between the docks and the buildings, then continued on toward Riva.

As soon as we had settled in I told the men to try to get some sleep, and that I wanted to do the same. Sergeant Miller volunteered to "mind the store," so I went upstairs in the deserted hotel, found a room with a nice bed in it and went to sleep. Several hours later I was awakened by the noise of a shell exploding close by, and I thought at first that the building had been hit. I contemplated moving to a safer place downstairs, then decided against it. I was on the far side of the building and there were still two floors above me so several shells would need to hit it before I was really in danger.

In the evening I came down quite refreshed, and Sergeant Miller excitedly told me about the shell explosion that had temporarily awakened me. He was in the open doorway of the aid Station watching as Colonel Darby, the division executive officer, and Colonel Cook were standing together on a stone walk near the lakeshore and conferring. Standing next to them were the regimental sergeant major, Sergeant John T. Evans, and Lieutenant James H. McLellan. Shortly before 6 p.m. a shell exploded overhead, and Sergeant Evans was killed instantly. The three officers were wounded. Colonel Darby was able to walk into the building, but died 45 minutes later. Lieutenant McLellan was treated and evacuated. Colonel Cook had received only a very minor wound, and remained on duty. These men did not come through our aid station, and although I didn't specifically ask, I assumed that they had been cared for at the regimental aid station, which had moved in with Regimental Headquarters. When the shell exploded Sergeant Miller was standing in the doorway of our 3rd Battalion Aid Station and the blast blew him backward into the room, but he wasn't hurt. The deaths of these two men was a newsworthy event, and for the next several days Sergeant Miller had to repeat his story many times.

That evening we moved again. Regimental Headquarters moved into Riva, and we, together with 3rd Battalion Headquarters moved into the village of San Alessandro, between Riva and Torbole, away from the lake, and a bit to the north. We installed the aid station in a schoolhouse in the middle of the village, and there for the first time in almost three weeks I was able to write a letter to my wife and to have a good night's sleep.

CHAPTER XIX

RESIA - THE AUSTRIAN BORDER

It seemed almost luxurious to sleep on the warm, wooden floor of the school-house in San Alessandro instead of out in the open on rocks and rubble, and it was wonderful to be able to sleep all night. I slept soundly and well, and didn't awaken until well after daylight.

After breakfast I thoroughly examined the town and our new quarters. We were in a wooden building with a single large classroom in its center and several smaller connecting rooms at each end. All had large windows with glass still intact, giving the whole interior of the building an appearance of lightness and airiness such as we had not seen in a long time. The floor of the building was a few feet above street level, and a wide stairway led up to the main entrance in the front. The surrounding houses were neat and clean, and had well kept grounds. Small vegetable and flower gardens were evident everywhere. The grass was green, and even though the nights were still cold, roses and other flowers were in bloom. Nestled in the mountains, San Alessandro was a pretty little village, and it had not been damaged by the War.

On this day (May 1) our living conditions improved dramatically. Field kitchens were set up and served steak for the first evening meal. Clean cloth-ing, and sleeping bags arrived. I was able to get a haircut and a shave in a local barbershop, and I bought stationery and picture postcards. Most of us were catching up on sleep. The officers in our unit even managed to obtain a bedroom in a private home across the street from the aid station.   The di-vision was licking its wounds, re-supplying, regrouping and getting ready to chase the enemy all of the way to the Brenner Pass. Rumors of peace and German surrender had been building up frequently for a week, and were now circulating everywhere, but the men had by now suffered through previous false alarms often enough so that they no longer paid much attention to them.

Late in the day word was received that Italian Partisans were holding the town of Arco at the northern end of the valley, but that the Germans were massing to attack and retake it. The Partisan leader asked for military help, and Company L was chosen to advance the next morning to relieve the situation. Air cover was requested for this advance, but was refused. This was unusual, and it raised our suspicions that something in the nature of a truce might be in the wind.

The following morning (May 2) Company L advanced into Arco without meeting any Germans, and at the same time Company F advanced into Albergo, also without opposition. No signs of enemy activity were seen all day. At about 5 p.m. another hint that something was up, came in the form of an order from General Hayes to all units, that if any German emissaries bearing white flags appeared, they were not to be fired upon, and were to be taken promptly to Division Headquarters. About two hours later the official call announcing the end of the fighting came in to Captain Bailey at the Battalion Command Post.

THE WAR IN ITALY WAS OVER! The Italians knew it too, because a British broadcast had been interrupted to announce that all German Armies in Northern Italy had surrendered unconditionally. The scene we had witnessed in Verona just a week before now repeated itself in San Alessandro, and all over the valley church bells rang. People cheered and waved to each other; they rang cowbells, pounded on tubs and contrived other ways to make noise; they danced and sang in the streets, and vino bottles appeared everywhere as if by magic. An unbelievable number of weapons also appeared, and there was much exuberant firing of guns and even small cannons. This was not the time to be shot by some ecstatic Italian, and I warned my men to stay under cover.

Most of our soldiers didn't join in the revelry, but instead stood aside watching it, looking relieved, and, yes, even a little bit sheepish. Many looked as if they still didn't believe the news, and I think some felt, as I did, that this wild celebration might be dangerous. Blackout regulations were no longer needed, and that night, for the first time since we had been in Italy, points of light dotted the countryside all around us. The next morning (May 3, 1945) things were calmer, but the natives were still going about their business with an air of exuberance, and they scurried briskly about everywhere. On the street enthusiastic and cheerful greetings were heard frequently.

Early in the afternoon a motley group of some twenty Italian men came to the schoolhouse to tell us that they were on their way up the hill to capture and jail the "Dirty Fascist" who lived there. They warned us that they were determined to catch this "criminal," and that there would probably be casualties. Each man carried some kind of weapon. There were a couple of small caliber rifles, some shotguns, pistols, pitchforks, brickbats and ordinary clubs, and there was much brandishing of these weapons, accompanied by arm waving, clenching of fists, boasting and bragging. After a lengthy conversation with Consiglio, who was still acting as my interpreter, they departed to go up the hill. Consiglio started to laugh, and still grinning told me about the bragging that various individuals in the group had done about what they were going to do to that "Dirty Fascist."

In an hour the group returned, much quieter and looking rather cowed. They were seeking medical attention. Although they still carried their weapons, they were no longer brandishing them menacingly. Several of them had pellets of birdshot under their hides, and the man, whom Consiglio pointed out as the biggest braggart of the group, had collected the largest number, most of them in his rear end. So with local anesthetic, a knife and some hemostats, I picked the birdshot out of these fellows. It probably would have done no real harm to have left it, for the pellets weren't very deep under the skin, but I was curious to know what had happened; I wasn't busy, and the activity provided the time for me to hear their story.   I purposely left the man who had received most of the birdshot to be treated last, and as I had him lie on his stomach on a litter, I told Consiglio to try to find out more about what had happened. A lively dialogue followed in which most of the members of the group, often interrupting each other and speaking two or three at a time, unfolded the story to Consiglio, who in turn related it to me in bits and pieces:

The group had gone up the hill to the manor house, and spent about half an hour breaking down the garden gate. Then they approached the house, shouting insults, and demanding that the Dirty Fascist come out with his hands up. When nothing happened they started throwing stones at the house, and then, when still no one appeared, some of them started shooting at it. This produced an immediate response. The Dirty Fascist charged out onto his porch carrying a double-barreled shotgun, and without any warning, shot at them. Consiglio thought that this first shot must have been fired into the air, because it had been fired at close range, and none of the individuals in the group indicated that they had been wounded by the first shot. I was of the same opinion because all of the shot I had so far removed had barely penetrated the skin. At the sound of the shot the mob immediately turned and ran for the gate, and there they hesitated, but their departure was hastened again by a second shot from the porch. It was apparently this second shot which had inflicted the damage upon them. When we asked if they would go back after the man, they agreed that they would not. They would be satisfied to let the army or the police do it.

On the evening of May 3 our vehicles caught up with us, and we learned that the battalion had been named to act as still another task force, my fourth one since we left the Apennines. This one was to make a run for the Austrian border, to the rear of the German Armies still engaging the American Seventh Army. Our mission was to seal off the border in order to prevent any of the men from the surrendered German Armies in Italy from joining the German divisions in the north that were still fighting. Colonel Hay had been picked to command the task force, and I considered this a good omen for the outcome of the mission.

The sky was gray and overcast, and it looked as if rain would fall any minute when we marched back down toward Lake Garda and into Torbole early on the morning of May 4. Infantrymen boarded the waiting trucks, and battalion vehicles integrated themselves into their proper places along the column. This task force, like the others, was comprised not just of armor, artillery and infantry, but contained all of the ancillary services that might be needed if it encountered any opposition to its advance. I knew that a few of our vehicles had been brought across the water into Torbole, but when I saw the number of tanks and self-propelled guns now lined up along the road, I concluded that the engineers had completed repairs to the road and the tunnels along the shore at least well enough to handle these heavy vehicles.

After a short delay while the entire column established its proper marching order, we got under way, and started toward the East on the road to Rovereto. There were occasional delays while minor road damage was repaired, and one longer delay during which the engineers cleared a large rockslide. We soon passed small groups of fully armed German soldiers. After we reached Rovereto and turned north onto the main highway to Bolzano and the Brenner Pass, more and larger groups of them appeared, and in places it looked as if whole companies had lined up at the roadside to watch us go by. These German soldiers were all neat, well dressed, well disciplined, and stood erect and proud, in stark contrast to the miserable, dejected prisoners or wild-eyed fanatics we had been accustomed to seeing during combat. None of them spoke to us or waved, and their faces remained expressionless, but we weren't expecting smiles. Soon we were regularly passing German artillery pieces and armored vehicles, fully armed and ready for action, and this worried some of our men. I kept assuring them that, in spite of the fact that their leader was treacherous lunatic, I thought that the rank and file of the

German Army would now play by the rules.

Traffic congestion slowed us up considerably as we approached and passed through the sizeable city of Trento. There had been a few armed German soldiers directing traffic for us in Rovereto, but in Trento there were many more, and some of our men obviously felt ill at ease to now be guided by Germans who had been trying to kill us only a few days before. Crowds of Italians lined the streets to get a look at us and cheer us on, but wherever there were German soldiers standing nearby, the cheering remained subdued and reserved. As we left the city we passed slowly by the bombed-out rail yard, which had been completely devastated by our Air Force, and as soon as we reached the rural area again, we were able to advance more rapidly.

We were now following the main road to Bolzano, which became increasingly crowded and congested as we advanced. The closer to the city we came, the slower was our progress. German soldiers, with rifles slung across their backs, were soon directing traffic at every intersection, and we saw people who appeared to be refugees walking southward, apparently carrying with them all of the possessions they owned. Some, we learned, had come from slave labor camps where they had been taken by the Germans to work on roads and other construction projects. We also saw large numbers of Czechoslovakian Army soldiers along the way, wearing the distinctive green uniforms that marked their nationality. They were much more cheerful than the Germans, and often smiled and waved to us.

Late in the afternoon the head of our column entered the outskirts of Bolzano, and although we were still well out in the country, we had to slow down markedly. The number of German soldiers directing traffic kept increasing as we progressed into the city, and by the time we had reached the downtown area there was one at every intersection. The traffic congestion was horrendous, and we moved forward only a few feet at a time. As soon as it became obvious that we were headed into severe traffic congestion, someone cheerfully ventured the information that, because our column was eight miles long, at the rate we were going it would take all night to pass through the city. In the meantime the weather had turned colder. It was still overcast. Scattered flakes of snow hung in the air, and puddles of nearly frozen water were everywhere on the ground.

In spite of the cold weather and the long time it took for the column ahead of us to pass, Italians were still lined up along the streets of Bolzano to greet us, and cheer us on. The crowds were not as dense as they had been in the Po Valley, and the demonstrations were not nearly as boisterous, probably because there were armed German soldiers directing traffic on almost every street corner. Nevertheless, these people seemed genuinely glad to see us, and happy to have been freed from German rule.

On one occasion, while the column was stopped, I remember the chaplain trying to give a particularly skinny, hungry looking little boy a can of meat and vegetable stew which he had saved from his C Rations. The chaplain kept pointing to the olive drab can and saying, *"Carne et Vegetabili"* over and over again. The youngster looked frightened, and didn't appear to understand. Finally the chaplain said something in Italian that I took to mean, "Take it to your mother." The kid then grabbed the can, and quickly disappeared into the crowd.

When we emerged from the other side of the city it was already well after dark, and we found that we were no longer on the road to the Brenner Pass, but were headed toward Merano. The road kept gradually climbing, and the weather turned colder as we gained altitude. Wet snow began to fall in large quantities. According to our maps the distance to the Austrian border on this route was much longer than the distance from Bolzano to the Brenner Pass, so we resigned ourselves to a trip that would last for the rest of the night.

Then something happened that none of us had ever expected to see. We were traveling under the usual blackout conditions when some of the trucks in front of us and behind us turned on their headlights. Soon word was passed along that the blackout had been lifted, and within minutes every vehicle in the column had its headlights shining. To the drivers, who less than a month before were risking life and limb driving the goat trails and cliff edges in the Apennines, this must have been something like heaven. As the falling snowflakes reflected their light in all directions, the beams from all of those headlights lit up the sky, and the entire column was quickly engulfed in a sea of light, which was several hundred feet high. We passed through Merano at about midnight, and were thankful that the route through this city was not as long and as tedious as our passage through Bolzano had been. It surprised me that, even at that late hour, people came outside or opened their windows to wave to us and watch us go by. Nighttime military convoys must have been common here for years, but this was probably the first one they had seen coming through with headlights burning brightly. After Merano the roadway, but not the road itself, became narrower, and there were more and sharper curves, which afforded glimpses of the column ahead and behind in all its lighted splendor. We continued to gain altitude as we moved forward, and it continued to snow.

At about 5 a.m. the column halted, and all of the vehicles pulled off of the road onto the shoulder. This time we remained stationary for a long time, and I surmised, correctly, that the head of the column had reached the Austrian border. What I didn't know was that some delicate negotiations were going on between our task force commander and German officers on both sides of it. The German Armies in Austria were still fighting, and had already turned some of their artillery around to bear upon us, but were deterred from firing by the huge display of light in the sky. They apparently thought that we were a much larger army than we actually were, a concept that our side tried hard not to dispel. Why else would we come up to the pass with lights ablaze? The German officers later admitted that they also thought something might have happened that they didn't know about, and therefore did not let loose with their artillery.

In the end the Germans were convinced that we wouldn't come across the border, and that we were entitled to be on the Italian side. What might have been a disaster for us was averted.

At daylight, while we continued to wait at the roadside, it stopped snowing, but the sky remained overcast and the fields all around us remained covered with an inch or more of new snow. A short distance to our left on the shore of a small lake was a large, nice looking building, and when I saw the sign in large letters painted on its side which read, *"ALBERGO al LAGO di RESIA"* (Lake Resia Hotel), I knew that it had been a resort hotel. When it was light enough to make out the road ahead I saw that it continued its upward climb as the valley narrowed. We were within the approach to Passo di Resia, the only pass through the Alps from Italy into Austria West of the Brenner Pass.

The snow in the fields was already beginning to melt when word was passed along the column that we had arrived, and would occupy this beautiful territory indefinitely. Battalion Headquarters was being established up ahead in the village of Resia, and now I had to find a suitable place in which to establish the aid station. My eye fell upon the hotel at the lakeshore, and I decided to look there first.

We were now in German speaking territory, and I didn't think I would need Consiglio, so I went alone. As I approached it, the building kept looking better and better. I walked up a few steps onto a small porch, and knocked on the door. It opened almost immediately, and there stood a German soldier in an immaculate full dress uniform. Showing no expression on his face, he raised his arm smartly, clicked his heels and said, "Heil Hitler." I didn't return the salute, and I don't believe he expected me to return it, for he lowered his arm immediately.

Actually I was astounded by this development, but did my best not to show surprise and to appear calm and confident. The German soldier of course didn't know that I could understand German, and he now stepped backward and to one side while motioning for me to come in and then to follow him. We passed quickly through what appeared to be a small hotel lobby. At the far end he opened a door and indicated that I should enter. Once again I was surprised, but I instantly recognized the scene that greeted me, for I had seen it many times before in war movies. I was in the office of the Kommandant, the commanding officer of whatever unit it was that was occupying the building.

Behind a large desk sat a German captain facing the door through which I had just entered. On the wall behind him was a large picture of Hitler, and Nazi flags, on flagstaffs, stood in stands on each side of it. Also in the room, standing at attention, were about half a dozen other Germans in uniform, but I don't remember them very well, nor do I remember their ranks. I had barely entered the room when the Captain arose from his chair, and threw me my second snappy Nazi salute. I didn't answer this one either, but looked around the neat, orderly room, and at the Germans in their spotless uniforms and highly polished boots. Then I looked down at my own dirty coat, still wet from melting snow, and my mud flecked combat boots, and thought, "What a contrast!"

For about twenty seconds nothing happened. Then the German Captain unsnapped the holster at his side and pulled out his pistol. I felt a moment of panic as I thought, "My God, he's going to shoot me!" However, he didn't shoot. Instead, he handed the pistol to me butt first, and tried to tell me, in English, that he was surrendering his hospital to the United States Army. His English was so poor that it became quickly apparent that he would be unable to carry on a satisfactory conversation with it, so as I slipped the pistol into my coat pocket, I said to him, *"Sie können es alles auf Deutsch sagen, aber langsam bitte."* (*"You* may say everything in German, but slowly please.") This broke the ice, and as I looked around the room again, I noted expressions of relief on some of the other faces. There was even the hint of a smile or two.

The German captain explained that he was in command of a German Army Field Hospital, and that about one hundred patients were still housed in the building. He obviously recognized my Cadeuceus emblem, which was worn by all Army doctors and which I wore on my collar, and he quickly asked, "Can you operate?" I replied that I could, but would do so only if absolutely necessary. First he should brief me about his hospital and its operation. Then we should make rounds together, and I would look at his patients and inspect the hospital. So we went into the main dining room, where I was able to see the patient records and ask questions, and after that we went through most of the building together.

The *Albergo al Lago di Resia* had been a very nice resort hotel before the War, and early during the conflict it had been taken over by the German Army for use as a Hospital. It had often been overcrowded with patients, but now was just filled to capacity. There were no longer any doctors present, because all of them, all of the Army nurses, and most of the medical technicians had been called up into Austria. There were a few civilian nurses working there, and other civilian workers were doing the menial chores. Most of the soldiers stationed there had little medical training. Supplies had become very scarce, and food was sometimes hard to come by. For several weeks now, they had no longer been able to evacuate patients to the fatherland, and they were doing the best they could with what they had.

We looked at the kitchens and at the medical and other supplies. We made rounds to the bedsides of most of the patients, but I didn't linger anywhere, and passed rapidly from one bed to the next.

Most of the patients had suffered combat wounds, and the situation with many of these men was not pretty. Although the rooms and the beds were clean, bandages were scarce and those that were available were made of crude, tan, crepe paper, and they were being used well beyond their capacity to soak up pus. Neoprontosil, the red antibiotic dye, which was the precursor of our sulfanilamide, was being used, but in spite of this, most of the wounds had been too long neglected, and were infected. I noticed that there were no abdominal or chest wounds among these patients, and had to assume that all who had suffered such wounds had already died. The worst cases I saw were those with open fractures of the legs and arms, where bone infection had set in, and there were several of these in which the limb beyond the fracture had become gangrenous, but had not been amputated. I could smell these as I approached the bed.

The patients all knew I was an American doctor, and I sensed that they were all glad to see me. Before I left each bedside I noticed that expressions of hopelessness and despair seemed to disappear. Just by appearing, I had given each of them some new hope for survival and perhaps even a return to a normal life.

After completing the rounds, I told the German captain to continue operating the hospital exactly as he had been doing, and that I would recommend to the American Military Government that his patients be transferred to our hospitals for specific treatment. He and his men would probably be prisoners of war, but I didn't think it would be for long, because the War was almost over. I told him too that German Army units to the south were cooperating with us and were even being allowed to keep some of their weapons in order to protect themselves from the Italians. Then I left to rejoin my men.

When I returned to them, the men were understandably disappointed that the hotel building was occupied and we couldn't stay there. Although we had to look elsewhere for quarters, I first made a quick trip to Battalion Headquarters in Resia to report the surrender of the German hospital, explain the situation there, and present my recommendations for taking care of the patients. I pointed out that there were about a hundred wounded Germans there, many of whom needed specific and definitive surgical treatment, and that the most practical way to accomplish this would be to ship them south to our hospitals.

On the way back to my men I started to look for quarters again. There wasn't anything suitable in Resia that hadn't already been taken, and we had driven almost back to the lake, before I noticed some clusters of buildings on the other side of it that looked promising. We detoured onto the only road leading in that direction, and soon had to stop, blocked by some cows that an elderly farmer was herding into the lane leading to his barn. He spoke German to his cattle, and I began to recognize words and expressions that I had not heard in years. He apologized for delaying us, and seemed extraordinarily pleased that I could answer him in German. He was the first civilian with whom I conversed in German, and he spoke with a similar accent and used the same idioms that I had been accustomed to as a child. I kept hearing German expressions that I had not heard since I was small. Above all, I was most happy to be able to easily understand everything he said. I told him that we were a medical unit of some thirty men, and were looking for somewhere to stay, and he told me that there were no houses big enough on his side of the lake, but his barn was large and was dry inside, and there was still a lot of hay left in the hayloft. We were welcome to stay there until we found something better. So we followed the cows up the lane to look at the barn. We had lived in worse places many times, so we moved in, set up the aid station, and slept in the hayloft.

We stayed in the barn that night and the next, and the following morning I stopped in at the German hospital, to find the building empty. All of the patients and staff had been evacuated. I hurried back to our barn, and we promptly moved into the *"Albergo al Lago di Resia"* where we stayed in comfort until the time came for the battalion to leave the area.

In the meantime our task force had turned into an extensive border patrol, and because there was not much for the infantry to do, training sessions began once again.

The command posts for our task force, for our battalion and for the German units doing similar patrolling were all close together in the village, but we were half a mile out of town and isolated from all of this hustle and bustle. We didn't participate in any training, but held a formal sick call daily, and we were available for emergencies whenever they occurred. We also carried on a large civilian practice, which included many young children. We slept a lot, and ate well because we now had kitchen facilities, plus otherwise idle litter bearers who were good cooks.

Before the War this hotel must have been a very lovely place in which to stay. There were good-sized guest rooms on all three floors. A large, single story, glassed-in dining room at one end of the building extended out toward the lake, and had a large sun deck as its roof. Underneath the dining room the large walk-out basement opened close to the water's edge, and in it rowboats were stored for the winter. There was a swimming area and a bathhouse, but while we were there the water in the lake was much too cold for us to be able to swim. The building stood at the water's edge, several hundred feet from the main road, and had a private driveway, which joined the main road quite some distance away in both directions.

In the basement of the hotel I found a supply of picture post cards, which the hotel management had apparently supplied to its guests. These showed several views of the building and the surrounding countryside, and the winter scenes indicated that this had also been a popular center for winter sports. I still have about a dozen of these pictures in my possession.

For the medical detachment, the week spent at Passo di Resia was a pleasant one of rest and recuperation. We were occupied only with our own housekeeping chores, and the daily sick call, which was never very busy. We only occasionally treated a German soldier, but we did see and treat a lot of civilians, so those of us who ran the aid station were the busiest. I never turned down anyone who came asking for medical help.

Most of the people living in the area were blond, blue-eyed, and spoke German, but many insisted emphatically that they were Austrian. Some spoke a dialect that I could barely understand, but these people could understand me very well, and many of them were also able to speak the German I knew in addition to their dialect. Although orders against fraternization had been issued, they were almost impossible to enforce. I enjoyed talking to the people, and perhaps had more opportunity to do so than anyone else in the battalion, because so many of them came, with their families, to see me as patients.

Infantry units that were not directly involved in patrolling the border held training exercises every day, but there was also time for recreational activities. Local and German Army equipment for skiing and mountain climbing appeared as if by magic, and some of the men participated in these sports. Others played volleyball and softball. There was also time for just loafing around.

We were in a broad, open valley filled with cultivated fields, dotted here and there with small clusters of buildings. It was spring in the mountains and the grass was already green. Buds everywhere had burst, and tiny new leaves were showing. The valley was rimmed with evergreen forests covering the foothills, and beyond them the mountain peaks, composed of rock, were gleaming white where they were covered with ice and snow. Fed by snowmelt from the peaks and glaciers, a chain of three small, clear blue lakes, ran down the center of the valley, and the northernmost one of these was Lago di Resia, on the shore of which we were now staying. It was such a nice place in which to be, that we would all have been satisfied to have stayed as occupying forces until it was time to go home.

Long after the War, on a visit to Austria in 1971, my wife and I rented a car and drove southward through Resia late one afternoon to look for the *Albergo at Lago di Resia.* There were more buildings in the area than I had remembered, and I thought I recognized the lake, but wasn't sure because there was no building on the shore. We drove farther until I was certain that we had passed it by, and stopped for the night at an inn called *"Der Schwartzer Adler"* (The Black Eagle). The proprietor's wife spoke German, and when I asked her about the hotel I was looking for, she said she knew it well, and told us the following story about it:

Before the War the hotel was owned by a man who operated it with the help of his two sons, but soon after the War began, the Nazis came one night and took him away, never to be heard from again. Soon afterward the German Army confiscated the hotel and turned it into a hospital. The sons survived the war, and returned to operate the hotel again, but were so saddened by the loss of their father that they tore the building down and rebuilt the hotel up on the main road away from the lake. The original building was no longer there, and that was why I didn't recognize the spot. I couldn't recognize the new building either, because it had not been there during the War. The next morning we drove back, but it was during the off-season and the hotel was closed, so we weren't able to go inside or talk to anyone there.

In the fall of 1988 we retraced our route from Austria into Italy through

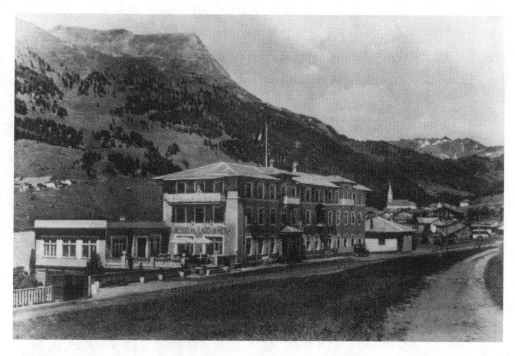

THE RESORT HOTEL, ALBERGO al LAGO di RESIA
Used by the enemy as a field hospital throughout the War, it was still filled with wounded German soldiers when its Kommandant formally surrendered it to the author in the spring of 1945.

Resia, and found the new building without difficulty, but again it was closed. This time there was a lot more new construction evident all around. The blacktop road was new and wider, and dams had been built so that the three lakes at the head of the valley had grown larger and merged into one much bigger body of water. Lago di Resia, as I had known it, didn't exist anymore, and the site of the old *Albergo al Lago di Resia* was now underwater.

CHAPTER XX

OCCUPATION PERIOD

On April 28 at about the time that I was making the amphibious journey around the blown tunnels on Lake Garda, the Italian dictator, Benito Mussolini, and his mistress were shot to death by Italian Partisans somewhere in the foothills West of Lake Como. Rumors of this event reached us soon after we entered Torbole on April 30, and were quickly confirmed. It was also reported that the Partisans had taken the bodies to Milan where they had hung them upside down in public for all to view, and that they would remain on display there for several more days. Several of our officers talked about making the trip to view the spectacle, but I don't know of anyone who went, because orders creating the task force to Resia arrived at about that same time.

Two days after Mussolini was killed, the German dictator, Adolf Hitler, committed suicide in his bunker in Berlin. The news of this event also first reached us as a rumor, but it was also quickly confirmed. Later when the total German surrender was signed on May 7, we heard about that through our military channels on the same day. The next day President Truman declared VE Day, and the War in Europe was officially over.

Almost immediately dozens of new and widely differing rumors regarding the future of our division began to circulate, and our newly acquired idleness allowed them to build upon themselves. All kinds of ramifications evolved freely and rapidly: "We were the only Mountain Troops in the U.S. Army, so we would occupy the Alpine regions indefinitely. We had been the last division to be sent to Europe, so we would be one of the last to leave. We would be the first to leave, and would be sent through the Suez Canal to join the War in the Pacific. We would get to the Pacific by going through the Panama Canal to the West Coast, where we would re-supply ourselves before going into combat." There were many, many more, and most of them had us fighting the Japanese sooner rather than later.

After VE Day I was able to do some sightseeing, but it wasn't possible to go far. I went into Austria to see more of that beautiful country and talk to the people. I found the Austrians to be more resentful of our presence than were the Italians, but their resentment was not so much directed at us personally as it was at the fact that they had lost the War. To me this was understandable. War casualty lists posted in the cities and villages were large in proportion to their populations; there were hardly any physically unimpaired young men left, and toward the end, even boys 15 and 16 years of age had been forced to serve at the various fronts. The people had been given a lot of propaganda and false information about how well the War was going for Germany, and now suddenly all was lost. They had no idea what the victors might do to them. From their viewpoint the outlook for the future was bleak indeed.

On one of my short sightseeing excursions we drove up into the mountains and walked to the marker, which designated the border between Italy, Austria and Switzerland, and I was able to stand upon the exact spot. The surrounding area was filled with fortifications, pillboxes and permanent dugouts which could not be seen from the valley below, and which had been left from previous wars. Later I visited the spot for a second time when I was called to care for a soldier who had injured himself while standing guard in that area.

On May 12 the battalion received orders to leave Passo di Resia. We were being replaced as occupation forces, and we left the Austrian border the following morning, on what turned out to be another long and tedious trip in a military convoy, headed back the way we had come. We didn't stop when we arrived in Riva, but went on southward along the east side of Lake Garda through the tunnels that had posed such problems for us two weeks before. We continued for the full length of the lake and around its southern end into the Po Valley, and late that night finally turned into a large open field in which we set up camp. The men slept in pup tents, using their shelter halves again for the first time since we had left the bivouac area near Pisa. Battalion Headquarters, the field kitchens and the aid station were set up in pyramidal tents, which were already on the scene when we arrived.

In the morning we found that we were camped in what had been a German airfield, one of a series of such airfields, which had been laid out with well-camouflaged runways oriented randomly in many different directions. We were near the town of Castenedolo, not far from Brescia, and compared to the pleasant temperatures in the mountains, it was hot and oppressive.

Military courtesy and garrison rules, including mandatory saluting, were reinstated, and started a lot of grumbling and complaining.

We soon noted that the whole division had been moved into the area. Our official mission was to receive and guard prisoners, but the situation with prisoners was already well in hand, and this seemed like a trivial job for the whole division to be doing. I was particularly skeptical about the mission because where we were camped I saw very few German prisoners. Another peculiar thing was the absence of formal training sessions. The Army, at least in our division, always filled any spare working hours with some kind of training program. Instead the men now spent all of their time engaged in sports such as softball and volleyball; there were trips to the south shore of Lake Garda for swimming, and passes to Brescia were issued liberally.

The stay near Castenedolo also marked the beginning of another unusual but pleasant practice. The distribution of the booty from the liquor warehouse in the Po Valley was begun, and every man got either a bottle of fine French champagne or cognac every other day. From then on the distribution continued at intervals until the supply was gone, and in all I received six or seven bottles, three of which I saved and eventually carried home in my duffle bag.

Equipment was being repaired or replaced. Some of our winter equipment was exchanged for summer gear, and there were some showdown inspections to make sure that all equipment was in good condition and properly maintained. Briefings and "poop sheets," which is what the mimeographed bulletins from higher headquarters were called, hinted strongly that we were in the early stages of redeployment to the Pacific without actually saying it in so many words. Most of the officers were resigned to the inevitability of such a move, and it appeared to me that the process had already begun. Censorship, which had totally ended a week or so previously was now, on May 16, reimposed, and all unit censors received orders that it was to be strictly enforced.

On May 17 the regiment was alerted to be ready to move, but to everyone's surprise, it was not a move for redeployment. We had been chosen for a possible combat mission. The Italians and the Yugoslavs were shooting at each other in the area North of Trieste. Both countries claimed a strip of land along the border, and Marshall Tito's men refused to leave territory that had previously been Italian. Signs of hostility had increased, and if it continued, the 10th Mountain Division would move in and control the area to keep the two sides apart. Everything else in the Division was put on hold. Rations and ammunition were distributed, and everyone made ready for combat again.

Were we actually going to fight? None of us could be sure.

The order to move came on May 19, and the division started immediately in a motorized column headed toward Udine and points east. Since our battalion was scheduled to be the last to leave, we didn't start until the morning of the 20th, and began what turned out to be another long, tedious trip in military convoy.

After passing through the city of Udine we began to see Yugoslav soldiers wearing the red star on their uniforms. There we also saw two kinds of Italian Partisans, Christian Democrats who wore green scarves, and Communists who wore red ones. The red star was displayed everywhere, graffiti style, particularly on the sides of buildings and on road signs.

We soon began making frequent stops, and I learned later that we had been held up by frequent new orders that kept changing our final destination. We had originally been scheduled to occupy the valley east of Udine in the vicinity of Cividale, but instead of going there, we kept heading northward, passing through small towns where people appeared to be celebrating and where partisan banners were being displayed. In time we passed by the 2nd Battalion and Regimental Headquarters in Cave del Predil, the 1st Battalion at Bretto di Soto, and finally ended up in a wild and rugged mountain pass named Passo di Predil. We set up the aid station in a building at the roadside, and the companies spread out in front of us and behind us to set up camps with pup tents and foxholes. We had passed through the entire division to become its spearhead once again, and found ourselves farther North and farther East than any of the other battalions.

Our mission was a delicate one. We were to keep any additional Yugoslavian soldiers or civilians from entering the disputed territory, and try to get those already there to leave by peaceful means. The men were warned over and over again never to go anywhere unarmed, to use tact and judgment, and above all to avoid any acts that could precipitate armed conflict. We must have done this well, because while we were there we never witnessed any armed aggression, although during our first few nights in the pass, we sometimes heard shots being exchanged high in the hills. Later we persuaded a large number of Yugoslavian soldiers to return across the line into Yugoslavia, and even gave them a ride in our quartermaster trucks. I was surprised to see that they were completely agreeable, and even waved goodbye to us with smiles on their faces as their convoy left.

Passo di Predil cut through the Julian Alps 3,000 feet above sea level, and the mountains surrounding it were the most rugged I had yet seen. Compared to the Apennines or the Southern Alps, the slopes were steeper, the cliffs were higher and the forests much wilder. Even though it rained for a short time almost every day, the cool weather was a welcome relief from the oppressive heat and humidity in the Po Valley. This was ideal country for rock climbing, and ample snow on the higher slopes offered excellent skiing. Instruction in both of these activities was soon under way, with old 10th Mountain veterans offering lessons to the newer men.

On the morning of May 22nd I received orders, which granted me, together with two other battalion officers, a leave for rest and recuperation at the 5th Army Officers' Rest Hotel in Stresa on the shore of Lake Maggiore. These orders came as a complete surprise because none of us had asked for leave, and when they arrived we had neither made arrangements to leave nor were we packed and ready to go. It was noon before we finally departed.

Stresa was three-quarters of the way across Northern Italy, and we again endured another long, tedious ride in a Jeep. Upon arrival late in the evening, we were assigned to private rooms. First I took a luxurious bath in a real bathtub, then crawled into bed on an innerspring mattress, between white sheets, and had an excellent night's sleep.

After breakfast in the hotel dining room the following morning, I took stock of my surroundings. The hotel was the *"Grande Albergo E Delle Isole Borromee,"* and it was located on the shore of Lago di Maggiore on the outskirts of Stresa. It was a wonderful place, a famous resort hotel where, before the War, only the truly rich could afford to stay. My room was in the middle of the building on the third floor. It had a private bath and a balcony overlooking the hotel's formal gardens and the lake. Just offshore stood one of the Borromean Islands with a picturesque chalet, or perhaps it was a small castle, standing on it. The hotel employees all spoke excellent English, but the waiters in the dining room were French, and the menus were all in French. This created a problem for me, because I knew no French at all, but I managed very well by using the finger pointing method of ordering; that is, I would point to one item in each section of the menu, and then wait to see what arrived at the table. This seemed to work very well, and the meals I received were excellent, until one evening I tried to install some "system" into my ordering, by pointing to the items with the longest French names in each section of the menu. The entree I chose that evening took up two whole lines, but when the food arrived I was disappointed, because the plate contained a plain boiled potato with a sprig of parsley on it, and three thin slices of Spam.

The hotel grounds were elegantly landscaped with pines growing next to palms. The shrubs were all precisely trimmed, and the gardens well kept.

Tennis, golf, horseback riding, swimming facilities, and fishing boat rentals were offered at fees over and above what we were entitled to as army officers, but the charges for these things were steep, and I didn't participate in any of them. I was still changing my Army lira into pennies and sending them home.

One afternoon the three of us drove all of the way around the beautiful Lake Maggiore. Another day I took a walk into Stresa with the intention of buying a present for my wife for her June birthday, but was again deterred by the exorbitant prices. Instead, for a few pennies, I bought some fishhooks and a hand line, and spent the afternoon on the hotel dock, where I caught and released a few small trout, some fish that resembled our Great Lakes Perch, and another small fish that I didn't recognize.

I also spent time in the tavern at the hotel, where a motley assortment of mixed drinks, none of which I cared for, was being offered. However, the locally brewed beer was good, and the price was reasonable, so beer was what I always ordered. I was intrigued by the bottles too, because I had seen similar ones when I was a very small child and had watched my grandfather make home brew. Instead of the familiar bottle caps we use today, these bottles were sealed with rubber washers encircling glass plugs that were held tightly in place by a heavy wire harness. I also remember that some of the early mason jars, used in my family for canning fruits and vegetables at home, used the same principle for sealing the contents against contamination.

When the vacation ended, I knew that the jeep ride back to Passo di Predil would be long and tedious, and I didn't look forward to it with any enthusiasm. We left in the afternoon, and got as far as Vicenza by evening. From there we called ahead and received permission to stay overnight. We also obtained permission to take an extra day in order to visit Venice, which was not far out of our way, and because there were no government accommodations in Vicenza we got permission to stay in an Italian hotel. The hotel turned out to be one of the worst in which I had ever stayed, and we were glad to leave it early the next morning.

As we drove toward Venice, we decided to try for a better breakfast than C Rations, and stopped at a farmhouse out in the country. Although we were now somewhat experienced in using single words with gestures when dickering with the natives, it took a little time to make the farmer and his wife understand what we wanted. Finally the woman understood, and agreed to make us a breakfast of eggs and toast in return for our unopened C Ration cans. She seemed happy to have the cans for a possible future food emergency, because they would keep more or less indefinitely. So the three of us were invited into the kitchen, where we sat at a large wooden table to watch the preparations.

I had seen Italian farm women cook before, and the process always fascinated me. We were in a typical farm kitchen, a large room with thick stone walls, small windows and a huge fireplace with a wide hearth. The walls and ceiling were blackened by smoke, which had not always completely risen up the chimney in the past. Typical of the fireplaces I had seen in other Italian farmhouses, this one seemed shallow from front to back, and had a huge opening. In a few minutes the farmer came in with some eggs he had apparently just gathered, and his wife went out briefly to get the fuel with which to cook our breakfast. When she returned, she carried two bundles of twigs, 6 to 8 inches long, about 4 inches in diameter, and tied up with a few long strands of dried grass. Each contained dozens of tiny twigs taken from trees and bushes, and most of them were not much thicker than matchsticks. These little bundles were the typical cooking fuel all over rural Italy, and I had seen them used before in small cookstoves and sometimes out in the open, but most often in fireplaces such as this one. The woman produced a large loaf of homemade bread and sliced off several pieces, which she stood on edge against the sides of a small rack in the center of which she had put one of the bundles of twigs. On the top of the rack she set a metal pot of water, which would be heated for making up the instant coffee we had with us, instead of the tea, which she would normally have brewed. She lit the bundle of twigs, blew on it with a small bellows to get it burning briskly, and using this heat source, she made toast. As each piece was done, she buttered it with home churned butter. In the meantime the water continued to heat. Next she produced a frying pan, broke six fresh eggs, with yolks standing high, into it, added several generous chunks of butter and a tablespoon of water, placed a lid over the pan, and cooked them over the second bundle of twigs. The remains of that second fire then continued to heat our water while she served the breakfast, which consisted of two delicately cooked eggs, some hard salami or summer sausage, toast with butter and jam, and coffee. It was a simple but truly memorable breakfast. Everything was delicious, and I was so pleased with it, that as we said our goodbyes, I slipped the farm couple a package of cigarettes.

We stayed in Venice almost the whole day, and spent most of the morning in a gondola with a gondolier who spoke excellent English and gave us an excellent tour of the city. We walked about in St. Mark's Square, had lunch at the Allied Officers' Club, and visited a number of shops. Once again I didn't buy anything because of the high prices. Before leaving the city in the afternoon, we took another gondola ride for an hour or so. I particularly remember being disappointed by the canals for the second time that day, because sewage and garbage floated everywhere, and an offensive smell permeated the whole city. I have never been back, but whenever I see a travelogue about Venice, I often wonder if it still smells like that.

That evening we stopped at an Army evacuation hospital north of Udine for supper, and once again I had a chance to talk to professionals on the hospital staff. We made it back to the battalion before dark, and learned that while we were gone, things had remained calm and settled in the area, and no longer was there any shooting in the hills at night. Training sessions had started again, and extensive field exercises were being planned in which the medical detachments were expected to participate.

My daily routine now became quite a bit like it had been when we first arrived at the front in January except that we no longer had to operate under blackout conditions, and the troops were now engaged in training and recreational activities instead of combat. The line companies were spread out in the pass with the platoons and squads scattered here and there, but the distances weren't so long, and I didn't have to travel as far to visit them. Usually I would make rounds in the jeep each morning, and while making them, I also inspected kitchens, latrines, water supplies and sanitation practices. Occasionally I was required to give a lecture on some medical subject. I also held a daily sick call at the aid station, and when an injury occurred, I would sometimes see someone out in the field. I also remained responsible for checking the immunization records of all of the men, and administering the necessary shots to be sure that everyone was currently adequately immunized.

Before beginning sick call daily at 1 p.m. I regularly ate lunch at the Battalion Officers' Mess. The sick call usually did not last long because few of our men were ever sick, but afterward I would usually spend time seeing and treating civilians. These sessions usually ended about 3 p.m., and the rest of the day was devoted to sports and recreation. Medical emergencies, both military and civilian, were treated anytime day or night, and occasionally interrupted this routine. Later during our stay, I occasionally made house calls on civilian patients in the evenings.

The regimental and battalion histories state that on June 3 we were visited and heard a speech by Field Marshall Sir Harold Alexander, the Supreme Commander of the Mediterranean Theater of Operations, but I don't remember it at all. I clearly remember the speech by General Mark Clark two months before, and I am sure that I would have remembered Field Marshall Alexander, if I had been there to hear his speech. I have since seen a picture of this occasion, taken while he was speaking, which also shows his audience, and it appears to me that not all of the battalion was present. The rest of the men must have been still deployed out in the pass, and I was probably somewhere out there with them.

Sometime about the end of the first week in June the 2nd and 3rd Battalions switched territories, and we moved from the pass into the town of Cave del Predil where Regimental Headquarters had been established in a very nice hotel. Battalion Headquarters was there too. The aid station was located about a block down the street, and the back room there was a popular place for junior officers to spend time away from the higher brass. It became sort of a day room where they would gather for conversation, reading or to play cards. Our daily routine didn't change very much, and we were now even more comfortable than we had been before. The headquarters hotel had a gymnasium with excellent showers; there were tennis and handball courts, and also pool tables for our use.

Softball was very popular. Diamonds were laid out and the various units had teams that played each other. I soon became the regular pitcher for the officers' team, and the catcher for the medical detachment team, and often played one game before supper and another after supper. The medical detachment team was good, and won more often than it lost. Occasionally some officer would express his disapproval that I was playing ball with the enlisted men, because he felt that I was losing their respect by fraternizing too much. I didn't see it that way, however. I liked these men, and I was quite sure that they liked me. I considered them to be friends, not inferiors.

Swimming had always been my best sport, and now I became the coach of the regimental swimming team. We drove to the town of Villach in Austria, where there was a swimming pool in which we could practice, and where we held a few meets. I didn't enter any of the races myself, because there were quite a few very good swimmers on the team. Later in the summer when the weather was warmer, we often drove up to a small lake near Hermagor, also in Austria, for recreational swimming, and I especially enjoyed this because as we swam we mingled with the natives. The bathhouse facilities were well kept and clean, as were the beaches and the docks. Small children, up to the age of six or seven, swam nude. For most of us this was unheard of, and it took a little time before we were comfortable with it, but the older children and adults didn't disturb us, because all wore bathing suits like the ones we had been accustomed to seeing on our beaches at home.

On one of these swimming trips an incident occurred which illustrates a main difference between the German Military and our Army. A small group of us were swimming from one of the docks, and were joined by about a dozen 8 to 12-year-old Austrian boys. I could tell from their conversation that they held us in awe, even bordering on hero worship, because we were Americans and we were soldiers. At first they were shy, and kept their distance, but as time went by, they became bolder and came closer. We were discussing a swimming meet, and it was obvious that although they were listening, they didn't understand what we were saying. Then one bright youngster caught on to the fact that the men were regularly calling me "Sir," and said to the others in German,

"They treat him like an officer sometimes, but he can't be, because no officer associates with the common soldiers like this."

They were astonished when I spoke to them in German, and assured them that I was indeed an officer, but that most American officers were not haughty and conceited *(hochmütig und eingebildet)* like the German officers, and American soldiers obeyed orders because they had confidence in their officers, not because they were afraid of them. After several visits to this same swimming spot, many of the native regulars had seen me and other officers in uniform. They knew we were officers, and continued to act surprised that we would swim with the enlisted men.

I also went on a trip with a group of our men to the city of Klagenfurt, which is a transportation hub in Southern Austria. The railroad yards had been completely wrecked by bombing raids, but one building at the edge of the area still stood. It appeared to be a passenger station with several sets of rails running parallel in front of it, and it appeared to have suffered only minor exterior damage. Several of us went inside and found that the safe in the office had been blown, but still contained a large quantity of fancy banknotes in huge denominations of marks. They had been printed on high quality currency paper, bright orange on one side, and gray with possibly another color on the opposite side. I had collected stamps as a child, and recognized the numbers on these bills as being the same as those on some of the German stamps from the runaway inflation era that followed World War I. This was currency left over from that hyperinfiationary time, and it no longer had any monetary value. I knew that a *"milliarde"* was one billion, and here were bills for one hundred, five hundred, one thousand *"milliarden"* and higher.

At the end of June I received another rest leave, this time to Milan, one of the largest cities in Northern Italy. Lieutenant Wilkinson from K Company and I went together, and this time I had my own jeep and driver for transportation, which allowed us a lot of freedom to take side trips. The drive to

Milan took all day, but was not quite as long as the trip to Stresa had been five weeks before. The *Albergo Diana* was a nice, big city hotel in the downtown area, but it was not nearly as fancy as the hotel at Stresa. Again I had a private room. I spent a lot of time in the hotel, reading the American magazines that were there. I considered it a treat to have both the time and the magazines. I also spent a lot of time walking about downtown, and shopping for gifts to send home. All of the shops had heavy iron grates or shutters over the doors and windows, which were closed and locked overnight to prevent break-ins and robberies. Again I didn't buy much. The fact that I could turn my lira into pennies, send them home, and thus would be able to buy twenty or more times what I could buy with them in Italy, was a great deterrent. I did, however, have some pictures taken of myself, and although I thought at the time that they also were too expensive, I am glad to have them. Of the ones that I still have, two were taken outdoors, and one portrait type picture was taken inside the photographer's shop.

With the *Albergo Diana* in Milan as our headquarters, we made three lengthy side trips. On June 30 we went to the city of Como, and drove along the lakeshore for some distance. On the way back we stopped in town to shop for an hour or so, and I finally bought a present for my wife. It was a nice looking purse made of white plastic, which was something that was not yet common at home. The idea was good, but the plastic wasn't, because soon after she received the purse, the plastic deteriorated and crumbled. My money had been wasted. I don't believe my wife ever got to carry that purse before it had to be discarded.

On July 1 we went to *Genova* (Genoa) on the Ligurian Sea. Stores were closed and there was little activity because it was a Sunday, but we drove along the waterfront. The harbor, like the one in Naples, had been heavily bombed and appeared wrecked, but the bathing beaches were nice and were filled with people. Most of the buildings were white and reflected the bright sunshine, and many of them seemed to be modern apartment dwellings.

On the Fourth of July we took a side trip to *Torino* (Turin), and I was impressed that this was the cleanest and best kept of the larger cities in Italy. Almost all of the stores were open, and the prices were better, but nevertheless the merchandise seemed shoddy, and not worth the prices being asked.

For me the highlight of the vacation in Milan was an evening at the opera. None of my officer friends cared about opera, but I had had extensive exposure to it in high school, where I had sung in the chorus in a number of operatic presentations, and had been encouraged to attend a number of professionally presented operas at Orchestra Hall in downtown Detroit. I had a good voice and during my senior year, was picked to sing on stage there in the chorus of Verdi's "Requiem," and enjoyed the thrill of being on the same stage with Lily Pons, Ezio Pinza and Rosa Tentoni, who were among. the top opera stars of the time. My high school music teachers even wanted me to consider singing as a career, but my mind had long been made up. I remained determined to become a doctor.

La Scala is the most famous opera house in Milan, but when I was there it was not in operation because of damage caused by bombing raids. There were a number of other opera houses in the city, but on the evening I wanted to attend, all but one of them were closed for one reason or another, so I went to the only one that was open, the *Teatro Puccini,* and saw *"Lucia di Lammermoor."*

The opera house was about three blocks from the hotel. I walked to get there, and when I arrived at the ticket window the only seats left were the expensive ones on the main floor near the front and the very cheap ones in the 3rd or 4th balcony. I bought the expensive one, and was glad that I had, because I sat among well dressed gentlemen and elegantly clad, perfumed ladies while the patrons in the upper balconies appeared so shabby and un- washed that I wondered what it smelled like up there. There were a few Brit- ish soldiers in the audience, but I didn't see any other American military people.

The bomb damage to La Scala was repaired and it opened again in 1946, a year or so after I had been in Milan. Since then I have seen pictures of its interior in publications, in movies and on television. The interior of the Teatro Puccini looked very much like the pictures of La Scala, with a relatively small, steeply sloped main floor, theater boxes along the side walls, and sev- eral balconies across the back extending all of the way up to the high domed ceiling. There was standing room only in the back of the top balcony, and the people there looked, for the most part, like street beggars. There was a large bar in the lobby on the main floor, where the elite of Milan fortified them- selves during the intermissions, of which there were three during the three- hour performance. One thing that I didn't like was that the people in the audience, instead of going out into the lobby to smoke during intermissions, did so right in their seats. However no one smoked during the performance.

The opera was beautifully presented, and the singers, none of whose names I recognized, all had excellent voices. The performance was better than anything I had ever attended in the United States. The singer who played Lucia had an exceptional voice, and with my eyes closed I had no trouble visualizing the beautiful heroine, but when I looked at the scenes on the stage,

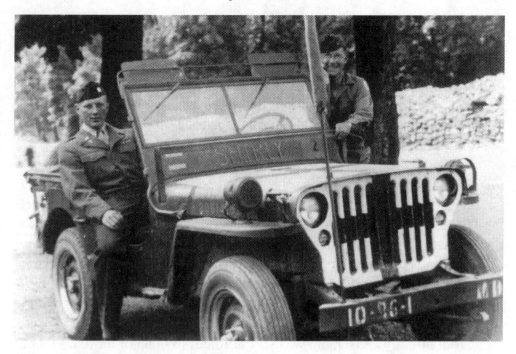

THE AUTHOR AND HIS DRIVER, PFC. CHARLES ARGYLE, WITH THE MEDICAL DETACHMENT JEEP

the incongruity of the situation was almost comical, because the diva, who sang Lucia, was built like a linebacker on a professional football team. However, even though she dwarfed the rest of the cast, her voice was beautiful and had been excellently trained.

On Friday, July 6th we left to return to the battalion, and had gone some 30 miles to Bergamo, when Lieutenant Wilkinson realized that he had forgotten to bring along the expensive fly rod, which he had purchased in Milan. By this time we had picked up two of our headquarters company men who were hitchhiking back from their leaves, so the three of us stayed in Bergamo for a couple of hours, while Lieutenant Wilkinson and our driver returned to the hotel to retrieve the pole. During this time I treated myself to a professional shave, complete with perfumed after shave lotion, for which I paid all of twenty lira in a fancy barber shop, and I bartered in a jewelry store for several pieces of jewelry which I managed to obtain for some cigarettes. By 2:00 p.m. we were all together again, and continued on our journey. We stopped at the Red Cross tent in Verona for coffee and doughnuts, arrived back at the battalion about 11:00 p.m., and I went to bed immediately.

In the morning I found that the whole camp was in a state of doom and gloom. While I was gone the division had been told that it had been assigned to permanently occupy the Trieste area for at least the next year. Then the next day it had been alerted to be ready to move for immediate, direct redeployment to China, and now several more days had passed, but nothing more had been heard. I became suspicious that something big might be happening in the War with Japan, and that the War Department in Washington was trying to make rapid decisions as the situation changed.

We were left hanging indecisively for another week while the division rumor mill worked overtime, but then the immediate fate of the division was definitely decided. The 34th Division had been assigned the task of occupying the Trieste area, and would relieve us. We would be redeployed to the Pacific, but would go through the United States, where we would be re-equipped and retrained. We had been the last division to reach Europe; now we would be the first division from Europe to leave and engage the Japanese. We should reach the U.S. sometime during the latter half of August, and the first thing in store for us was a leave for everyone in the division.

Strict military censorship was still in force, so none of us could let our families know we were coming home, but I managed to get the message across in the next letter to my wife. Birthdays had always been important in my family, and whenever one came around in the immediate family, it was celebrated with gifts, special dinners and other nice things. My father's birthday was August 19, and I wrote several things about the upcoming celebration of his birthday and about his birthday gifts. Then I concluded with, "and I'm sure Aunt Clara will also be pleased with her birthday gift this year." Aunt Clara was a great aunt, who lived near us, but we never celebrated her birthday in our immediate family, and we never had exchanged birthday gifts. At first my wife was puzzled when she read this, but when my mother heard this statement over the phone, she knew immediately that I was expecting to be home at least by Aunt Clara's birthday, which was August 25th.

On the morning of July 16, as we watched the men of the 34th Division move happily into our positions, we boarded trucks and left the area for good. The convoy went to Udine, where the infantrymen were loaded onto trains for the rest of the journey. Our regimental and battalion vehicles continued to our final destination which was Florence, and there we stayed for a time, in neat rows of tents on the banks of the Arno River.

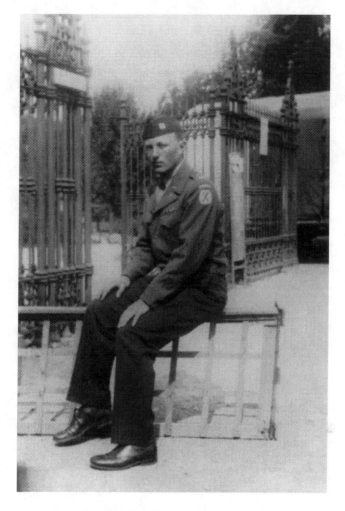

THE AUTHOR IN NORTHERN ITALY IN 1945.

CHAPTER XXI

CIVILIAN MEDICAL PRACTICE

In previous chapters I have described a few of the civilian medical problems I saw while I was in Italy: a youth with a severe nephrotic syndrome, an epidemic of diphtheria, and the extraction of rotten civilian teeth. Much of the time I actually did carry on a large civilian practice, and I believe it was common practice along most of the front for the medical units there to give medical care freely to civilians whenever the combat situation allowed.

Until now I have left most of the tales of civilian medical practice out of this narrative because some readers might not care for the subject matter and its inclusion in a random fashion might spoil the story. I also tried to avoid interruption of the continuity of the war stories with seemingly irrelevant details. Because I had many encounters with civilians and my memory of most of them is not completely clear, it is impossible for me to include each of the incidents I remember at exactly its correct time and place in the sequence of events. Many were short, one-time consultations in which the patient only needed reassurance rather than medicine or medical treatment, and most of these have escaped my memory completely. Nevertheless, non-military medicine was such a large part of my life in Italy that it deserves a place in my book, and I have therefore chosen to detail some of it separately in this chapter.

I rarely saw an elderly patient, but saw and treated many children, and also quite a few young adults. We did not have the new antibiotic, penicillin, at the front but we did have a plentiful supply of sulfanilamide and sulfadiazine, and at the time these were indeed miracle drugs for many of the infections, which were common in the civilian population. I also didn't see many civilian war casualties while we were engaged in actual fighting at the front. This is not surprising, because I was usually in the far forward area of the combat zone and civilians usually vacated these areas before the serious shooting started. War type wounds among civilians were more common in the areas behind us, and were mainly caused by long-range artillery, mines, unexploded shells and booby traps. Bombing raids had previously caused many similar wounds earlier in the War, but by the time I reached Italy the enemy had already been rendered incapable of doing much bombing. I have forgotten the first civilian patient I saw in Italy, and don't even remember where the encounter took place. It may perhaps have been in Bagnoli north of Naples, but more likely it was in San Marcello when we first went into the front line.

Until after we got into the German speaking areas of Italy where I could handle the language myself, I always needed my interpreter when I examined or treated civilians. He was needed and came along whenever I made the equivalent of housecalls to the smaller units of the battalion, because I so often treated both soldiers and civilians on these trips. In time I learned to say such things as *"Due ogne quattro ore, con molta aqua."* (Two every four hours, with much water.), but I always relied upon him to relay the patient's history to me and had him explain the treatment to each patient in detail. I also let him screen the civilians asking for medical help, and asked him to keep trying to learn from them any information that might be of use to us. Most of the time he was the one who brought the need for seeing a civilian to my attention, and during the course of his activities I believe he often went out of his way to find an extra patient or two.

Occasionally I was asked to look at a wound that had previously been surgically treated at one of our Army medical installations. These always seemed to have healed well, and any problem would be minor, such as a suture knot working its way to the surface through the scar. I also saw a lot of old wounds that had not been treated at all, except for the application of household remedies commonly used by the country folk. Some of these were infected, but a surprising number were not, and from watching some of them over a period of time, I learned that even huge tissue defects would heal by granulation, scar formation, and contraction, if given sufficient time. The infected wounds usually responded well to local treatment, which we usually taught the patient or someone in the family to carryout. Local application of sulfanilamide powder was helpful.

Twice, when the battalion was in a reserve status and we were a little farther than usual from the front, I was called upon because a woman was having difficulty with childbirth. The cases were almost identical, and taught me some principles, which I was to remember throughout the rest of my medical career. Both women were young and having their first babies, and both had probably been in labor over 24 hours before I arrived on the scene.

In each place a middle-aged Italian woman seemed to be in charge, but I couldn't be sure if she was a midwife or just a relative or friend who had had some previous experience assisting with childbirth. In each case, I could hear the woman in labor crying and carrying on well before I arrived at the bedside, and I also could hear the voices of other women urging the mother-to-be to bear down and push the baby out.

As I entered the room for the first of these obstetrical cases, something occurred which I was to witness many times later in my career and which improved the situation immediately. I was the authority, the *"Dottore Americano,"* and just my arrival had changed the situation from one of near panic, to one of confidence and hope. The laboring mother-to-be settled down. The ladies in waiting stopped yelling, and even started to smile a little. In my subsequent practice I was to witness this same phenomenon many times, whenever, under similar circumstances, a respected obstetrical consultant entered a labor or delivery room to help with a problem. After examining the patient and checking the fetal heart sounds, I found nothing seriously wrong, and thought that this was probably a case of moderately prolonged but otherwise normal labor. In fact my arrival at the bedside had been delayed long enough for nature to accomplish its work, because the baby's head was already beginning to crown. The mother looked tired but was in good condition, and I found that the baby's heart tones remained excellent through several labor contractions. Sanitation in the dingy bedroom wasn't the best, so I chose to delay delivery of the head to allow the perineum to stretch out completely. If possible, I would try to complete the delivery without the need for stitches.

Through Consiglio I told the patient when to bear down, not to push too hard, and when to rest. The crowning increased; more and more of the baby's head appeared during each succeeding contraction, and after about a dozen more pains, she delivered a vigorous, healthy baby boy. There were no perineal tears, and no stitches were needed. When the placenta came, I made sure that it was intact and all there, before I finished up, and went into the next room where the men of the family were waiting.

An older man, whom I presumed was a grandfather of the new baby, came into the room carrying several dark and dusty bottles. Some fine looking crystal glasses appeared, and soon everyone drank a toast to the new baby with some truly excellent wine. It was certainly a far cry from the watered down *"vino rosa"* that was for sale in the local shops.

The second delivery was almost a repeat performance of the first, except that I arrived a little earlier, the baby was a girl, and the mother did sustain a few tiny perineal lacerations, which fell together so well, that again I did not use any sutures. The wine offered to celebrate this blessed event was equally as good as the first had been.

Near the beginning of the time during which we stayed with the "Duke" in the rear area near Lucca, Consiglio came to me to say that a family had approached him and asked for medical help for one of its girls, who was very ill and had a high fever. We went together to see her, and found the home to be nicely furnished, well kept and clean. The parents met us at the door, and took us upstairs into an attractive, bright, sunny bedroom. The large bed was made up with brilliantly clean, white bedding, and lying in the center of it, wearing a spotless white nightgown, was an unusually beautiful, dark eyed, black haired, 19-year-old Italian girl. She had been having chills and fever for three days, and, since the very beginning, had experienced burning on urination. Now she was urinating in only very small amounts, and it still burned.

She looked sick. Her temperature was over 104 Degrees F., and her face was flushed, but my examination turned up nothing else of real significance, except for some tenderness in the costovertebral angles over the kidneys. I requested a urine specimen, and while the patient obliged with the help of her mother the rest of us left the room. We had only the simplest of laboratory facilities, but in this case I only needed to look at the specimen to know that it was full of pus. This girl had a severe pyelonephritis.

Consiglio interpreted as I explained the diagnosis to her parents in some detail. Then I left some aspirin compound to be taken for high fever and backache, and specified that it was not to be taken unless it was needed. I also gave her a loading dose of sulfadiazine on the spot, and left enough for a week's treatment, to be taken two tablets every four hours around the clock, regardless of how she felt. I also warned about the dangers of not drinking enough water. When the medicine was all gone, I would return to see her again, and at that time the urine should be re-examined. However, if she didn't seem to be getting better someone should come and let me know, and if we had to move out of the area too soon for her to finish the medicine, I promised to see her again just before we left.

We did stay in the area long enough for me to make the followup visit, and as we entered the bedroom this time I was once again struck by the extraordinary beauty of this Italian girl. She appeared quite well now, and was sitting propped up in bed with extra pillows, wearing a white lace nightgown and bedjacket. Not a hair was out of place. She wore no makeup, but there was no need for any. Her facial features were symmetrical and pleasant to look at, and her smooth, fair complexion was made even fairer by contrast to her jet-black hair and very dark eyes.

She said she felt fine. There was no problem with urination. The specimen had been saved just before I arrived, and when I looked at it in the sunlight streaming into the window it looked clear, but when I shook the glass container I could see that there were many tiny crystals in it that glinted in the sunlight. They were obviously sulfonamide crystals, which had formed in the urine. Being in the specimen, they were also probably in the renal tubules, and if they stayed there very long, they could cause irreversible kidney damage. My patient had taken all but six of the sulfa tablets I had left, and I told her not to take them, but to continue drinking as much water as possible. I also asked her parents to bring another urine sample to the aid station in 24 hours, which they did. This second specimen was light in color, clear and contained no crystals, and when I checked it for protein, there was none. I was quite sure there had been no kidney damage.

When it came time to leave the girl's house on this second visit, Consiglio stopped me at the door, saying that her parents had asked if I could do anything for another daughter who had a problem, and I agreed to have a look at her. She was 14 years old, and was a small, thin, mousy looking girl, who didn't look at all like her sister. Her story was that she had not started to menstruate until she was 13, but now, for about a year, she had been menstruating too much. Her periods were not heavy, but each one lasted for several weeks. She had angular features; her skin was poor and rough, and there was a definite greenish tinge to her complexion. Her mucous membranes were extremely pale, and it was obvious to me that she was very anemic.

These findings fit a condition which I had read about in medical school, but which I had never seen, called chlorosis, which had been relatively common among pioneer women on the American frontier after a hard winter with a poor diet. It was essentially a dietary anemia of such a severe degree, that the complexion developed a greenish cast, hence the name. It normally affected only women, because their menstrual blood loss each month deepened the underlying dietary anemia. For this girl I would normally have prescribed ferrous sulfate and a multivitamin, and perhaps a very small daily dose of dessicated thyroid, as was common practice at the time, to try to influence the endocrine cycles toward more normal menstrual periods. None of these medicines were available to a battalion aid station in a combat situation, but I remembered that chlorosis had been successfully treated in the old days with hefty doses of sulfur and molasses. The sulfur was more or less inert, but molasses, the darker the better, was rich in iron and the B vitamins. The family understood what molasses was, and said they could get some, so I prescribed an ounce (30 c.c.) at least twice a day. I also recommended 1/4 grain of dessicated thyroid daily for three months, and wrote this out in case they could locate a pharmacy or pharmacist who could supply it. I also advised that if she didn't improve by summer, they should try to get the girl to a specialist (gynecologist) who might relieve the problem by scraping out the womb (D & C).

After we left the house that day I never saw any of this family again. I can only hope that what I did for these girls resulted in permanent improvement, and that things eventually turned out well for them.

In the late winter and spring I saw a lot of children with children's diseases, particularly measles and chicken pox. These were self-limiting diseases, but the incidence of complications such as tonsillitis, middle ear infections and pneumonia was high compared to what I had seen in the U.S. I never hesitated to treat the complications with sulfonamides, and in those days these drugs were very effective.

One day an 8-year-old boy was brought in to the aid station by his parents. He had been chopping wood, and had managed to chop his left thumb through the proximal phalanx, in such a fashion that it was almost completely severed. I thought that it wasn't salvageable and said so immediately, but I wasn't very busy at the time, so, using some local anesthetic, I decided to see what could be done with it. After blocking that side of the hand with novocaine, I looked at the situation more closely. The bone had been completely transected, and so had most of the soft tissues, but on the palmar side there remained a small bridge of skin, a few threads of intact flexor tendon, and a questionably intact vascular bundle. The digital artery looked as if it had been stretched, mauled and badly beaten up. I couldn't detect any pulsation in it, and I couldn't be sure that any blood was flowing through it.

The stable in which we were working was no hospital operating room, and I was under no illusions about the sterility of my surroundings, but nevertheless I decided to put the thumb back on, and see how things went. I didn't want to use catgut sutures because I knew that catgut was easily infected, and I didn't want to leave non-absorbable sutures in the wound because I had already seen a number of wounds repaired with them, which had become infected. Such wounds keep extruding the non-absorbable suture materials piecemeal, and seem to take forever to heal, because the healing process is never completed until all of the foreign material is gone. In this case the severed bone had been exposed and could easily become infected (osteomyelitis). The tissues of the severed thumb would also be exceptionally prone to becoming infected because their blood supply was completely or almost completely gone. The situation was so critical that if infection of any kind were to start in this wound, the thumb could not possibly be saved.

I decided to use a monofilament, non-absorbable suture material and tied each stitch on the outside of the skin in such a manner that at the first sign of infection in any one of them, the offending stitch could be removed immediately. I kept the repair simple. Nothing was done to the bone, and six long sutures were placed through the tendons, well away from the severed ends, three on each side of the wound. Each of these sutures was carried across and brought out through the skin on the opposite side of the wound and well away from it. The proximal ties were made through three small shirt buttons which had been sterilized by soaking them in alcohol for a while, and the distal ties, out on the thumb, were made over small gauze pledgets. These were precautionary measures to keep the suture from cutting into the skin. Many very fine non-absorbable sutures were now placed deeply through the skin edges to include much of the non-tendon tissue underneath, and all of these were tied on the outside of the skin in such a way that any one could be removed at the first sign of infection without completely disrupting the wound.

The medical technicians had not seen anything like this before, and were duly impressed as I explained to them that if infection got started at any of the stitches, I could cure it by pulling the offending stitch out, and that I could remove at least half of them early without jeopardizing the overall repair. In time all of the sutures would be removed, and there would be no foreign material left anywhere in the wound to work its way to the surface or to breed infection.

After dressing the wound, I splinted the fracture securely with the thumb in a more or less neutral position, and I also immobilized the wrist in order to minimize any effect that the forearm muscles might have on the wound site. Then with the help of Consiglio, I gave the family instructions. I had used sulfa powder in the wound, and I now prescribed sulfadiazine and medication for pain to be taken orally for a few days. They should report the boy's progress to Consiglio every day, and he would let me know of any problems. I should see him every two or three days, and the boy should keep the hand elevated most of the time. They should leave the splint and dressing alone, no matter how bad it looked or smelled, but they should also try to keep it as clean as possible.

During the following week I saw the boy three or four times, He had remarkably little pain, and had no fever, so I didn't remove the dressing until it was over a week old. When the dressing came off, the thumb didn't look pretty, but it was still alive; there was no sign of gangrene. I removed all of the skin stitches, and carefully replaced the bandage and the splints. In spite of the fact that the battalion was doing a lot of moving around, I saw the boy several times after that. He always came in to the aid station with his grandfather, who usually brought us two or three fresh eggs in payment for the service, but I have no idea how the grandfather found out where I was each time. At three weeks I removed the deep sutures that I had placed in the tendons, and with the buttons and gauze pledgets gone, the thumb looked much better. The splints remained in place for a total of six weeks, after which I showed the boy how to remove them to exercise the thumb and wrist, and how to replace them in order to protect the fracture for several more weeks. At this time he could easily oppose the thumb against his other four fingers, and the joint in the thumb had about half of its normal range of motion. I was extremely pleased with the result and was satisfied that this would remain a very useful thumb.

Shortly after his last visit we went on the attack to break out into the Po Valley, and I never saw the boy again, but I have thought about him often, and continue to hope that the thumb has served him well. A few years later, in private practice at home, I had a similar case in a young man of about the same age; I treated it in the same manner, and the result was equally satisfying.

I also remember a 2-or 3-year-old girl who was brought in after she had pulled a pot of boiling water over onto herself from the top of the stove. The child was crying loudly, and the family was in a state near panic. The burn seemed to be severe second degree, and it involved quite a large area, which included the front of the chest and abdomen, one shoulder and the corresponding flank. We treated it with an occlusive burn dressing, snugly taped so that it was almost like a body cast, and provided medication for pain relief. As in the previous case I told the family to try to keep the bandage clean, and not to remove it no matter how sloppy or smelly it became, but if the child became ill and feverish, I should see her immediately. Otherwise I would personally remove the bandage in about ten days. When the time was up and the child returned, I was faced with the dirtiest, sloppiest, smelliest, sopping wet dressing I had ever seen. The stench was incredible. There appeared to be pus running out from under the edges everywhere, but when I cut the bandage off, all of this came with it. Underneath this horrible dressing, new, pink, healthy looking skin appeared. It was painless, and there was no evidence anywhere that there would be any scarring. This was in sharp contrast to burns I had previously seen, where daily dressings had been done and, in spite of sterile technique, infection had set in. I had to conclude privately, that the practice of doing painful burn dressings daily, very popular at the time, might be doing more harm than good. Later, in civilian practice, I used this method of treating severe second-degree burns regularly with good success. The most severely burned of my post-war cases was a 3-year-old child who had fallen from a tabletop into a tub full of boiling laundry water which her mother had just removed from the stovetop and placed on the floor. Fortunately the mother was able to snatch the child out of the hot water and drop her into a tub full of cold rinse water standing nearby. Still the child had second-degree burns, with huge blisters, of the trunk, buttocks and thighs. This time, after I applied the snug occlusive dressing, I put the child in a plaster body cast, which included both thighs, for two weeks, and when the time came to remove it I relived my experience with the burned child in Italy all over again. The dressing and the plaster had become soaked, and the smell was exceptionally bad, but the skin underneath was beautiful, and this child also had no scarring anywhere.

After the fighting in Europe ceased, my practice among the civilian populace increased tremendously, and it also changed quite a bit. We were in German speaking areas all of the time, and I no longer needed Consiglio to interpret. There were fewer injuries and more illnesses, and I usually saw more civilians on a day-today basis than I saw soldiers. The civilians always seemed grateful for whatever I could do for them, or for someone in their family, and they invariably thanked me whenever I did anything at all. In a letter dated June 24, 1945 I wrote to my wife:

"Also being the only Doctor in the area, I make a round of calls on the civilian population every evening, and have seen some very interesting cases, and done quite a bit of good in curing people of their illnesses. The people are universally very grateful, more than even I had realized, for our commanding officer told me that the local mayor had told him how glad they were that I was around. "Next to God, Himself, they consider him the most important figure here." I'd never thought of it that way, but it certainly makes me feel good to know that the extra hours I put in are appreciated."

Soon after we moved from Passo di Predil into the town of Cave del Predil, I saw a soldier with sore throat, fever and a stiff neck, and immediately suspected meningitis, so I sent him back to the hospital for more investigation and treatment. Later that same day I saw another one with the same symptoms, and evacuated him too. That evening I saw an older child who was quite ill with fever and who also had a stiff neck, and a young adult with similar, but not so severe, symptoms. I treated the civilians on the spot with full doses of sulfadiazine, and when I checked on them the next morning, both were much improved. In the afternoon I saw several more soldiers with the same but milder symptoms, and also started them on sulfadiazine. Later in the day I received word from the hospital that our men had meningiococcus meningitis, and I now knew the correct diagnosis with certainty. We were having an epidemic, so I began treating everyone that I suspected might be starting with this infection with sulfadiazine, which in those days worked wonderfully well against the meningiococcus.

I had been taught in medical school that an epidemic caused by this organism could be quickly stopped by giving each patient's contacts a single prophylactic dose of sulfadiazine promptly, and since I was now stationed near Regimental Headquarters, I discussed this with the regimental commander and the regimental surgeon. I suggested that we give every man in the regiment the prophylactic dose, rather than wait for someone higher up in the chain of command to order us to do it. They agreed, and we decided to go ahead. Now the problem was to get enough sulfadiazine for the project, and I had to make a 200 mile overnight trip to get it. The next day every man in the regiment more or less willingly took the prophylactic dose, and I had enough additional sulfadiazine to provide the same to everyone in the immediate family and other close contacts of the civilians I was treating for the disease. After that there were no new cases, and in a few days I felt sure that the epidemic had been stopped.

Of the civilian patients I treated overseas, I liked the smaller children best, and I saw a lot of them. Since then there have always been a lot of children in my medical practice, and I have always enjoyed having them as patients. This enjoyment really began with the children I treated overseas, and is perhaps the reason that during my career I have given hundreds of sports physicals to school children free of charge, and have never charged a fee for giving an immunization injection, but charged only for the cost of the materials used. I don't remember the last civilian patient I treated overseas, but I know it was in Cave del Predil, and it could have been a child. At least I like to think so.

CHAPTER XXII

THE RETURN

"July 18, 1945
Florence, Italy

Dearest —,

I'm coming home, Honey! Although it's terribly hard for me to believe it yet. I've known it for almost a week, but couldn't write you because censorship was in effect, but has now been lifted."

Our departure from Italy was only a week away, and I was finally writing the letter that for months I had dreamed of writing. I was ecstatic. I didn't care that the trip from the Yugoslavian border had been long and tiresome and that the conditions of our stay in Florence were miserable. It was abominably hot. The temperatures hovered near the one hundred degree mark every afternoon, and to make matters worse we weren't wearing the summer khaki that would have been normal in such a climate, but were still wearing the woolen winter uniforms we wore up in the mountains. As if that weren't aggravation enough, we were under strict orders to wear our steel helmets over helmet liners at all times, and were required to wear ties. Everyone sweltered, and there was much complaining.

The time to turn in our equipment soon arrived. The aid station equipment posed no problem because we had taken good care of it, and had regularly replaced things as needed. However the first aid kits carried by every medic were another matter. As commanding officer of the medical detachment I was responsible for 41 of these kits, complete with instruments and supplies, and when we rounded them up only about half were complete. Some were missing altogether. Barney Summers and several of the enlisted men took care of this problem. I don't know how they did it, but when all was settled, we had been given credit for turning in all of them. Whenever I tried to bring up the subject of how it was done, they would just shrug and say, "Don't ask." Much of the equipment was probably certified as lost in combat, but it crossed my mind that some of these kits may possibly have been turned in more than once.

Turning in my jeep posed another problem. Many Army vehicles, including mine, had been altered during the course of the War, and when the order came to turn such vehicles in, it specified that all of them must be returned in government issue condition, free of all modifications and unauthorized decorations. Many alterations and modifications had been made to many Army vehicles when repairs were needed and the proper parts weren't immediately available. It was common practice to scavenge from enemy wrecks and civilian vehicles, especially during combat, when parts were difficult to obtain. Changes were also often made to improve comfort, or to make someone's vehicle look distinctive.

Early in combat the steering wheel of my jeep had been shattered by a shell fragment, and our mechanics had replaced it with the steering wheel from a 1937 European Ford. Both of the hard front seats had been replaced with soft upholstered ones taken from a passenger sedan somewhere along the line. The siren from a German tank had been mounted on a front fender, and the name "SHIRLY" (my driver's wife's first name) had been painted under the windshield. There were other, more minor alterations. Many Army vehicles had had regulation seats removed in favor of softer seating, and so many of the original seats had been lost or discarded, that it now seemed impossible to get the pair needed to restore my jeep to an acceptable condition. I was resigned that in the end I would have to pay Uncle Sam for two seats at least.

Pfc. Charles Argyle had been my jeep driver since our vehicles were first issued, and had been involved with all of the alterations, which had been made in it. With only about 36 hours left before we had to turn it in, he asked me to turn him loose with the jeep to scavenge the countryside, and made me promise to ask no questions when he returned. I let him go, and he returned just before the deadline with an intact, unaltered jeep, which we turned in without any problem.

Once the disposition of equipment was behind us, the time in Florence dragged. Our camp was close enough to downtown so that I could walk along the Arno River, and visit some of the bridges, which had shops on them, but again I didn't buy anything. The level of the water in the river was low; there was very little current, and the river didn't smell at all wholesome, so a walk along the riverbank was not really pleasant.

An officer from the 87th told me that there was a BAR Gunner with the same last name as mine in his regiment, so one afternoon I went to look for him. I found him without much trouble, and was surprised that he had very dark hair, dark eyes and an almost swarthy complexion, because most of my family were blue-eyed blonds or redheads. He too came from Detroit but his family was small. He had not been aware of my family, and showed no interest in getting to know us. So our conversation ended quickly, and I have never seen or talked to him again.

On July 26 we finally left Florence for *Livorno* (Leghorn), and before evening, boarded the ship that would take us back to the U.S. It was a new ship named *Westbrook Victory,* and although it was similar to the ship, which had brought me to Italy, it was nicer because it was new and had been specifically designed to carry troops. Although we were crowded on board, and some men slept on cots on deck and on the hatches, most agreed that this journey was more pleasant than the passage to Italy on the *ARGENTINA* had been.

The dispensary and sick bay were spacious, new and well equipped, and were located at the level of the main deck, instead of below somewhere in the bowels of the ship. All of the medical officers in the regiment were on board, so sick call was not a major chore for anyone, and medical services operated smoothly and uneventfully until about four days before we were scheduled to land, when one of the men presented at sick call with abdominal pain and nausea. He was quickly put to bed in the sick bay, and all of the doctors on board had a look at him. Two of us thought that he had appendicitis, and the other three weren't so sure. A blood count might help clinch the diagnosis.

There was a microscope in the dispensary, but we could find no stains or microscope slides, nor could we find the counting chamber needed for doing the blood count. So after giving the problem some thought, I removed the glass disc from a flashlight to use as a microscope slide, made a smear of the patient's blood on it, fixed it with gentle heat, and stained it with the gentian violet that we normally applied topically to treat yeast and fungal infections. Under the microscope it was easy to see that, although we could not make an accurate count of them, this smear contained many more white blood cells than are found in a normal smear and that most of them were polymorphonuclear leucocytes, indicating that an intense inflammatory process was going on somewhere in the patient. There was now complete agreement that acute appendicitis was the most probable diagnosis, and that an operation as soon as possible was necessary.

Under normal circumstances this patient would have been evacuated to a hospital where a surgical team could perform the operation, but such a transfer was not possible from where we were in the middle of the Atlantic. The man was gradually becoming sicker, and to wait for landfall was to risk perforation, peritonitis and perhaps a fatal final outcome. We would have to do it ourselves with the personnel and equipment available.

We first had to see what equipment we had with which to do the job. There was a set of brand new surgical instruments in the dispensary, and an autoclave in which to sterilize them. There were some cans of ether and some ether masks, but no anesthesia machine. There was plenty of suture material of all kinds, and there was also some penicillin on board. The surgical instruments were still in their original packaging, and it took all of two hours to clean the grease from them and sterilize them.

While this was going on, we took stock of the surgical manpower that was available. Dr. Sam Randall, the regimental surgeon was a dermatologist, and had had no major surgical training. The rest of us had been taken into the Army after a mere nine-month internship, which had followed immediately after our graduation from medical school. One of us, Dr. Kilian Meyer, had had part of a surgical residency. He and I were the only ones who had previously done any significant abdominal surgery on our own, and I was the only one in the group with any real experience at all in anesthesia. After a short discussion we decided that Dr. Meyer would be the surgeon, Dr. Ellsworth Miller would assist, and I would administer the anesthetic. We all agreed that this was the best and most experienced surgical team that we could muster on board the ship.

The operation actually began with a hefty preanesthetic injection of a barbiturate, and another of morphine and atropine an hour ahead of time. Anesthesia consisted of ether dripped upon an ether mask, from a can with a safety pin placed through the seal to let it trickle out. When properly administered open drop ether is a safe and effective anesthetic, but in modern times the art of its administration has been largely lost with the advent of much more sophisticated equipment and systems of anesthesia. As soon as the actual operation began, the captain turned his ship into the wind to minimize its rolling and pitching. The surgery went well, and a gangrenous but not quite perforated appendix was removed. I stayed with the patient until he was fully awake again, and then returned with him to the sick bay to observe his progress a little longer. He recovered well, and had no postoperative problems.

After dark on the evening before we landed, lights on the shore of our homeland became visible, and the next morning, August 7, we docked at

Hampton Roads at the same berth, I believe, from which I had left the previous December. A crowd of people stood behind a fence separating them from the dock area, and waved greetings to us. At dockside the first soldier I saw was a sergeant who greeted us as we were lined up along the ship's rail, and I was pleased to note that on his chest he was wearing overseas ribbons with battle stars. Before any of us got off of the ship, our appendectomy patient was sent down on a cable from the ship to the dock in a basket litter rigged with ropes and pulleys. As he progressed down the cable he smiled and waved, and the men on board and the civilians on shore cheered. The cheers continued as he was quickly loaded into a waiting ambulance, and driven off to the station hospital. I am now compelled to smile every time I recall this scene, because, although the surgical technique for a simple appendectomy has not changed through the years, today we would have made that man walk off of the ship under his own power.

In due time, loaded with rucksack and duffle bag, I walked down the gangplank toward the crowd of happy people on shore, and suddenly there was a lump in my throat, a tear in my eye, and I felt fiercely proud of my country, its people, and what they had accomplished. I understood the urge to kiss the ground that others under similar circumstances have often described. I didn't do it, but it would have been easy. Everything looked wonderful. I was ever so glad to be back, and for the next several days I particularly noticed the American flag wherever it was flown. I realized that the "Stars and Stripes" meant more to me now than it ever had before.

Processing through Camp Patrick Henry was remarkably rapid. This time we were well treated by the camp personnel, who were now almost all overseas veterans. What a contrast to the treatment I had received on my way out of the country! Everyone had expected a two-week leave, but now something else unusual happened. We were all placed on thirty days' "temporary duty" at home, after which we were to report in at Camp Carson near Colorado Springs, Colorado.

At 2 p.m. I sent a telegram to my wife:

"=ARRIVED SAFELY EXPECT TO SEE YOU SOON DONT ATTEMPT TO CONTACT OR WRITE ME HERE LOVE= =AL"

The first atomic bomb was dropped on Hiroshima on August 6, which was our last day at sea. It caused heretofore unheard of damage, and we all hoped that the Japanese would be persuaded to surrender, but even this momentous event seemed unimportant to me at the time, because I was on my way home to the wife I loved so much. I remember almost nothing of the trip from Camp Patrick Henry to Detroit, except that I went by train and the trip lasted overnight. The last part of the trip covered the same route that I had taken from Detroit to Carlisle Barracks a little more than a year before, and as we traveled along the shore of Lake Erie, I became most impatient. I was very anxious to get home, and it seemed to me as if I had already been on that train for an eternity.

Somewhere during the process of leaving Camp Patrick Henry, I must have been able to telephone ahead, because my wife and family met me at the station. My wife looked a bit tired, but her smile was radiant, and to me she was the most beautiful girl in the world. I couldn't keep from looking at her, and hardly noticed that dozens of other happy reunions between servicemen and their families were taking place all over the station. On the ride home we sat together in the car, holding hands. Something that had been missing from my life had now been put back. It was indeed a happy reunion!

Since we did not yet have a home of our own, my wife had been staying with her mother while I was away, and we had stayed there together for the duration of my previous leave. Now, together again, we stayed there once more. My father-in-law was still serving as a naval officer in the Pacific, and was not at home, but my wife's only sister also lived there. My family lived only three miles away, so there was much visiting back and forth. Together, we celebrated my return by drinking the champagne I had brought from Italy, an event that I had often imagined happening long before I arrived home.

The news of the day was all about the devastation that the first atomic bomb had wrought upon Hiroshima, and I felt some hope that Japan might soon surrender. The Japanese had also suffered severe defeats in earlier sea and air battles, and their homeland had suffered significant conventional bombing and shore bombardments by American warships. For some six or eight weeks they had been urged by the Allies to surrender, and had even been given a timetable for the destruction of Japanese cities by our B-29 bomber raids. On August 8th Russia, with over a million veteran troops available on their Asian front, declared war on Japan, and my hopes for peace rose another notch. The following day the news media reported that these Russian Armies launched an all out attack, and the second atomic bomb was dropped, this time on Nagasaki. This bomb also produced unprecedented destruction for a single bomb, and the Allies let Japan know immediately that there were more on the way if they didn't surrender immediately. On August 10 our newspaper headlines read "JAPS ASK PEACE," and the next day the Allies received and accepted an offer for the total surrender of the Japanese government, with the single condition being that the Allied Military Commander should govern the Japanese people through the authority of Emperor Hirohito. I was pretty sure that the War was over, but we still had to wait to see if both sides could officially agree upon the terms.

The War actually ended on August 14. My wife and I had gone the see the matinee showing of a movie at our neighborhood theatre, and when we emerged late in the afternoon, there were newspaper extras on the street with huge headlines declaring that the war had ended. Although we were miles from downtown, the sidewalks were filled with deliriously happy people, and it took a long time for us to walk the several blocks back to our house. I felt a huge sense of relief, because even though I had to serve another year in the Army, I knew now that I wouldn't be going into combat in the Pacific. I felt extremely lucky to be already at home with my wife, and I couldn't help but think of the men of the 34th Division who had gloated over the fact that we were being redeployed while they were replacing us as occupation forces in the Julian Alps. I was at home, but they were still over there.

CHAPTER XXIII

TERMINATION

After the signing of the Japanese Surrender Agreement and the announce-ment by President Truman proclaiming VJ Day on September 2, 1945, World War II was essentially over, but I was still under orders to report for duty at Camp Carson, near Colorado Springs, Colorado after my period of tempo-rary duty at home was finished. I had at least another year to serve in the Army.

My wife and I both realized that the combination of recent historical events had been incredibly fortunate for us, and we immediately started plan-ning for the future, knowing that I would probably not be required to leave the country again. This would make it possible for her to go with me on any future assignment, so we shopped for a car. Most of my Army pay had gone into the bank, and my entire card playing winnings had also been added to our savings account, so we had enough money to pay cash.

No new cars had been manufactured for the civilian market for four years, so only used cars were being offered for sale. Having lived all of our lives close to Livernois Avenue, which was then known as the "Avenue of Used Car Lots" in the Motor City, we confidently started to shop there, but it didn't take long for disappointment to set in. New tires for civilian cars had not been available for four years either, and the tires on the cars displayed for sale were generally bald. Many showed evidence of repeated vulcanization procedures, or other signs of multiple repairs. All of the cars that we looked at had tires that were bald or had been re-cut to make it look like there was some tread left. All of them had high odometer readings, loose joints, smoky motors, a lot of rust, and were generally in such poor condition that before the War most of them would have been sold by the pound for junk or scrap metal. We went the full length of the several miles of Livernois Avenue, and visited every used car lot along the way, but didn't find anything in which I wanted to chance driving to Colorado. We looked in other places in and around Detroit and found nothing even remotely suitable, so we decided to go to Lansing to see if anything better might be available there.

The next morning we left for Lansing in my father-in-law's car, and started making the rounds of car dealers and used car lots as soon as we arrived. Prices were higher, but the cars offered seemed to be in better condition and seemed to represent better value than those we had seen in Detroit. Early in the afternoon we walked into Al Hanson's Studebaker dealership on Michigan Avenue, less than a mile from Sparrow Hospital where I had interned. I had met Mr. Hanson once before, and looking through the open door to his office where he was sitting at his desk, I recognized him. I think he may have been influenced by the fact that I was in uniform, wearing my decorations and my Combat Medical Badge, because, when I explained that we were looking for a car that was good enough to take us to my next duty post in Colorado, a gleam came into his eye, a grin appeared on his face, and he said that something had just come in that might do.

He led us into the showroom and there stood a spotless, gleaming, blue-gray, 1941 Studebaker Champion, with overdrive. The car looked brand new, and the tread on the tires didn't appear worn. There were only 15,000 miles on the odometer. Mr. Hanson said that we could have it for $1,066.00. I produced my checkbook in a flash and wrote the check, and after the rest of the formalities had been completed and we actually owned the car, we learned more about it.

It had originally been purchased new from Mr. Hanson in 1941 by a man who was drafted into the service soon afterward. He had stored it, raised on blocks, in his garage before he was shipped overseas, because his wife didn't drive. When the time came for his discharge he decided to make a career of the Army, and re-enlisted. Now he was being sent overseas again to a place where he couldn't take the car, so he turned it in to be sold. It had only been in the dealership a few minutes when we bought it.

We were amazed, and a bit awestruck, by our incredible good fortune. Needless to say, in future years I bought a number of cars from Mr. Hanson.

We were now ready to drive to Camp Carson together, but new orders arrived in the mail that changed our plans. I was ordered to board a troop train in Rockford, Illinois, and make the balance of the trip to Colorado Springs on it. We could drive to Rockford together, but my wife didn't want to drive the rest of the way from there alone, so we asked my mother to join us. She was delighted at the invitation, and when the time came the three of us drove to Rockford, where we stayed in a hotel overnight. It was still necessary to conserve gasoline, so the wartime 35 mile per hour speed limit was still in effect, and made this a long, tedious journey.

The next day I joined the troop train, and was surprised to learn that because I was the ranking officer on board, I had been designated to be the Train Commander. Any infantry officer of any rank would have been more suited to this job than I, or any other medical officer for that matter, but there was at the time nowhere I could protest the appointment, so I resigned myself to heading what I expected would be a somewhat chaotic train trip.

A field kitchen had been installed in the baggage car, and when I arrived on the scene, food supplies were being loaded for which I had to sign. A mess sergeant appeared in the kitchen who told me not to worry, because he had already recruited all of the help he needed, and there should be no problems. I signed for the food, including an extra ration in case of emergency, and the train soon departed.

There was a problem with the food, however. All we had on board were the ingredients for a good vegetable beef stew, and that was what we ate, three times a day for the 48 hours and six meals that it took to reach our destination. There was a lot of grumbling about this, but in general the men took it good naturedly, and I kept telling everyone to "blame it on the guys in Chicago." At the end of the trip I was asked to turn in the emergency rations I had signed for, but when we looked for them the cupboard was bare. I certified that the emergency food was needed to replace the breakfast rations that we had not been given. The explanation was accepted, and I had once more slipped out of what could have been an unpleasant predicament.

In the meantime my wife, with my mother as her passenger, completed the drive to Colorado Springs, and rented a room in a motel on the route out of town toward Pike's Peak. They left word of their arrival at the post, and soon we were together again.

The first thing we did was to look for more suitable and more permanent lodgings, and we eventually found them in Manitou Springs near the entrance to "The Garden of the Gods." The house was set into a mountainside, was four stories high, and had entrances on several floors. My wife and I had a one-bedroom apartment on the third floor, which had an outside entrance at the ground level of the mountain in the back, and my mother had a sleeping room on the floor above. My mother stayed for three weeks, which she seemed to enjoy very much, after which we took her to board the train for her return to Detroit. Eventually John and Margaret Ninfo, Donovan Owen and his wife, and Emory Cain and his wife, all men from my battalion, rented apartments in the same building, and we had some pleasant times together.

In time we got to know our landlord and landlady, Mr. and Mrs. Havard, quite well, and some of the male tenants often played cards with Mr. Havard in the evening. He had a health problem, and one evening asked if I could be of any help. He had developed "shingles" (herpes zoster) in a band around the left side of his chest about three years previously, and it just wasn't getting well. John Ninfo and I both looked at it, and agreed that the diagnosis was correct. The affected band showed scarring, scabbing and, here and there, some active blisters. It wasn't very painful, but was extremely aggravating.

This disease is caused by a virus infection of a nerve trunk and its corresponding nerve endings in the skin, which in this case was an intercostal nerve, which coursed along one of the ribs. One of the treatments often used in those days was to administer a viral vaccine of some kind, the theory being that this would stimulate the body's immune system to overcome the herpes virus. The most popular vaccine to use was cowpox, the same vaccine that was used to immunize people against smallpox. When I inquired, Mr. Havard said he had never had a smallpox vaccination, but was willing to try anything.

So I brought a tube of the vaccine home one evening and vaccinated him on the left arm. He got a very severe and rapid "take" reaction. By the fifth day his entire upper arm was firey red, swollen to twice normal size, and there was a large gooey blister on the spot where I had given him the vaccination. He had a high fever for an elderly person, and was having chills intermittently. I became concerned about the spread of the cowpox virus to other parts of the body, and had to warn him against touching the blister on his arm and getting the blister fluid into the herpes lesions on his chest, or into a minor scratch, or into his eyes, because he might then develop vaccination scars at all such sites. There was nothing else I could do except offer adequate doses of aspirin for his fever and discomfort.

After three or four days of relatively high fever, the blister fluid at the vaccination site turned bloody and the blister started to form a scab, exactly as it was supposed to do. The swelling and redness in the arm receded gradually until the arm was again normal in appearance, and the fever was gone. Before the vaccination scab fell off to reveal the vaccination scar underneath, scabs from the herpetic area on the chest began falling away, and there were no longer any active blisters in the area. Four weeks later, there were no more scabs, and the entire area around his chest showed only the old scarring which had been caused by the old disease.

Today, vaccination treatment for herpes zoster is no longer acceptable, because modern studies have shown that cowpox vaccine has no effect on the herpes virus, but in my opinion there must have been something in the process which helped, because I had seen it used successfully before I used it on Mr. Havard, and I have used it with success quite a few times later.

When I first reported in at Camp Carson the whole division had not yet arrived, but more and more men kept coming in daily, and sometime during the last half of September the battalion was again in full operation. The ranks had thinned dramatically, however, because most of those men with a high number of service points had already been discharged. Almost immediately a lot of the men were given an extra two weeks off, plus travel time, and the rest were issued one pass after another. In another few days most of the rest of us were given extra time off, and only a small skeleton crew remained to operate the battalion.

The abundance of free time gave us a chance to enjoy Colorado that fall. We made many short trips in our car, often including one of the other couples living in our apartment building. We visited the Garden of the Gods, Leadville, Denver and Pueblo, and we drove up Pike's Peak. We visited the Royal Gorge, but couldn't drive out on the bridge because the wooden planking was rotten and was full of holes through which the bottom of the gorge nine hundred feet below could be seen. One of our favorite trips was a drive into the mountains on the Rampart Range Road. I even went deer hunting in this area without success, carrying an M 1 Rifle I had signed out from camp. At the foot of the hill where we lived there was a soda spring. I don't remember drinking any of the water, but we always told our friends to bring the Scotch when they came to visit, because we had a plentiful supply of soda.

On October 13, 1945 the War Department declared that the 10th Mountain Division would be inactivated as of October 25, and shortly before that date I was transferred to the staff of Carson General Hospital where I was put to work removing plates, wires and screws from orthopedic patients who had received them in the treatment of their fractures, and in whom this hardware was either causing some problem or had outlived its usefulness. I was no longer a part of the 10th Mountain Division, and within days the division itself, for all practical purposes, ceased to exist. My division had been important to me, more important than I had realized, and now that it was gone I felt sad. I didn't look forward to another year in the Army with any enthusiasm.

The rest of my tour of duty was most tedious, and offered absolutely nothing that might have induced me to stay in the service. Included in it were a number of absurdities, the most glaring one of which was an emergency move to Camp Crowder, Missouri where I had to take part in prolonging an epidemic of German measles, for which my superiors received glowing citations and commendations for their handling of the epidemic. In the process of closing down Camp Crowder late in the spring, I was the last officer on the post, and had to sign for everything. I owned the whole camp, lock, stock, barrel and Sherman tanks, and for a long time I feared that I might be held responsible for the loss of something that was out of my control and would have to repay the government for it. I dangled in this state of uncertainty far too long, but was finally relieved, and was sent to Fort Sheridan, Illinois to be "separated from the service" on July 29, 1946.

The procedure at the separation center was more complicated than I thought it would be, and involved a physical examination of sorts. One phase of the process was called counseling, but it should have been called recruiting. Everyone was urged to reenlist with the promise that he would retain his rank as a permanent one, but while I was there the only men I saw re-enlisting were privates.

As I waited for the final phase of my separation, I had time to reflect upon my military service and how it had affected the course of my life. I remembered how hard it had been to leave my wife, and my continual, deep longing to come back home to her, and the dread that I might not come back, and the ever-continuing hope that the War would end, and my belief that it might not end for years. Then I thought about how really lucky I had been in the two years past. I had married the right girl; I had received my license to practice medicine; the Army had assigned me to a most extraordinary division, and I had picked the right battalion in which to serve; while in combat I had had some close encounters with disaster, but had managed to escape the casualty list; the War in Italy had ended just a week before my unit would have been attacking some of the roughest, most easily defended mountain territory in Europe; by the time another week had gone by, the rest of the hostilities in Europe had ended; I had been among the first of the combat troops returned from Europe, expecting to be redeployed to the Pacific, and the War with Japan had ended only a week after I had arrived home; and for the last year of my service my wife and I had been together, and had been lucky enough to have lived in some very beautiful areas in our country.

I had time to think of the men with whom I had served, and of those who had died, and of the many wounded who had passed through my hands. Although I didn't realize it then, they had been a profound influence upon me, upon the way I would practice medicine, and the way I would live the rest of my life. I would always remember their sacrifices, and the constant mental and physical stress they suffered, and the prolonged discomforts and adversities they endured, and their always willing, unselfish support of each other. I would never forget those who were wounded, and the major and sometimes gruesome wounds that many had suffered with hardly a whimper and never any tears in my presence. Later, in my postwar civilian medical practice, these memories would make it difficult for me to muster much sympathy for patients with relatively minor illnesses or injuries, and would occasionally make it all but impossible for me to put up with some of their weepings and wailings. I would find it very difficult to treat many of the people who came to me without real disease, but who complained bitterly of relatively minor dis-eases or discomforts.

At the beginning of my tour of duty I had great doubts about myself, doubts that I would be able to serve with dignity and honor. I had no desire to die, or be any kind of a hero, and I had resented having to be away from my wife, my home, my family and my career. Now I was much more confident. I was quite sure that in a time of global warfare I had served my country well, and for that I was proud. I had not disgraced it, nor had I disgraced myself, and for that I was thankful, but I fervently hoped that I would never have to do anything like it, ever again. Now there would be new decisions to make, but they could wait for a time, while I became accustomed to no longer being a soldier.

END

APPENDIX A

Application For Unit Citation

COPY OF AN OFFICIAL APPLICATION FOR A UNIT CITATION FOR THE MEDICAL DETACHMENT OF THE 86TH MOUNTAIN INFANTRY REGIMENT

(Author's Note: A carbon copy of the following document on onionskin second sheets was found among the remaining papers of the Regimental Medical Detachment, and was kept in my possession, because I was the last officer transferred out of the detachment when the division was deactivated. I have reproduced it here exactly as it appears on the original sheets. Words in Italics placed in parentheses are not in the original document, but have been inserted to correct spelling and, where necessary, to clarify a passage. Some corrections of punctuation have also been made for the same reason.)

MEDICAL DETACHMENT
86th Mt. Infantry Regt.
APO 345, U.S. Army

7 July 45
SUBJECT: Information Requested For Meritorius Service Unit Plaque
TO: Division Surgeon, 10th Mountain Division

1. Military courtesy in the detachment has always been of exceptionally high standard. The personnel has consistently been neat in appearance and installations and equipment have, in general, been in good order. The great percentage of the men have always been enthusiastic in the execution of orders and have taken their medical duties most seriously.
2. Awards and decorations:

a. Combat Medical Badges   152
b. Bronze Star Medals   74
    Silver Star Medals   2
    Good Conduct Medals   139
    Purple Heart Medals   36

3. K.I.A. and W.I.A.:
a. Killed In Action   4
b. Wounded In Action   36

4. Total casualties evacuated:
a. Number of casualties thru Aid Station
    from 1 Feb. 45 to 2 May 45   871
b. Peak casualty days   70, 80, 50

1st Bn Sec – 70 Casualties were evacuated thru Aid Station 4 Mar 45 at Tamburini, Italy

2nd Bn Sec – 80 casualties were evacuated thru Aid Station 15 Apr 45 at Rocca Roffino, Italy

3rd Bn Sec – 75 casualties were evacuated thru Aid Station 24 Feb 45 at Mt. Della Torraccia, Italy.

5. Instances of exceptional service:

a. **Regimental Section**

On the night of 18 April 45, (*the*) Regimental Aid Station (*was*) established in a house near Calderino, Italy. Elements of the 2nd Battalion were receiving intense artillery fire and the Bn. Aid Station was under constant shelling. (*Author's Note: April 18th was the night that the 1st Battalion plus F Company of the 2nd Battalion were scaling Riva Ridge. The 2nd Battalion minus F Company was standing in reserve near the town of Vidiciatico. Once the battle on Riva Ridge began, the Germans shelled this area.*) So great a number of casualties over a short period of time beseiged the Bn. Aid Station that it was necessary to evacuate many of the wounded directly to (*the*) Regimental Aid Station during a period of six hours. Evacuation was extremely hazardous due to sniper fire and heavy artillery throughout the night. Due to the untiring effort and devotion to duty, all casualties were speedily evacuated.

b. **1st Battalion Aid Section**

On the night of 22 April 45, a convoy of the 1st Bn. Vehicles and men, including all medical personnel, was ambushed at a road junction by an enemy force just south of the Po River. Because of the confusion, a part of the convoy, including Hq. Co. and Aid Station personnel, were isolated from the forward elements of the convoy. Due to the element of surprise and unpreparedness, there was great confusion and excitement among our troops. Mortar, small arms fire, and grenades rained into the column causing many casualties and burning many vehicles. Some thirty minutes after the fire fight began, two enemy tanks appeared at the crossroads and fired point blank into the troops. Amid the fire fight the medics established two separate aid stations to take care of the dispersed casualties. All medical personnel under these harassing conditions performed their duties according to the tradition of the Medical Dept. and were responsible for the saving of many lives.

c. **2nd Battalion Aid Section**

On the morning of 29 April 45, the 2nd Bn. Aid Station was moving up the highway on the east side of Lake Garda behind leading elements of the 2nd Battalion. Approximately two miles south of Torbole an enemy 88 shell exploded well within the entrance of a tunnel, inflicting extremely heavy casualties on "M" Company (*of the 3rd. Bn.*) and the command group of the 2nd Battalion. In spite of heavy enemy shelling, the 2nd Bn. Aid Station set up within a nearby tunnel and proceeded to function with admirable speed and efficiency, thus saving many lives and hastening evacuation by two 3/4 ton amphibious vehicles to the collecting company.

d. **3rd Battalion Aid Section**

While the 3rd Battalion Aid Station was set up at Carge, Italy, 24 February 45, the personnel was hard pressed to handle the large number of casualties that resulted from an attack and counterattack on Mt. Tella Torraccio (*Monte della Torraccia*). At least 50 allied casualties flowed thru the Aid Station, 24 Feb 45, alone. In addition a large number of German prisoners were treated. One company aid man and one litter team leader were killed, while a dozen other men were temporarily removed from battle by exhaustion and wounds. During the hectic, bloody days at Carge, 23 Feb 45 to 3 Mar 45, the Aid Station was under heavy enemy artillery and mortar fire. Shells landed within 20 feet of the Aid Station. Occasionally enemy snipers fired on men in the close vicinity of the Aid Station. Throughout this trying time all personnel gave their utmost and gained the gratitude of all. The aid men were right up in the front with their companies and able to give prompt attention to the wounded, thus saving many lives. The litter teams made countless trips up the steep and often exposed flanks of the northern Apennines. Aid Station personnel, jeep drivers, and Battalion Surgeon treated wounded and evacuated them for 48 hours without sleep.

6. Locations and dates of all installations :

a. **Regimental Aid Section**

Location	From	To
San Marcello	1 Feb	5 Feb
San Cassiano di Morano	5 Feb	17 Feb
La Ca	17 Feb	20 Feb
Gaggio Montana (*Montano*)	20 Feb	2 Mar
Malandrone	2 Mar	4 Mar
Iola	4 Mar	5 Mar
Tambourini	5 Mar	5 Apr
Riola	6 Apr	15 Apr
Capponara	15 Apr	17 Apr
La Costa	17 Apr	18 Apr
Palestrina	18 Apr	19 Apr
Mongardino	19 Apr	20 Apr
Bomporto	20 Apr	22 Apr
San Benedetto (*San Benedetto Po*)	22 Apr	23 Apr
Governalo (*Governolo*)	23 Apr	24 Apr
Verona	24 Apr	26 Apr
Bussolengo	26 Apr	27 Apr
Torbole	27 Apr	28 Apr
Riva	28 Apr	2 May

b. **1st Battalion Aid Section**

Location	From	To
Doccia	1 Feb	2 Feb
Arcina	2 Feb	17 Feb
Forne	17 Feb	22 Feb
Gaggio Montana (*Gaggio Montano*)	22 Feb	1 Mar
Corge (*Carge*)	1 Mar	3 Mar
Tamburini	3 Mar	4 Mar
Sassomolare (*Sassamolare*)	4 Mar	16 Mar
Montecatini (*Montecatini Terme*)	16 Mar	19 Mar
Pietra di Cloroe (*Pietra Colora*)	19 Mar	21 Mar
Madovna di Brasa (*?Madna di Brasa*)	21 Mar	31 Mar
Prunetta	31 Mar	5 Apr
Pietra di Cloroe (*?Pietra Colora*)	5 Apr	6 Apr
Riola	6 Apr	15 Apr
Bortaloni (*?*)	15 Apr	17 Apr
La Costa	17 Apr	18 Apr

Mongardino (*?*)	18 Apr	20 Apr
Fondo Catara	21 Apr	23 Apr
Gargo	23 Apr	24 Apr
Governalo (*Governolo*)	24 Apr	25 Apr
Villa Franko (*Villafranca*)	25 Apr	26 Apr
Bussolengo	26 Apr	28 Apr
Tunnels (*at Lake Garda*)	28 Apr	29 Apr
Nago	30 Apr	2 May

c. **2nd Battalion Aid Section**

Location	From	To
Prunetta	1 Feb	4 Feb
Mutigliano (*Cutigliano*)	4 Feb	18 Feb
Torlaino (*?*)	18 Feb	19 Feb
Vidiciatico	19 Feb	1 Mar
To Possinoe (*?*)	1 Mar	4 Mar
Sassomolare (*Sassamolare*)	4 Mar	10 Mar
Modina di Brassa (*Madna di Brasa*)	10 Mar	25 Mar
Colora	25 Mar	26 Mar
Sassomolare (*Sassamolare*)	26 Mar	8 Apr
Coniali	8 Apr	14 Apr
Monte Sineitro	14 Apr	15 Apr
Rocca Rofeno	15 Apr	16 Apr
Monte Pastire (Montepastore)	16 Apr	18 Apr
Casa Vigo	18 Apr	19 Apr
Casa Bianco	19 Apr	20 Apr
Bomporto	20 Apr	24 Apr
Governale (Governolo)	24 Apr	27 Apr
Piano di Tempesta	27 Apr	29 Apr
Torbole	29 Apr	30 Apr
Riva	30 Apr	2 May

d. 3rd Battalion Aid Section

Location	From	To
Lizzano	1 Feb	7 Feb
Lucca	7 Feb	18 Feb
Il Palazzo	18 Feb	19 Feb
Gabba	19 Feb	20 Feb
Mazzacana (Mazzancana)	20 Feb	23 Feb
Carge	23 Feb	3 Mar
Terminale (Monte Terminale)	3 Mar	4 Mar

Iola	4 Mar	8 Mar
Campo Tizzoro	8 Mar	14 Mar
S. Maria	14 Mar	17 Mar
Sassomolare (Sassamolare)	17 Mar	22 Mar
Prunetta	22 Mar	28 Mar
S. Maria	28 Mar	30 Mar
Sassomolare (Sassamolare)	30 Mar	6 Apr
Ma'a di Brasa (?Madna di Brasa)	6 Apr	9 Apr
S. Maria di Lebante	9 Apr	12 Apr
Cereglia	12 Apr	13 Apr
Tole	13 Apr	14 Apr
Montepistore (Montepastore)	14 Apr	15 Apr
Badia	15 Apr	16 Apr
S. Lorenzo	16 Apr	18 Apr
Ponte Samoggia	18 Apr	19 Apr
Bomporto	19 Apr	20 Apr
Gorgo	20 Apr	22 Apr
Governalo (Governolo)	22 Apr	23 Apr
Verona	23 Apr	24 Apr
Bussolengo	24 Apr	25 Apr
Ponte di campagnano	25 Apr	26 Apr
Lake Garda (East Shore)	26 Apr	28 Apr
Torbole	28 Apr	29 Apr
S. Alessandro	29 Apr	2 May

7. AWOL,Court Martial, V.D. (*Venereal Disease*) Rate
 a. AWOL   1
 b. Court Martial   1
 c. V.D.   0

SAMUEL J. RANDALL
Capt. MC, 86th Mt Inf
Regimental Surgeon

AUTHOR'S NOTE: (*There are a number of minor discrepancies between this document and my story. They are easily understandable. This document was prepared after the fact, from Regimental records available at the time. Dates are sometimes off by a day or two, probably because those men producing the records did not care what the exact date was. Place name discrepancies may be explained, because battalion and regimental command post name places were probably taken from the records. The aid station may have been set up in a nearby building, which, as was the custom in Italy at the time, had an entirely different name.)*

MAPS OF THE COMBAT AREAS

The map overlays presented here came in a packet inserted into a copy of ***COMBAT HISTORY OF THE 10TH MOUNTAIN DIVISION***, which was purchased from the quartermaster of the 10th Mountain Division Association, Inc. The publication originally came from the Infantry School Library at Fort Benning, Georgia, where it was compiled from the 10th Mountain Division narrative and very minimally edited (to correct spelling and grammar only) by Charles M. Hauptman of Billings, Montana. Hauptman was in the headquarters complement of the 85th Mountain Infantry Regiment. Much of the work was done by his son while he was a young lieutenant stationed at Fort Benning and was able to spend a considerable amount of time in research of library records.

Like so many similar military narratives, this one probably had multiple unknown authors. It is most likely typewritten and mimeographed on very poor quality paper, as was the custom at the time, and very difficult to read. I can appreciate this, because such is the condition of my copy of the narrative written for my regiment and most of the other old military papers in my possession.

The Hauptmans issued their publication in 1977, and when I called Charles in 1991, he could not remember the exact origin of these map overlays, but agreed that I should include them in my book. They are now quite familiar to veterans of the division because, in addition to being presented as an insert with the division history book they have appeared in travel brochures and guidebooks for trips back to Italy to visit the division's scenes of combat. They have also appeared lately on placemats developed for use at 10th Mountain Division Association dinners and banquets.

The numbers on these map overlays refer to detailed maps adapted from map art of Armand Casini originally published in 1946. During combat Casini served with the Headquarters Company of the 86th Mountain Infantry Regiment.

Many of the place names referred to in the book do not appear on the overlays, but an adequate number of names from the book are included on them to enable the reader to follow the action.

Albert H. Meinke, Jr., M.D

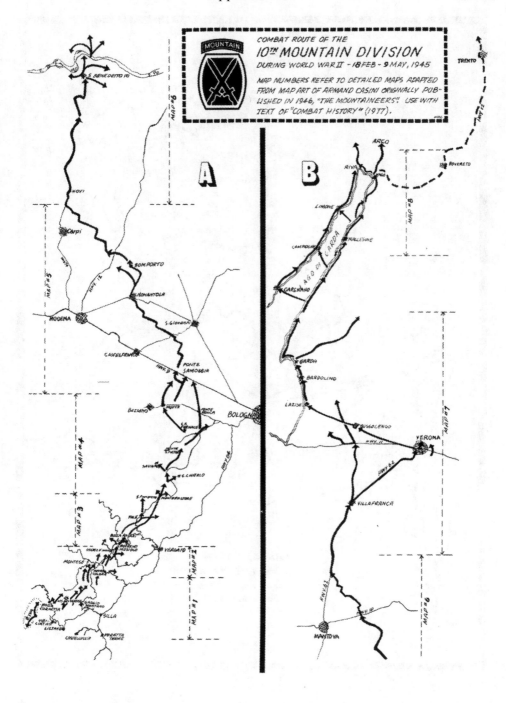

COMBAT ROUTE OF THE
10TH MOUNTAIN DIVISION
DURING WORLD WAR II - 18 FEB - 9 MAY, 1945

MAP NUMBERS REFER TO DETAILED MAPS ADAPTED
FROM MAP ART OF ARMAND CASINI ORIGINALLY PUB-
LISHED IN 1946, "THE MOUNTAINEERS". USE WITH
TEXT OF "COMBAT HISTORY" (1977).

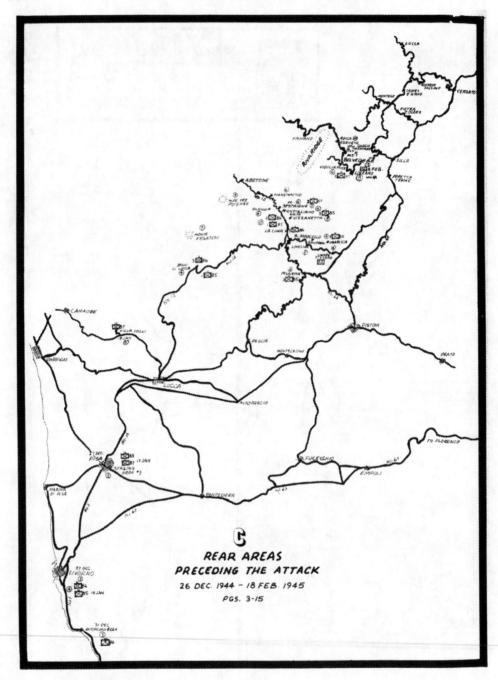

REAR AREAS
PRECEDING THE ATTACK
26 DEC. 1944 – 18 FEB. 1945
PGS. 3-15

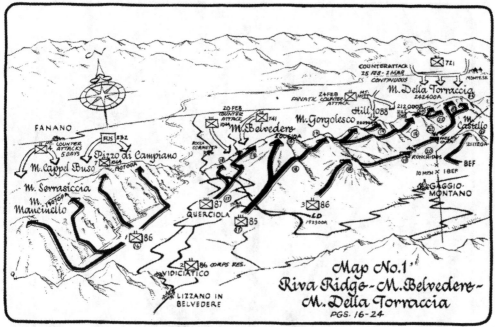

Map No. 1
Riva Ridge – M. Belvedere –
M. Della Torraccia
PGS. 16-24

LEGEND: XX - DIVISION ⊠ - INFANTRY REGIMENT ⊠ - BATTALION 06.1300 A
⊡ - ARMORED GROUP ⊠ - COMPANY DATE MILITARY TIME
(16) PAGE NUMBER REFERENCE IN "COMBAT HISTORY"

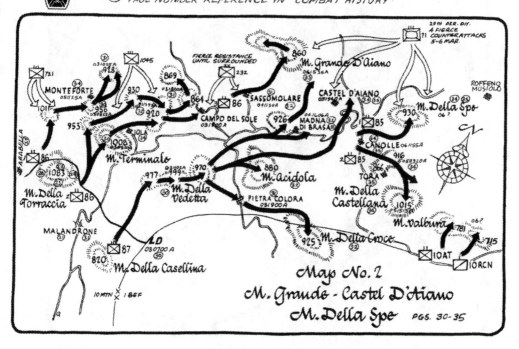

Map No. 2
M. Grande – Castel D'Aiano
M. Della Spe PGS. 30-35

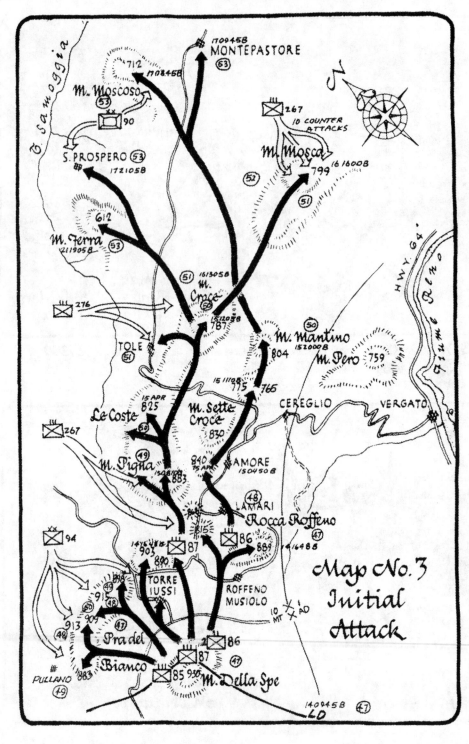

MONTEPASTORE
170945B
53
712
170845B
170845B
M. Moscoso
53
90
S. PROSPERO 53
172105B
267
10 COUNTER
ATTACKS
612
M. Mosca
M. Ferra 53
219058
52
799 161600B
51
51 161305B
51
M. Croce
787 151205B
M. Mantino
152000B
804
M. Pero 759
50
775 766
151110B
TOLE 51
CEREGLIO   VERGATO
276
Le Coste
825 15 APR
M. Sette
Croce
60
830
267
M. Pigna 49
AMORE
840
150450B
15 APR
150818/
883
LAMARI
Rocca Roffeno 48
815
47
94
86
889 141648B
147608B
903
87
890
TORRE
IUSSI
ROFFENO
MUSIOLO
49 88
915
48
50
909
913 909
48
Pra del
47
86
883 Bianco
87
47
PULLANO
85 935   M. Della Spe
49
140945B 47
LD

Map No. 3
Initial
Attack

HWY. 64

Fiume Reno

G. Samoggia

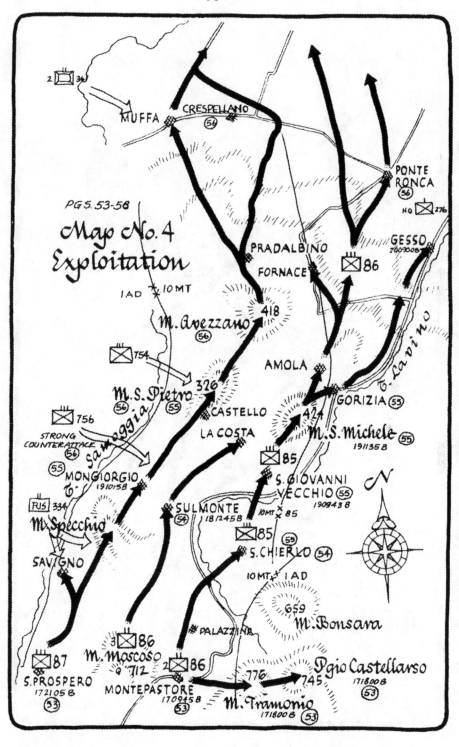

PGS. 53-58

Map No. 4
Exploitation

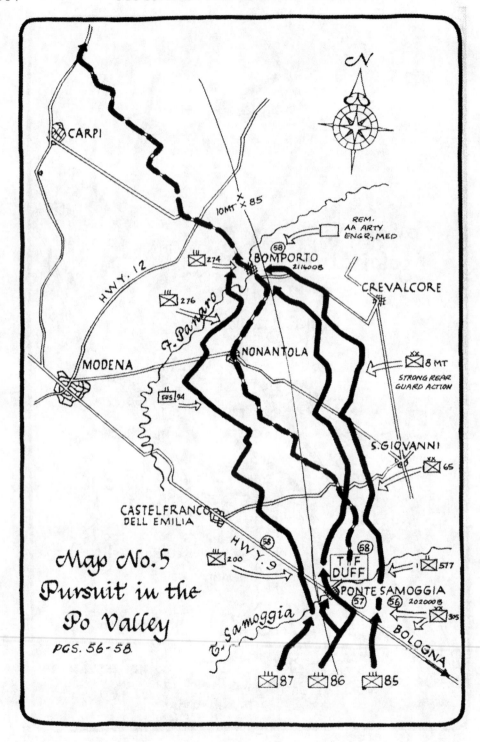

CARPI

10MT X X 85

REM.
AA ARTY
ENGR, MED

⊠ 274

BOMPORTO
58
2116008

CREVALCORE

HWY. 12

⊠ 276

F. Panaro

MODENA

NONANTOLA

⊠ 8 MT
STRONG REAR
GUARD ACTION

FUS 94

S. GIOVANNI

⊠ 65

CASTELFRANCO
DELL EMILIA

HWY. 9

58

T F
DUFF

58

⊠ 200

PONTE SAMOGGIA
57

56   2020008

⊠ 577

⊠ 305

Map No. 5
Pursuit in the
Po Valley
PGS. 56-58

E. Samoggia

BOLOGNA

⊠ 87   ⊠ 86   ⊠ 85

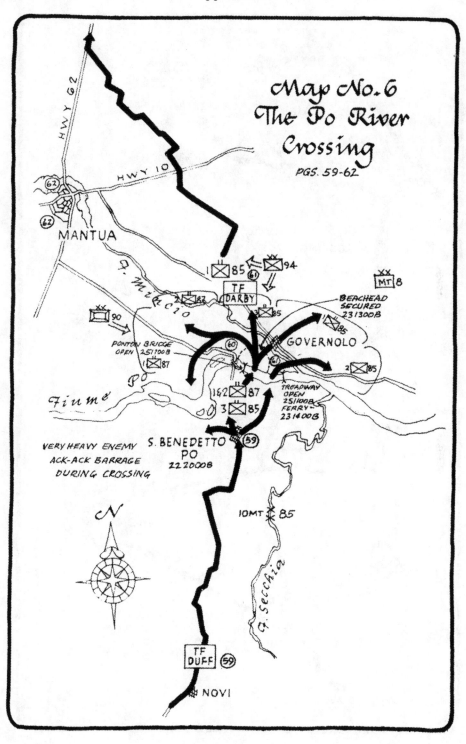

Map No. 6
The Po River
Crossing
PGS. 59-62

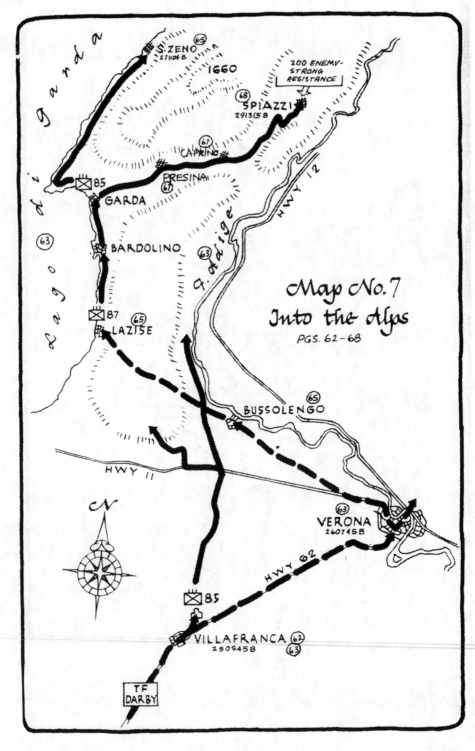

Map No. 7
Into the Alps
PGS. 62-68

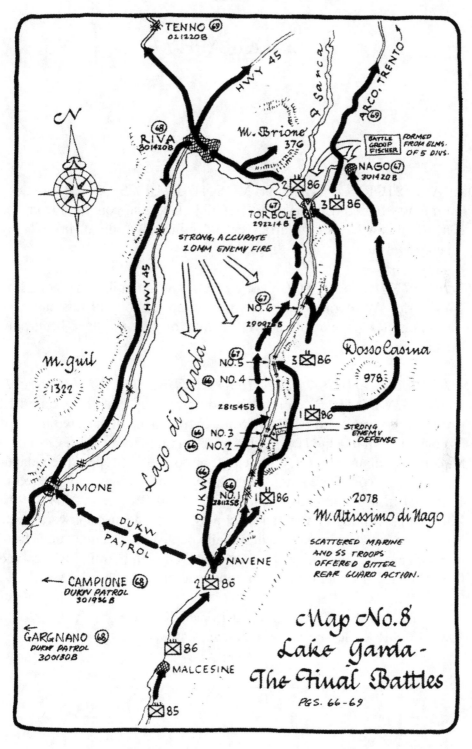

TENNO 69
011220B

HWY 45

Q Sarca

ARCO, TRENTO

RIVA 68
301420B

M. Brione
376

BATTLE GROUP FISCHER | FORMED FROM ELMS. OF 5 DIVS.

NAGO 67
301420 B

N

2 ☒ 86

3 ☒ 86

TORBOLE 67
292214 B

STRONG, ACCURATE
20MM ENEMY FIRE

HWY 45

NO. 6 67
290928B

Dosso Casina
978

M. guil
1322

NO. 5 67

3 ☒ 86

NO. 4 66

281545B

1 ☒ 86

STRONG ENEMY DEFENSE

Lago di Garda

NO. 3 66

NO. 2 66

DUKW 66

LIMONE

DUKW PATROL

NO. 1 66
281125B

1 ☒ 86

2078
M. Altissimo di Nago

SCATTERED MARINE
AND SS TROOPS
OFFERED BITTER
REAR GUARD ACTION.

CAMPIONE 68
DUKW PATROL
301936 B

NAVENE

2 ☒ 86

GARGNANO 68
DUKW PATROL
300130B

☒ 86

Map No. 8
Lake Garda -
The Final Battles
PGS. 66-69

MALCESINE

☒ 85

BIBLIOGRAPHY

COMBAT HISTORY OF THE 10TH MOUNTAIN DIVISION 1944-45 from the Infantry School Library, Fort Benning, Georgia, compiled from the 10th Mountain Division Narrative, and minimally edited, in 1977 by Charles M. Hauptman of Billings, Montana

HISTORY OF THE 86TH MOUNTAIN INFANTRY compiled and edited by T/4 Charles Wellborn. A tattered, mimeographed copy of this narrative was among the papers I had saved. It may or may not have been published.

REMOUNT BLUE - THE COMBAT STORY OF THE 3RD BATTALION, 86TH MOUNTAIN INFANTRY, compiled and narratively edited by David R. Brower, who was a 3rd Battalion Staff Officer and participated in all of its combat. I am indebted to Charles (Ed) Cochran, formerly of Company M, 86th Mountain Infantry Regiment, for a copy of the typewritten manuscript of this work. The manuscript indicates that it was copyrighted in 1948, but in a phone conversation with David Brower in May 1990 I learned that although a number of copies of the manuscript were made and distributed, it had never been formally published. The quotations from it, which are included in this book, were taken with permission received from David R. Brower during our conversation.

COMMMAND MISSIONS, by General Lucien K. Truscott, Jr.; Copyright 1987, 1988 R.R. Bowker; Ayer Company Publishers.

INDEX

A

Aid Station Personnel, duties,36-37
Aircraft, participation in combat, 93, 99, 184-186, 189, 192-193, 201
Aircraft, P-38 incident, 198
Aircraft, P-47 incidents, 185
Albergo (the village), 234
Albergo al Lago di Resia, 239-245
Albergo Diana, 257
Albergo E Delle Isole Borromee, 251
Alexander, Field Marshall, Sir Harold, 254
Albion College, 186
Alpini (Italian Mountain Troops), 107, 159
Ambulance Shuttle, 192, 195, 199
American Military Government, 63, 215-216, 241
Amphibious assault, Lake Garda, 218-222
Amputation, 111-113, 268-270
Anzola, 206
Apennine Mountains, 12, 47, 49, 127
Appendectomy on shipboard, 275-277
Arco, 234
Argyle, Charles, Pfc., 89, 133, 259, 274
Arno River, 260, 274
Artillery barrage, description, 98
Assault Boats, 206, 225
Atomic Bomb, 277-278

B

Bagni di Lucca, 52, 64, 66-67
Bagnoli, 27-28, 30
Bailey, Everett, Capt., 84, 225, 234

Baldo, Monte, 218
Belvedere, Monte, Chapter VII, 82-94
Bergamo, 259
Big Bertha, 200
Bivouac (Camp), 32, 36, 41, 43, 144, 202, 248
Black Market, Italian, 80, 81, 132
Bolzano, 237-238
Bomporto, 191, 194, 195
Brazilian Expeditionary Force, 53-56, 94
Breakfast, country style, Italian, 252-253
Brenner Pass, 209, 233, 236, 238-239
Brescia, 248-249
Bretto di Soto, 250
British Eighth Army, 53
Burn Treatment, 270-271
Bussolengo, 214, 216, 217

C

Ca di Bello, 165
Cable, Movement of casualties by, 89, 277
Camp Carson Colorado,161, 277, 281, 282, 285
Camp Crowder Missouri, 285-286
Camp Patrick Henry Virginia, 18, 277-278
Camp Swift, Texas, 32, 33, 37, 157
Campo del Sole, 117, 118, 129
Campo Tizzoro, 130,135, 159
Cappel Buso, Monte, 86
Captured enemy territory, 118
Car, used, purchase, 281-282
Carge, 96, 110, 115
Carpenter, Jack, Capt., 225
Carson General Hospital, 285

Casini, Armand, 297
Castenodolo, German airfield, 248
Casualty numbers & stories, 86-89, 91, 110, 225, 248
Cave del Predil, 250, 255, 271
Champagne & Cognac, 202, 249, 278
Chaplain, for Aid Station, 97, 104, 238
Check Point 50, 177-179, 181
Cheering civilians, 173, 196, 237
Childbirth, attendance at, 264-266
Children's Diseases, 268
Chlorosis, 267
Chow Line, procedure, 28
Churchill, Sir Winston, 12
Cividale, 250
Civilian Medical Practice, Chapter XXI, 263-272
Civilian Vigilantes, Italian, 235-236
Clark, Mark, General, 52, 139
Cloaca Magna in Rome, 146
Colorado Springs, Colorado, 281-283
Combat Exhaustion, Fatigue, 134-135
Combat Infantry Badge, 157
Combat Medical Badge, 157-158
Como, 247, 257
Company Aid Men, duties, 36
Consiglio, Vincenzo, Pfc., 51-52, 63, 66-67, 77-79, 190, 195, 235, 265, 266-267, 269, 271
Cook, Robert L. Col., 153, 155, 166, 226, 230
Crittenberger, Willis D., General, 52
Croce, Monte, 166-167
Crocette di Sotta, 135, 139
Currency exchange, 132
Custer, Franklin D. Lt., 127
Czech Soldiers, 237

D
Darby's Rangers, 209
Darby, William O., Col., 209, 229-231
DDT Powder, 67-68
Defensive Warfare, positions, 70-73
Della Torraccia, Monte, Chapter VIII, 82, 94, 95-114, 115, 116, 117, 129, 159,

162
Dinner, formal, 79-81
Diphtheria epidemic, 63
Division Supply Personnel, 215
Dole, Frederic, Capt., 84, 156, 179
Dole, Robert, Lt., 162
Dolomites, 13
Drake, William, Capt., Major, 84, 202, 225
Draper, Arthur, First Sergeant, 38, 42, 97
Duff, Robinson, Gen., 189, 191, 209
DUKWs, "Ducks," 219, 220, 222, 225

E
Egan, Thomas A. Capt., 73
Eighty-fifth Division, 216
Ely, Lawrence, Capt., 225.
Enemy plane incidents, 199, 206, 211
Evans, John T., Sgt., 229-230

F
Farmhouses, Italian, 61, 64-66
Ferguson, William E., T3, 43-44
Ferra, Monte, 167
First Armored Division, 53
Florence (Firenze), Italy, 132, 153, 260
Fort Sheridan, Separation Center, 286

G
Gabba, 91
Garda, Lake, Chapter XVII, 217-227, 13, 229
Genoa, 257
German Army, Medical practice in, 179
German Doctor, Medical Officer, 177-179, 181
German Measles epidemic, 285
Gibralter, Straits of, 23
Gorgolesco, Monte, 86, 87, 91-93, 98
Governolo, 207, 210
Grande Albergo e Delle Isole, 251-252
Grande D'Aiano, Monte, 136
Graves Registration Detail, 97, 105, 125, 171, 222
Gualandi di Sopra, di Sotta, 135-136

H

Hagan, Clarence, Lt., Chaplain, 43
Haircuts, 131-132
Hampton Roads, Virginia, 17, 277
Hampton, Colonel, 118
Hauptman, Charles M., 297
Hay, John, Maj., Col., 84-85, 102, 139, 155, 166, 174-175, 178, 191, 202, 228, 236
Hayes (Hays), Gen., Commanding, 10th Mounbtain Division
Hazen, Roy, P-47 pilot, 186
Hebrew Battalion, 56
Hermagor, Austria, 255
Herpes Zoster, "Shingles," treatment, 284-285
Highway 62, 209, 211
Highway 9, 159, 183, 187, 190
Hitler, Adolf, German dictator, 124, 180, 239-240, 247
Hives, during departure, 19
Hospital Visit, 133-134
Hospital, Italian, 69
Hyry, Walter, 92-93

I

II Corps, 53, 165
Inactivation of Division, 285
Italian Troopship, 30-31
IV Corps, 52-53, 206

J

Japanese-American soldiers, 53

K

Kitchen, Field, 28, 31, 41, 130, 182, 233, 256
Klagenfurt, Austria, 256

L

La Scala, 258
Ladd, Charles T.. T/5, 224
Lago di Resia, 239-245
Lake Como, 247,257

Lake Maggiore, 251-252
Laundry, Italian style, 69, 131
Lavino River, 182
Leghorn (Livorno), 31, 275
Lira, "Army Lira", 32, 252, 257
Litter Bearers, duties, 36-38
Lizzano, 69, 74
Louis, "The Duke," 78-82
Lucca, 77, 88, 266

M

M.A.S.H., Television Program, 14
Malcesine, 218, 219
Mancinello, Monte, 69, 86
Mantino, Monte, 164-166
Mantua (Mantova), 207, 209
Martin, George A., Capt., 127
Mauldin, Bill, Cartoonist, 14, 29, 158
Mazzancana, 93-96
McLellan, James H. Lieut., 230
Medical vehicles, 39, 49
Medical Detachment, Battalion, structure, 35
Medical Detachment, Regimental, structure, 35
Mediterranean Sea, 23
Meningitis epidemic, 271-272
Merano, 238
Meyer, Kilian, Capt., 276
Michigan, University of, 11, 73, 179, 310
Milan, 247, 256-258
Miller, Ellsworth, Capt., 276
Miller, Irving "Chuck," Sergeant, 38, 97, 230-231
Mincio River, 267
Mine Explosion, casualties, 42-46
Minefield, 164
Mittenwald Division (German), 106, 110
Montepastore, 182
Mosco, Monte, 166-167
Moscoso, Monte, 166-167
Mountain Infantry Regiment, 85th, 18, 57
Mountain Infantry Regiment, 86th, 18, 57
Mountain Infantry Regiment, 87th, 18, 57
Mules as Division Transport, 33, 107,

115, 127, 169-161, 163, 169
Mushroom Cloud, 212
Mussolini, Benito, Italian Dictator, 247

N
Nago, 226, 228, 229
Naples, Italy, 23, 24-25, 27
National Ski Patrol, 57
Navene, 217, 218, 219, 221
Ninetieth Panzer Grenadier Division
    (German), 181
Ninety-second Division, 30, 41, 53
Ninfo, John, Lt., Capt., 161, 283-284
Nisei Regiment, 53

O
Okumoto, Dr. Pete, Lt., Capt., 133, 157
Opera in Milan, 257-259
Oran, Algeria, 24

P
Panaro River, 191
Partisans, Italian, 107, 197, 198, 200,
    214, 234, 247, 250
Passo di Predil, 250, 271
Passo di Resia, 239, 243, 248
Patch, Shoulder, 58
Patti, Thomas J., Pfc., 93
Patton, Herbert, Ofc., 160
Pfaelzer, Major, 166
Pisa, 32, 37, 39
Pizzo di Campiano, 86
Po River, Chapter XVI, 205-208, 13, 195,
    196, 197, 200, 209
Po Valley, 12, 41, 85, 120, 126, 159, 160,
    166, 182, 183-184, 187, 189, 205, 206,
    248
Ponte Ronca, 183
Ponte Samoggia, 184, 187, 190, 192, 193,
    206
Prisoner, German SS Trooper, 180, 181
Prisoners, German, use of, 121, 124, 166,

171, 174-176
Prisoners, unguarded, 193, 197
Promotion, 156-157
Propaganda leaflets, 119, 136
Propaganda, verbal, 119
Prunetta, 138-139
Pyelonephritis, 266-267

Q
Quercianella, 41, 42, 46, 47

R
Raabe, Max H., Lt. Capt., 73, 74, 79
Radio, Field, SCR-300, 55, 105, 178
Randall, Samuel J., Capt., 153, 276, 294
Rations, 10 in 1, 140
Rations, C, 40, 107, 126, 140, 215
Rations, D, 40
Rations, German, 40
Rations K, 40, 88, 95, 107, 194, 215
Red Cross Services, 27, 28, 107, 259
Refugees, 237
Resia, 233, 239, 242, 244, 245
Riva, 223, 229, 230, 231
Riva Ridge, Chapter VII, 83-93, 129
Rocca Roffeno, 162, 164
Rogers, William E. "Ed," Lt., 97
Roosevelt, Pres. Franklin D., 162
Rovereto, 236
Rowland, Harold E., Pvt., 160
Rucksack, Mountain, 19, 95, 116, 175,
    190, 207, 214, 220, 222, 277
Ruffner, General, 209

S
San Alessandro, 231, 233, 234
San Benedetto Po, 196, 202, 205
San Lorenzo, 184
San Marcello, 49-52, 64
San Maria Delabante, 161, 162
San Prospero, 167
San Zeno, 217

Sarca River, 229
Sasso Baldino, 141
Scheuerman, Dr. Wally, Capt., 133
Schuh mine (German), 111
Seamans, John, Maj., 89, 225
Seasickness, 23
Serrasiccia, Monte, 86
Sette Croce, Monte, 165
Ship, troop, 22
Shoulder Patch, 10th Mountain Division, 58
Sikh soldiers, 56
Sixth South African Division, 53
Slit Trench, 144, 145, 146
Snipers, 63, 136, 164
Stresa, 251, 252, 257
Sulmonte, 177
Summers, Byron P., Lt., 38, 42. 68, 79, 83, 97, 108, 131, 137, 141, 159, 273
Surrender of German Army Hospital, 240
Swados, Harrison, T/4, 110
Syphilis, on shipboard, 21, 22, 23

T
Task Force 45, 30, 52, 77
Task Force Darby - Verona, Chapter XVII, 209-216
Task Force Duff, Chapter XV, 189-204
Task Force to Resia, 236-245
Teatro Puccini, 258
Tenth Mountain Division, 11, 17, 34, 52, 56
Tenth Mountain Division, structure of, 17
Thirty-fourth Division, 260, 279
Toilet, Public Street Corner Booth, 148
Toilet, Public, "The Pit," 149-150
Toilets, Destruction by explosion, 150-152
Toilets, evolution of, 146-148
Tole, 167
Tomlinson, Clarence M., Col., 139, 153, 155, 157, 166
Torbole, 221, 223, 226, 228, 229, 231, 236
Trench foot, 76

Trento, 237
Troop Train, 282-283
Troopship, Westbrook Victory, 271
Truman, U.S. President, 247, 281
Truscott, Lucien K., Gen., 54
Tunnels, battles for, 221-227
Turin, 257

U
Udine, 250, 254, 260
Unit Citation Application – Appendix A, 289-295
Urinals, 150

V
Vehicle & Equipment turn in, 273-274
Venereal Diseases, 21, 138-139, 294
Venice, 252-254
Verona, see Task Force Darby, 205-216, 234, 259
Vicenza, 252
Vidiciatico, 87
Villach, Austria, 255
Villsfranca Airfield, 210

W
Watson, "Duke," Capt., 84
Webb, 1st Sergeant, 137
Whiskey, Army issue, 153-155
Wilkinson, Lieut., 256, 259
Wounds, described, 75, 92, 100, 108, 111-113, 180, 182, 212-214, 241, 264, 268-270

Y
Yugoslav Border, Trieste, 249

ABOUT THE AUTHOR

Dr. Meinke was born and grew up in Detroit, Michigan where he was graduated from Thomas M. Cooley High School. In 1940 he completed pre-medical studies at Albion College and entered medical school at the University of Michigan. In 1941 he received his A.B. degree from Albion, and, because of a sharply accelerated program brought about by the entry of the United States into World War II, received his M.D. degree in October 1943. After an abbreviated internship he entered the service on August 2,1944.

Twice decorated, Dr. Meinke was awarded the Bronze Star Medal for his participation in the battle for Monte Della Torraccia, and later received a Bronze Oak Leaf Cluster for outstanding service in the clearing of casualties from the tunnel disaster on the shore of Lake Garda. He also holds the Combat Medical Badge, which is the equivalent of the Combat Infantry Badge awarded to infantry men for participation in front-line combat.

While in medical school he met Edmere L. Bondesen, a lovely girl from Detroit who was also attending the University, and near the end of July 1944, only a few days before Dr. Meinke entered the Army, they were married. With military service completed, they settled in Eaton Rapids, Michigan and started their family. There are four children: Albert H. Meinke, III, M.D., William B. Meinke, M.D., James A. Meinke and Joanna Meinke Ballard.

Dr. Meinke then entered into general medical practice in Eaton Rapids, but soon leaned toward general surgery, obstetrics and emergency medicine. He was deeply involved in the establishment and operation of the Eaton Rapids Community Hospital, and for many years served as its medical director, chief of surgery, and head of emergency services. He also served on its governing board for a time. In 1948 he helped to establish the Eaton Rapids Medical Clinic, one of the first group practices in Michigan, and later served as its president for many years. In 1984, after forty years in practice, he retired. He and his wife now reside in a lovely home on the west shore of Torch Lake in northern Lower Michigan.

ISBN 155369600-X

9 781553 696001

Printed in the United States
By Bookmasters